MEDICAL MASTERCLASS

EDITOR-IN-CHIEF

JOHN D FIRTH DM FRCP
Consultant Physician and Nephrologist
Addenbrooke's Hospital
Cambridge

CLINICAL SKILLS

EDITORS

JOHN D FIRTH DM FRCP
Consultant Physician and Nephrologist
Addenbrooke's Hospital
Cambridge

CLAIRE G NICHOLL FRCP
Consultant Physician and Clinical Director
Addenbrooke's Hospital
Cambridge

DEE C TRAUE MRCP(UK)
Macmillan Consultant in Palliative Medicine
Addenbrooke's Hospital
Cambridge

Second Edition

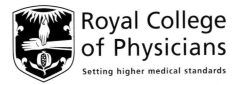

Royal College
of Physicians
Setting higher medical standards

Disclaimer

Although every effort has been made to ensure that drug doses and other information are presented accurately in this publication, the ultimate responsibility rests with the prescribing physician. Neither the publishers nor the authors can be held responsible for any consequences arising from the use of information contained herein. Any product mentioned in this publication should be used in accordance with the prescribing information prepared by the manufacturers.

The information presented in this publication reflects the opinions of its contributors and should not be taken to represent the policy and views of the Royal College of Physicians of London, unless this is specifically stated.

Every effort has been made by the contributors to contact holders of copyright to obtain permission to reproduce copyrighted material. However, if any have been inadvertently overlooked, the publisher will be pleased to make the necessary arrangements at the first opportunity.

LIST OF CONTRIBUTORS

Dr JD Firth DM FRCP
Consultant Physician and Nephrologist
Addenbrooke's Hospital
Cambridge

Dr R Morgan BSc FRCP
Consultant Physician and Postgraduate Clinical Tutor
Medicine for the Elderly
Arrowe Park Hospital
Wirral

Dr CG Nicholl FRCP
Consultant Physician and Clinical Director
Medicine for the Elderly
Addenbrooke's Hospital
Cambridge

Dr JR Ross PhD MRCP(UK)
Consultant in Palliative Medicine
St Joseph's Hospice
London

Dr DC Traue MRCP(UK)
Macmillan Consultant in Palliative Medicine
Palliative Care Team
Addenbrooke's Hospital
Cambridge

Dr KJ Wilson FRCP
Consultant Physician
Medicine for the Elderly
Addenbrooke's Hospital
Cambridge

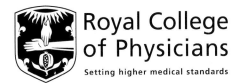
Royal College
of Physicians
Setting higher medical standards

© 2008, 2010 Royal College of Physicians of London

Published by:
Royal College of Physicians of London
11 St. Andrews Place
Regent's Park
London NW1 4LE
United Kingdom

Set and printed by Graphicraft Limited, Hong Kong

First edition published 2001
Reprinted 2004
Second edition published 2008
This module updated and reprinted 2010

ISBN: 978-1-86016-266-4 (this book)
ISBN: 978-1-86016-260-2 (set)

Distribution Information:
Jerwood Medical Education Resource Centre
Royal College of Physicians of London
11 St. Andrews Place
Regent's Park
London NW1 4LE
United Kingdom
Tel: +44 (0)207 935 1174 ext 422/490
Fax: +44 (0)207 486 6653
Email: merc@rcplondon.ac.uk
Web: http://www.rcplondon.ac.uk/

CONTENTS

List of contributors iii
Foreword vii
Preface viii
Acknowledgements x
Key features xi

CLINICAL SKILLS FOR PACES

Introduction 3

History-taking for PACES (Station 2) 6

Communication Skills and Ethics for PACES (Station 4) 10

Examination for PACES Stations 1, 3 and 5: General Considerations 12

Station 1: Respiratory System 15

Station 1: Abdominal System 20

Station 3: Cardiovascular System 26

Station 3: Central Nervous System 35

Station 5: Brief Clinical Consulations 53

PAIN RELIEF AND PALLIATIVE CARE

PACES Stations and Acute Scenarios 61

1.1 History-taking 61
  1.1.1 Pain 61
  1.1.2 Constipation/bowel obstruction 63
1.2 Communication skills and ethics 65
  1.2.1 Pain 65
  1.2.2 Breathlessness 66
  1.2.3 Nausea and vomiting 67
  1.2.4 Bowel obstruction 69
  1.2.5 End of life 70
1.3 Acute scenarios 71
  1.3.1 Pain 71
  1.3.2 Breathlessness 74
  1.3.3 Nausea and vomiting 76
  1.3.4 Bowel obstruction 79

Diseases and Treatments 82

2.1 Pain 82
2.2 Breathlessness 87
2.3 Nausea and vomiting 88
2.4 Constipation 89
2.5 Bowel obstruction 90
2.6 Anxiety and depression 91
2.7 Confusion 93
2.8 End-of-life care: the dying patient 94
2.9 Specialist palliative care services 96

Self-assessment 98

3.1 Self-assessment questions 98
3.2 Self-assessment answers 101

MEDICINE FOR THE ELDERLY

PACES Stations and Acute Scenarios 107

1.1 History-taking 107
  1.1.1 Frequent falls 107
  1.1.2 Recent onset of confusion 110
  1.1.3 Urinary incontinence and immobility 114
  1.1.4 Collapse 116
  1.1.5 Vague aches and pains 119
  1.1.6 Swollen legs and back pain 121
  1.1.7 Failure to thrive: gradual decline and weight loss 127
1.2 Clinical examination 129
  1.2.1 Confusion (respiratory) 129
  1.2.2 Confusion (abdominal) 130
  1.2.3 Failure to thrive (abdominal) 131
  1.2.4 Frequent falls (cardiovascular) 131
  1.2.5 Confusion (cardiovascular) 132
  1.2.6 Frequent falls (neurological) 132
  1.2.7 Confusion (neurological) 134
  1.2.8 Impaired mobility (neurological) 135
  1.2.9 Confusion (skin) 135
  1.2.10 Frequent falls (locomotor) 136
  1.2.11 Confusion (endocrine) 136
  1.2.12 Confusion (eye) 136

CONTENTS

1.3 **Communication skills and ethics 137**
- 1.3.1 Frequent falls 137
- 1.3.2 Confusion 138
- 1.3.3 Collapse 139

1.4 **Acute scenarios 141**
- 1.4.1 Sudden onset of confusion 141
- 1.4.2 Collapse 143

Diseases and Treatments 147

2.1 **Why elderly patients are different 147**

2.2 **General approach to management 149**

2.3 **Falls 151**

2.4 **Urinary and faecal incontinence 155**
- 2.4.1 Urinary incontinence 155
- 2.4.2 Faecal incontinence 157

2.5 **Hypothermia 158**

2.6 **Drugs in elderly people 161**

2.7 **Dementia 162**

2.8 **Rehabilitation 165**

2.9 **Aids, appliances and assistive technology 166**

2.10 **Hearing impairment 168**

2.11 **Nutrition 170**

2.12 **Benefits 174**

2.13 **Legal aspects of elderly care 175**

Investigations and Practical Procedures 178

3.1 **Diagnosis vs common sense 178**

3.2 **Assessment of cognition, mood and function 178**

Self-assessment 181

4.1 **Self-assessment questions 181**

4.2 **Self-assessment answers 185**

The Medical Masterclass Series 188
Index 204

FOREWORD

Since its initial publication in 2001, *Medical Masterclass* has been regarded as a key learning and teaching resource for physicians around the world. The resource was produced in part to meet the vision of the Royal College of Physicians: *'Doctors of the highest quality, serving patients well'*. This vision continues and, along with advances in clinical practice and changes in the format of the MRCP(UK) exam, has justified the publication of this second edition.

The MRCP(UK) is an international examination that seeks to advance the learning of and enhance the training process for physicians worldwide. On passing the exam physicians are recognised as having attained the required knowledge, skills and manner appropriate for training at a specialist level. However, passing the exam is a challenge. The pass rate at each sitting of the written papers is about 40%. Even the most prominent consultants have had to sit each part of the exam more than once in order to pass. With this challenge in mind, the College has produced *Medical Masterclass*, a comprehensive learning resource to help candidates with the preparation that is key to making the grade.

Medical Masterclass has been produced by the Education Department of the College. A work of this size represents a formidable amount of effort by the Editor-in-Chief – Dr John Firth – and his team of editors and authors. I would like to thank our colleagues for this wonderful educational product and wholeheartedly recommend it as an invaluable learning resource for all physicians preparing for their MRCP(UK) examination.

Professor Ian Gilmore MD PRCP
President of the Royal College of Physicians

PREFACE

The second edition of *Medical Masterclass* is produced and published by the Education Department of the Royal College of Physicians of London. It comprises 12 textbooks, a companion interactive website and two CD-ROMs. Its aim is to help doctors in their first few years of training to improve their medical knowledge and skills; and in particular to (a) learn how to deal with patients who are acutely ill, and (b) pass postgraduate examinations, such as the MRCP(UK) or European Diploma in Internal Medicine.

The 12 textbooks are divided as follows: two cover the scientific background to medicine, one is devoted to general clinical skills [including specific guidance on exam technique for PACES, the practical assessment of clinical examination skills that is the final part of the MRCP(UK) exam], one deals with acute medicine and the other eight cover the range of medical specialties.

The core material of each of the medical specialties is dealt with in seven sections:

- Case histories – you are presented with letters of referral commonly received in each specialty and led through the ways in which the patients' histories should be explored, and what should then follow in the way of investigation and/or treatment.

- Physical examination scenarios – these emphasise the logical analysis of physical signs and sensible clinical reasoning: 'having found this, what would you do?'

- Communication and ethical scenarios – what are the difficult issues that commonly arise in each specialty? What do you actually say to the 'frequently asked (but still very difficult) questions?'

- Acute presentations – what are the priorities if you are the doctor seeing the patient in the Emergency Department or the Medical Admissions Unit?

- Diseases and treatments – structured concise notes.

- Investigations and practical procedures – more short and to-the-point notes.

- Self assessment questions – in the form used in the MRCP(UK) Part 1 and Part 2 exams.

The companion website – which is continually updated – enables you to take mock MRCP(UK) Part 1 or Part 2 exams, or to be selective in the questions you tackle (if you want to do ten questions on cardiology, or any other specialty, you can do). For every question you complete you can see how your score compares with that of others who have logged onto the site and attempted it. The two CD-ROMs each contain 30 interactive cases requiring diagnosis and treatment.

I hope that you enjoy using *Medical Masterclass* to learn more about medicine, which – whatever is happening politically to primary care, hospitals and medical career structures – remains a wonderful occupation. It is sometimes intellectually and/or emotionally very challenging, and also sometimes extremely rewarding, particularly when reduced to the essential of a doctor trying to provide best care for a patient.

John Firth DM FRCP
Editor-in-Chief

ACKNOWLEDGEMENTS

Medical Masterclass has been produced by a team. The names of those who have written or edited material are clearly indicated elsewhere, but without the support of many other people it would not exist. Naming names is risky, but those worthy of particular note include: Sir Richard Thompson (College Treasurer) and Mrs Winnie Wade (Director of Education), who steered the project through committees that are traditionally described as labyrinthine, and which certainly seem so to me; and also Arthur Wadsworth (Project Co-ordinator) and Don Liu in the College Education Department office. Don is a veteran of the first edition of *Medical Masterclass*, and it would be fair to say that without his great efforts a second edition might not have seen the light of day.

John Firth DM FRCP
Editor-in-Chief

We have created a range of icon boxes that sit among the text of the various *Medical Masterclass* modules. They are there to help you identify key information and to make learning easier and more enjoyable. Here is a brief explanation:

> Iron-deficiency anaemia with a change in bowel habit in a middle-aged or older patient means colonic malignancy until proved otherwise.

This icon is used to highlight points of particular importance.

> Dietary deficiency is very rarely, if ever, the sole cause of iron-deficiency anaemia.

This icon is used to indicate common or important drug interactions, pitfalls of practical procedures, or when to take symptoms or signs particularly seriously.

> A man with a renal transplant is immunosuppressed with ciclosporin, azathioprine and prednisolone. He develops recurrent gout and is started on allopurinol. Four weeks later he is admitted with septicaemia and found to be profoundly leucopenic. The problem is that allopurinol, by inhibiting xanthine oxidase, has inhibited the metabolism of azathioprine, rendering a 'normal dose' toxic.

Case examples/case histories are used to demonstrate why and how an understanding of the scientific background to medicine helps in the practice of clinical medicine.

CLINICAL SKILLS FOR PACES

Author:

JD Firth

Editor:

JD Firth

Editor-in-Chief:

JD Firth

How the PACES exam works

The Practical Assessment of Clinical Examination Skills (PACES) comprises five stations, each lasting 20 minutes, as shown in Table 1. Candidates are allocated to start at any one of the stations and then rotate round the 'carousel' of stations (as it is called) until they have completed all five.

At each station the candidate meets two different examiners who score independently. Go to http://www.mrcpuk.org/ to see what the mark sheets look like. Two are completed by each examiner for station 1, 3 and 5, hence by the time a candidate has finished they have had eight mark sheets completed by each of two examiners at each station, making a total of sixteen mark sheets in all.

As they move through the PACES carousel, the candidates' performance is judged against seven clinical skills, as described and shown in Table 2. Following each encounter each examiner scores the candidate for those clinical skills that are assessed during that encounter on a three point scale: unsatisfactory, 0 points; borderline, 1 point; satisfactory, 2 points.

Why is the PACES exam the way it is now?

The format of the MRCP clinical exam has developed and been refined over many years, remaining widely accepted by physicians – both trainees and consultants – as a valid and appropriate test of clinical knowledge, technique and application. However, one particular problem perceived by some was that, until the most recent changes (2010/3 diet onwards – the exam is run three times per year, each running of the exam being called a diet), the exam did not explicitly separate the testing of competencies in different clinical skills. Whilst to pass a candidate needed to obtain 'pass' or 'clear pass' overall judgement scores from most if not all of 10 examiners (diets up to 2009/2), or many scores of 'satisfactory' for the various clinical skills (all diets from 2009/3 to 2010/2), the exam did not explicitly separate the testing of competencies in different clinical skills. This meant that a candidate who scored highly in some skills could compensate for deficient performance in others, e.g. they might be poor at communication, but pass the exam because they were very good at physical examination.

The PACES exam now requires candidates to demonstrate that they are (1) competent across the full range of clinical skills, with Table 2 showing the likely pass mark that must be achieved for each of the seven, and (2) attain a minimum total score across the whole assessment of (provisionally) 130/172. Consistent with historical practice, it is intended that the same proportion of candidates will pass each diet as have done so historically (which has been a very stable figure of about 45%).

There is one caveat to the above, which relates to clinical skill G, 'maintaining patient welfare'. This is the domain in which 'roughness' is indicated, and if an examiner thinks that a candidate hurts a patient and causes them pain, then they would score this as 'unsatisfactory' for that encounter, with two such scores probably resulting in an outright fail of the entire examination. However, remember that the examiners are all experienced and sensible doctors, and don't allow this to make you frightened to actually touch the patient. A patient in the exam will not uncommonly say or indicate that something is a bit uncomfortable or painful when, for example, you are examining their abdomen. This does not mean that the examiner will fail you, as long as you behave appropriately, which means that

TABLE 1 – THE PACES CAROUSEL

Station	
1	Respiratory system examination (10 minutes) Abdominal system examination (10 minutes)
2	History taking skills (20 minutes)
3	Cardiovascular system examination (10 minutes) Central nervous system examination (10 minutes)
4	Communication skills and ethics (20 minutes)
5	Brief Clinical Consultations (2 × 10 minutes)

TABLE 2 – ASSESSMENT OF CLINICAL SKILLS

Station	Encounter	Physical examination	Identifying Physical signs	Clinical communication	Differential Diagnosis	Clinical judgement	Managing patient's concerns	Managing patient welfare	Marks
1	Respiratory	✓	✓		✓	✓		✓	0–20
1	Abdomen	✓	✓		✓	✓		✓	0–20
2	History			✓	✓	✓	✓	✓	0–20
3	Cardiovascular	✓	✓		✓	✓		✓	0–20
3	Nervous system	✓	✓		✓	✓		✓	0–20
4	Communication			✓		✓	✓	✓	0–16
5	Brief consultation 1	✓	✓	✓	✓	✓	✓	✓	0–28
5	Brief consultation 2	✓	✓	✓	✓	✓	✓	✓	0–28
Pass mark		14/24	14/24	10/16	16/28	18/32	10/16	28/32	130/172

Physical examination	A systematic/focused and appropriate technique is required, conducted in a fluent and professional manner.
Identifying physical signs	Those that are present should be identified, and physical signs that are not present should not be found!
Clinical communication	Histories should be elicited in a systematic/focused, appropriate, fluent and professional manner. Relevant clinical information should be explained in an accurate, clear, comprehensive, fluent and professional manner.
Differential diagnosis	A sensible differential diagnosis is required.
Clinical judgement	A sensible and appropriate plan for investigation and/or management is required, demonstrating clinical knowledge – including of law and ethics – relevant to the case.
Managing patients' concerns	The patient/relative must be listened to in an empathetic manner. Their understanding of matters under discussion must be confirmed, and their concerns sought, detected and acknowledged.
Maintaining patient welfare	The patient/relative must be treated in a manner that ensures their comfort, safety and dignity.

you acknowledge the discomfort and back off, as I hope you would in your routine practice.

What are PACES examiners really looking for?

PACES examiners are looking for someone with a 'safe pair of hands'.

The stations of the PACES exam replicate the things that a doctor pursuing clinical practice as a physician has to do in their daily work. In the Medical Admissions Unit, the ward or the outpatient clinic you typically have about ten to fifteen minutes to talk to a patient to find out what's wrong. You need to be able to perform a clinical examination of any system in a few minutes and produce a sensible interpretation of the findings. You need to be able to formulate a reasonable plan for investigation and management, which needs to be explained to and discussed with the

patient. Sometimes you need to talk about difficult things with patients and relatives: few welcome diseases or uncertainty or death, and many get confused or angry in their presence, particularly if the wonders of modern medicine cannot help. Sometimes the initiation or continuation of active medical treatments would cause more misery than good, and to pursue them would not be kind or sensible. These issues need to be explained, and to do so well requires skill, and like most things can be improved by practice.

As an experienced physician, the PACES examiner should be able to do all of the above him- or her-self. Given that the MRCP exam is the entry point into specialist medical training, and that many of those taking the exam are seeking to pursue a career as a physician, the main thought in the examiner's mind is 'would I be happy if this doctor was my specialty registrar, working in my outpatient clinic, on my ward, or in the Medical Admissions Unit on take?'. If after observing your

performance during an encounter they think 'yes', then they will score you satisfactory on most if not all of the clinical skills tested, and if they think 'no', then they won't. So what, in general terms, makes them think 'yes' or 'no'?

Candidates who score satisfactory for the clinical skills are those who seem to be a 'safe pair of hands'. The PACES exam is not a test of erudite knowledge. What is important is that candidates have an obviously reproducible and effective method of taking histories from patients and examining them, can interpret the findings to construct a sensible differential diagnosis, that they can plan a reasonable strategy for investigation and management, and that – if there are difficult matters to discuss – they will do so in a caring and effective manner that is likely to leave patients and relatives reassured that a good doctor and health care team are doing and will do everything that they can reasonably and sensibly be expected to do, even if the outlook is bleak.

Four 'rules of thumb':

> **Rules of thumb for PACES**
> - **Develop solid and reproducible methods.**
> - **Do not confabulate.**
> - **Be logical and sensible.**
> - **Remember that common things are common.**

1) Develop solid and reproducible methods

There is, or should be, no such thing as a 'way you take a history for PACES' or 'way you examine a system for PACES' that is distinct from your routine clinical practice. If there is, you will come unstuck one way or another. The candidate who pauses at every stage of their history taking or examination of a system because they are thinking 'what should I do next?' is not going to do well. It stands out a mile. If you don't have a method that is second nature, what is going to happen when you're doing a shift on a busy Medical Admissions Unit and the pressure is on? So develop and use a correct method in your routine practice and it will stand you in good stead in the exam. When someone suggested to the great golfer Gary Player that he was lucky, he is said to have replied, 'the more I practice, the luckier I get'. Clinical medicine is the same.

2) Do not confabulate

When the examiners ask you about the history you have taken in station 2, it may be that they will explore some aspect that you did not cover in detail. It is fatal if you try to pretend that you did pursue a point when you did not: the examiners heard every word that was said. Admit it instantly: 'I did not pursue that line in detail'.

Some physical signs are obvious and some are not. The examiners know this. Before a candidate sees any case, they will both have examined the patient and agreed what the signs are, dividing these into those that are clearly present and those that are subtle or debatable. You are expected to correctly identify the abnormalities that are obvious, and if you recognize those that are subtle the examiners will approve, but if you make things up, then you are in trouble.

Matters of fact may arise in the ethics and communication skills scenario that you are unsure of. Say to the patient or relative 'I'm not sure about that', and – if it is an important matter – 'I will find out and let you know'.

The worst sort of registrar for a consultant to have to deal with is one who confabulates, who simply makes things up. If you do, then the examiner will certainly score you unsatisfactory. Never confabulate.

3) Be logical and sensible

When you have summarized the history, the physical findings, or the communication or ethical issue, discussion with the examiners will move on. If the history suggests that the patient has ischaemic cardiac chest pain, then an ECG should be the first thing that you ask for, not some sophisticated radionuclide scan. To suggest something like this would indicate a lack of contact with the real world, and examiners don't want a registrar whose feet are not planted reasonably firmly on planet Earth.

4) Remember that common things are common

If a man is breathless, looks blue and has a few crackles and wheezes in his chest, then the most likely diagnosis by far is that he has chronic obstructive pulmonary disease, the most relevant question that could be asked would relate to his smoking history, and sensible investigations to request initially would be peak flow, spirometry/lung function tests, a chest radiograph and arterial blood gases. This is bread-and-butter stuff, and the candidate who says this would very rapidly have the examiner scoring them satisfactory in all domains. Only make a diagnosis of fibrosing alveolitis or bronchiectasis if the patient is obviously clubbed with a large number of crackles in the chest. Examiners become wary if a candidate makes a succession of relatively rare diagnoses on the basis of flimsy evidence, when virtually every outpatient clinic or ward round they have ever done themselves has been heavily populated by patients who have not had exotic things wrong with them. Common things are common.

A bit of practical advice

For the PACES exam, wear sensible working clothes and shoes that conform to current standards relating to prevention of hospital-acquired infections. There are no regulations that stipulate a dress code for PACES, but some candidates do not help themselves to perform optimally by their choice of attire. 'Dressing up' for the exam can be a mistake. The best suit, comprising tight-fitting jacket and trousers, or the pencil skirt, may be just the thing in some circumstances, but they make it difficult to move around freely. You are unlikely to be able to palpate the abdomen to best effect if you cannot courch down easily. Wear the neatest and tidiest clothes that you wear for work. If you are worried that these might be too scruffy or casual for the exam, then you might reflect on their suitability as day to day professional garb.

In about five minutes some patients will give a lucid chronological account of all their symptoms, specify precisely what their problems are now, contrasting this with their previous state of health, say what treatments they are taking and have taken in the past, give a concise statement of their past medical history, mention relevant risk factors for disease, including family history, and volunteer any particular reasons they have for concern. Very few patients are able to do this, but after taking a history the doctor should be able to do so on their behalf.

In the five minutes before starting the history taking station the candidate is given written instructions in the form of a letter from the patient's GP (Table 3). Fourteen minutes are allowed for the history taking, after which the patient or surrogate (hereafter simply called the patient) is asked to leave the station. The examiners say when two minutes of the fourteen are left so that the consultation can be wound up in a controlled manner. There is then one minute for the candidate to collect their thoughts, followed by five minutes of discussion with the examiners.

Be aware of the details of the marksheet that the examiner will be looking at as you talk (Table 4).

'Always listen to the patient; they might be telling you the diagnosis' is one of many aphorisms attributed to Osler. There is merit in the saying, whether or not it came from the great man. To take a good history requires the doctor to be able to listen well, meaning more than simply an absence of deafness, but that they are quick to spot important nuances in the story and able to explore them in a manner that extracts maximum information without lingering. The most experienced practitioners are able to do this without the patient noticing that the flow of their conversation has been interrupted, perhaps by little more than a nod of the head which indicates 'tell me more about that'. Since time is constrained both in routine clinical practice and in PACES, it is important that the doctor is able to steer the conversation productively, identifying the key issues and keeping discussion focused upon them. It is more difficult to do this with some patients than with others.

Beginning the consultation

Establish what the main problems are.

Introduce yourself to the patient and establish how old they are, what their job is, and what the main problem is. For instance, if the case is a cardiological one, 'I am Dr Brown, a doctor working in the cardiology clinic . . . I have a letter from your general practitioner, Dr Smith, who tells me that you are 28 years old and work as a secretary (wait for nod or comment of

TABLE 3 HISTORY TAKING FOR PACES – FORMAT OF STATION 2

Time	
5 minutes before starting station	Read the scenario very carefully. What is the main task? – working out the diagnosis?; sorting out a plan for investigation or management?; often both of these are required. Write down any points that you want to be sure of covering.
0–12 minutes	Take history from patient (1). Examiner reminds 'two minutes to go' at 12 minutes.
12–14 minutes	Wind up discussion before patient leaves the room (2).
14–15 minutes	Reflection. What will be your opening statement about the case? What are the main diagnoses/options for investigation or treatment that you are considering?
15–20 minutes	Discussion with examiners.

Notes
(1) The history taking station may involve a 'real' patient or a surrogate, but the tendency is more and more often to use surrogates.
(2) It is not stated explicitly in the examiner's instructions that the candidate should agree a plan for investigation/management with patient before they leave after 14 minutes, but it is a natural way to terminate discussion and is recognized as such by many examiners.

TABLE 4 KEY FEATURES OF THE EXAMINER'S MARKSHEET FOR HISTORY TAKING SKILLS

Clinical skill	To score satisfactory	To score unsatisfactory
Clinical communication skills	Elicits the presenting complaint and conducts other elements of the history (systems review and past/family/medication history are specifically noted) in a thorough, systematic, fluent and professional manner. Assesses the impact of symptoms on the patient's occupation, lifestyle and activities of daily living. Explains relevant clinical information in an accurate, clear, structured, comprehensive, fluent and professional manner.	Omits important areas of the history and/or appears unsystematic, unpractised or unprofessional. When trying to explain things to the patient either omits important information, gives inaccurate information, uses jargon, or conducts the discussion in a manner that is poorly structured, appears unpractised or is unprofessional.
Managing patient's concerns	Listens and is empathetic. Seeks, detects and attempts to address the patient's concerns. Confirms the patient's knowledge and understanding.	Does not listen well and/or is not empathetic. Overlooks patient's concerns. Does not check the patient's knowledge and understanding.
Differential diagnosis	Sensible, and includes the correct diagnosis	Poor, and fails to consider the correct diagnosis
Clinical judgement	Offers a sensible and appropriate management plan.	Offers an inappropriate management plan.
Maintaining patient welfare	Treats the patient in an appropriate manner.	Causes the patient physical or emotional discomfort, or treats them in an unsafe manner.

confirmation) and that there is concern because you have been getting dizzy turns (or whatever the problem is) . . . is that right? Is that the main problem?'

Assuming that you have read the instructions correctly, it should not happen in **PACES** that the patient will say 'no, that's not the main problem', but in real life it is not at all uncommon for the situation to have changed between the time that a letter of referral is written and the time a patient arrives in the clinic. It is frustrating to embark on several minutes of history taking, only to have the patient say 'but that's not the real problem now . . . the trouble now is . . .' To begin the consultation by confirming the main problem gives the patient confidence that you are going to tackle their problems, which might not be precisely the same as those written down, and it immediately signals to the examiner that you have been through the mill, you know what you are doing.

Having established the main problem, you then need to find out right at the beginning if there are other problems that the patient thinks need to be considered. 'Are there any other problems that we need to deal with?' The patient may volunteer these immediately, but if they do not, then you should use any information present in the letter of referral: 'Dr Smith says that you have also been getting some pain in the chest? . . . is that right?'

The business of checking information with the patient is a recurrent theme in good history taking: if this is neglected, then it is possible for the conversation to wander off course.

By establishing the main problem or problems at the start, you have the right framework for the consultation.

Exploring the main problems

 Focus on each problem in turn, thinking about likely diagnoses as you talk.

Having confirmed what the main problem is, ask the patient to tell you about it: 'what happens when you get one of your dizzy turns?'

Give them a minute or two, making encouraging noises if necessary to keep them going. If the story is making sense, keep quiet and let the patient continue. But if it isn't, then you need to intervene. Say something like 'can I just make sure that I understand things properly?' This is more generous than saying something which implies 'you are rambling in an incoherent manner', since it suggests that the difficulty is yours and not the patients.

Be particular and not general.

If the history is proving difficult to follow, a useful device is to focus on a particular episode and avoid generalizations. In this case, 'tell me about the worst episode of dizziness that you have had . . . when did it happen? . . . exactly what were you doing when it started? Standing up? Sitting down?' 'What was the first thing that you noticed?' 'What happened next?' 'And after that?' After getting as much information as possible about the episode by such open questioning, you should then proceed to ask directed questions that might lead you to a particular diagnosis. From the moment that you meet any patient, you should be thinking 'what is the diagnosis?' In this case appropriate questions would explore the possibilities of vasovagal, cardiac or epileptiform episodes.

After getting clear details about the worst episode, you can then go on to ask about the others: 'how many attacks have you had in all?' 'Were they the same as this one or were they different?'

Check that you understand each problem before going on to the next one.

If the patient tries to go off at a tangent, or talk about one of their other problems before you have finished your exploration of the first, do not allow them to do so: 'can we talk about that in a moment? . . . I want to make sure that I understand about the dizzy spells first'. If you don't do this, you will land up with a mish mash of a history that will be much more difficult to put together, and the examiner will think you've lost the plot, which you will have done. Check that you have got things right about the dizziness before progressing to explore the next problem in a similarly focused manner.

Make sure that you deal with each of the main problems in turn before moving on to other aspects of the history: it suggests a scatter-brained approach if you don't.

Avoid letting the patient make assumptions.

Some patients will have decided that they know what the diagnosis is already. The man with chest pain may have decided that it is due to indigestion and be reluctant to consider any other possibility. If you ask 'what is the pain like?' the reply comes 'like indigestion'. If you then ask 'how do you know it's indigestion?' the response is 'because it feels like it'. Such issues are not infrequent in real life and commonly feature in PACES scenarios because the ability to tease out the nature of the symptom separates those who can take a good history from those who cannot. The key thing in this context is to avoid opportunity for the word indigestion to be used:

• 'Where is the pain worst? . . . point to the spot'.

• 'Does it go anywhere else?'

• 'Does anything bring it on? . . . eating?, exercise?'

This line of enquiry may reveal that, whilst the pain can be brought on by eating a heavy meal, it can also be provoked by exercise and the cause is likely to be cardiac ischaemia. The candidate who cannot get past the 'it's-like-indigestion' barrier will not get onto the right track, fail to get the diagnosis, and fail to score the satisfactories that they hope for.

Find out if the patient has particular concerns.

Detailed exploration and discussion of patient's or relative's concerns are mainly conducted in Station 4, but it is always important to find out if the patient has any particular concerns about issues under discussion in Station 2. A man with chest pain that seems trivial and not at all typical of coronary ischaemia may be extremely concerned about it if

his brother has recently dropped dead of a heart attack. If this information is not elicited by the doctor, simply by asking 'is there any particular reason that you are worried about these pains?', then it is unlikely that the patient will be reassured by the consultation.

Explore social implications of the main problems.

In many cases this is not an important matter, but when it is, it is absolutely crucial to explore social aspects thoroughly. An apparently minor symptom can become of major significance if it acts as 'the straw that breaks the camel's back'. A simple enquiry along the lines 'does the pain (or whatever the symptom is) stop you doing anything that you need to do?' will usually do the trick.

Other aspects of the history

Use all the information in the referral letter.

Some details of the patient's medical and social background will have been given in the letter of referral, but some important issues will deliberately not have been included. Hence, having talked through the main problems, you need to have an efficient method of eliciting the rest of the information required for a proper medical history. Use a structured approach and draw on all information in the GP's letter, checking that it is correct as you go along. There is no proscribed sequence in which information should be elicited, i.e. there is no strict order in which you have to move from past medical history to drugs to functional enquiry etc.

As a general rule it is sensible to talk about things in order of their importance to the case. What you must be able to demonstrate to the examiners is that you can cover the ground in a reasonably smooth and polished manner, without too many pauses where it is obvious that you are thinking 'what am I supposed to be asking about now?' A reasonable sequence of questions in a case where there are no great social issues or family history to explore would be as follows:

Past medical history:
'Your doctor's letter says that you have had x and y in the past . . . is this correct? . . . have you had any other operations or medical problems that have taken you into hospital?'

Medication:
'The letter says that you are on the following drugs . . . is this correct? . . . are you taking any other medications that your doctor has prescribed at the moment? . . . or any other things that you have bought over-the-counter?' Aside from the importance of knowing what medications a patient takes, their list of drugs is a useful clue as to what other diagnoses they have been given in the past and should prompt discussion if any are unexplained: 'why are you using the inhalers?' etc. It will also be sensible at this point to check 'are you allergic to any medicines you've been given in the past? . . . what happened?'.

Functional enquiry:
'Aside from the things that we have talked about already, have you had any other problems with your heart or chest? . . . what is the most exercise you can do? . . . what stops you doing more?' 'Have you had any problems with indigestion or your bowels?' 'Have you had any

problems with your urine, bladder or kidneys?' 'Have you had any problems with dizziness (already discussed in this case), funny turns, fits or faints? . . . or depression or any other psychiatric problems?'

Social history:
'Do you smoke? . . . how many? . . . have you smoked in the past? . . . how many and for how long?' 'Do you drink alcohol? . . . how much? . . . have you been a heavy drinker in the past?'

Other social information:
'Do you live on your own or with someone else?' will frequently elicit the response 'I live with my wife and children', or somesuch, and further discussion of this nature will not be needed. If the context of the case is different, such that social factors are clearly important, then you will almost certainly have explored these earlier than now, the requirement being to find out how the patient's condition or concerns affects their life. Using common sense as a guide (always invaluable) you will probably already have asked how the patient's main problem(s) affect what they can do: 'how far can you walk?', 'do you use a stick or a frame?', 'can you get up stairs?', 'can you get out of the house?', 'who does the shopping?' etc. as appropriate.

Family history:
This will almost certainly have come up before now in any case where it is relevant, but all patients should be asked 'are there any diseases or illnesses that run in the family?', and 'do (or did) your mother and father, or your brothers and sisters have any serious medical problems?' If it looks as though the patient might have an uncommon genetic condition, ask 'are (or were) your parents related?', 'were they cousins?' (autosomal recessive conditions likely with consanguinity).

'Sensitive' issues
Many patients will be sensitive about some issues, including infections associated with particular behaviours, alcohol/drug abuse and psychiatric illness. Detailed exploration of these should be left until the end of the history, by which time you will hopefully have established some rapport with the patient. In the context of the PACES exam your ability to deal with such things is tested in station 4, but some aspects of history taking will draw on similar skills.

Concluding discussion with the patient
The examiner will signal two minutes before the end of your time for taking the history. If you have paced the consultation correctly you will already have covered virtually all of the ground detailed above. Things will not go well if you find yourself spending this time firing a rapid stream of questions at the patient, each demanding a 'yes/no' answer. Because it may reveal something important, both in routine clinical practice and in PACES, it is always worth asking the patient, 'is there anything else you would like to tell me before we conclude?' And to summarise the plan of action with the patient is an appropriate and polished way to finish with them, even if not specifically demanded by the station instructions.

One minute for thinking
What was the task that was set in the letter of referral? What are the main diagnoses to consider? What would be the most likely causes of the problem, remembering that common things are common? How would you pursue investigation? Imagine yourself sitting behind the desk in the outpatient clinic: what would you order in 'real life'? What treatment options are available?

- Speak clearly and simply.
- Be empathetic.
- Be honest.
- Be comforting and compassionate (but not unrealistic).
- Be firm when necessary.
- Stay calm.

Teaching of communication skills is now a standard element of medical school training and of some postgraduate courses. This is a good thing, but courses on communication skills can only get you so far. To become proficient at dealing with the difficult situations that commonly arise in clinical practice there is no substitute for personal experience, but – as in all other aspects of life – it is important that this experience does not amount to making the same mistakes repeatedly. Make a deliberate point of observing closely how experienced colleagues that you respect handle things: when they are going to talk with the angry or distressed patient or relative, ask if you can join them as a 'fly on the wall'. After dealing with or observing a difficult situation, reflect upon it: what went well? What went badly? How might things have been handled differently? If a turn of phrase was used that seemed effective, file it away for future reference; if something was said that caused things to go awry, then avoid repeating the error.

Very few PACES examiners have been on courses to learn communication skills, but all will have spent many hours talking through problems with patients, relatives, carers and other health professionals over the years. Some of this time will have been needed to sort out issues that were caused or exacerbated by junior doctors who behaved sub-optimally, or made a mess of explaining things in one way or another. They don't want a registrar who they think is likely to cause a queue of disaffected patients, relatives and others to be heading down to the 'patient satisfaction' office or contacting their secretary to ask for an appointment. When listening to candidates in PACES, the ones who have 'clocked up the miles' and have some experience of dealing with conversations that are difficult are very obvious and are appropriately rewarded in the scores that they obtain.

The format of PACES station 4 is shown in Table 5. Note the details of the marksheet that the examiner will be looking at as you talk (Table 6). Although the structure of the discussion is less easily formalized than that for history taking (because there are fewer standard areas to be covered, such as past medical history, medications, allergies etc), there are a few key things that you should always do in your routine clinical practice and in the exam (Table 7).

TABLE 5 COMMUNICATION SKILLS AND ETHICS FOR **PACES** – FORMAT OF STATION **4**

Time	
5 minutes before starting station	Read the scenario very carefully. What is the main task? Write down any points that you want to be sure of covering.
0–15 minutes	Discussion with surrogate (1)
15–20 minutes	Discussion with examiners

Notes
(1) Communication skills and ethics stations always use a surrogate.

TABLE 6 KEY FEATURES OF EXAMINER'S MARKSHEET FOR THE COMMUNICATION SKILLS AND ETHICS STATION

Clinical skill	To score satisfactory	To score unsatisfactory
Clinical communication skills	Explains relevant clinical information in an accurate, clear, structured, comprehensive, fluent and professional manner.	When trying to explain things to the patient either omits important information, gives inaccurate or unclear information, uses jargon, or conducts the discussion in a manner that is poorly structured, appears unpractised or is unprofessional.
Managing patient's concerns	Listens and is empathetic. Seeks, detects and attempts to address the patient's or relative's concerns. Confirms the patient's knowledge and understanding.	Does not listen well and/or is not empathetic. Overlooks patient's or relative's concerns. Does not check the patient's or relative's knowledge and understanding.
Clinical judgement	Selects or negotiates a sensible and appropriate management plan.	Selects or negotiates an inappropriate, incomplete or incorrect management plan.
Maintaining patient welfare	Treats the patient or relative in an appropriate manner.	Causes the patient or relative physical or emotional discomfort, or treats them in an unsafe manner.

TABLE 7 KEY REQUIREMENTS FOR THE COMMUNICATION SKILLS AND ETHICS STATION

Beginning the discussion	Greet the person. Explain who you are. Confirm who they are. Confirm the reason for the meeting – 'I understand that you wanted to speak to me about . . . , is that right?'; 'I wanted to speak to you about . . .' Find out what they know already – 'how much do you know about the situation?'; 'have any other doctors had chance to speak to you about things?'
General approach	Establish and maintain good rapport. Be polite and courteous, even in the face of an aggressive response. Speak quietly but clearly. Do not give long speeches and do not hurry – use short phrases and allow time for information to sink in. Develop a dialogue – 'would you like to know exactly what's going on?'; 'have you got any questions about that?' Give information gradually – 'the chest X-ray showed a shadow on the lung . . . this was confirmed on the CT scan'. Maintain eye contact.
Be emphathetic	'I can see why you think that'. 'I can see why you are concerned about that'.
Be honest	'I'm afraid I don't know, but I will find out for you'. 'I am sorry, we made a mistake'. 'This is not good news'. 'We cannot cure this and make it go away completely'. Do not promise things that cannot be delivered.
Do not destroy hope, but do not be unrealistic	'The outlook is uncertain, but there are treatments that can help this condition'. 'Symptoms can be relieved'.
Correct misunderstandings: be firm when necessary	'No, I don't think that's right, my understanding is that . . .' 'No, I am not allowed to hide information from a patient if they want to know . . . but I certainly won't force anything on to them that they don't want to hear'. 'I am afraid that it is a legal requirement that you are not able to drive for one year after having a fit . . . I have to advise you that you must tell the DVLA and your insurance company . . . and I have to write in your notes that I have told you this'.
Offer further discussion	'I can meet you again to talk over things some more if that would be helpful'. 'Do you think it would be helpful if we were to meet together with your father/mother (as appropriate) to talk things over?' 'If you would like to meet my consultant to discuss things, then I can help make arrangements'.

> **Learn how to examine each of the respiratory, abdominal, cardiovascular and neurological systems in between six and seven minutes – not more and not less. Use a watch to time yourself when you are practicing for PACES.**

Ten minutes of station 1 are allocated for examination of the respiratory system and ten minutes for the abdominal system; in station 3 there are ten minutes each for cardiovascular and neurological examinations; station 5 provides ten minutes for each of two brief clinical encounters. In stations 1 and 3 you are undoubtedly going to have to perform thorough clinical examinations of the respiratory, abdominal and cardiovascular systems, and some part of the neurological system. Station 5 will require focused history taking, focused examination and discussion with the patient.

Given that the examiners need time to question you – even if you would prefer that they didn't – you must make sure that you can perform each of the necessary examinations in stations 1 and 3 in six minutes, seven at the most. It is extremely important that you learn how to do this. If you seem to be going too slowly, the examiner will either have to encourage you to hurry up, or stop you before you have finished, and neither circumstance is likely to help you think clearly about what the examination is revealing and then give a lucid account of your

findings. A less common problem, but also best avoided, arises if you race through an examination very quickly. This leaves a lot of time for a lot of questions, which may not be in your best interest, and if you have missed anything, then the examiner will almost certainly think 'well, it's not a surprise, they were rushing and didn't notice . . . they need to settle down . . . perhaps they should come back and try the exam again another time'. By contrast, if you performed a well paced examination, then the examiner may think 'well, the sign they missed was rather difficult . . . and their technique looked pretty sound . . . I'll score physical examination as satisfactory and identifying physical signs as borderline instead of unsatisfactory'. And on such decisions can pass or fail depend. Use a watch to time yourself when you are practicing for PACES.

> **Read the instructions.**

The examiner will begin by asking you to read the written instructions that are displayed next to the patient. These are always very simple, for instance, 'this man is breathless on exertion, please examine his respiratory system'. But I can still remember a particularly nervous candidate who began to perform a cardiovascular examination on the respiratory station, and then looked as though they were about to have a

cardiorespiratory arrest themselves when after about 60 seconds I recognized the error that they had made and directed them to read the instructions again and examine the respiratory system. To their considerable credit, they then managed to perform reasonably well and I scored them as such.

> **Always perform a thorough examination unless told not to do so by the examiner.**

Although the examiners seek to avoid this, on some occasions the instructions for the candidate can be open to varied interpretation. If the instruction says 'examine the respiratory system', then there is no doubt that a full examination of the respiratory system is required: but if it says 'examine the chest', then does this mean a full respiratory examination beginning with general inspection from the foot of the bed, then moving on to the hands etc, or that the candidate should move directly to the chest itself? The default position should always be that you perform a full examination of the relevant system, beginning with general inspection. An enormous amount of information can be gleaned from the foot of the bed, but don't stand there frozen in a Parkinsonian posture for a minute. If the examiner wants you to truncate things and move directly on to a more limited examination, perhaps just of the chest itself, then they will tell you so and thereby take responsibility for the 'cutting of corners'.

> There is no single 'right way' to perform a physical examination, but avoid eccentricities.

Many candidates are worried that there is a particular 'RCP-approved' method of performing a physical examination and that if they vary from this they will inevitably fail. This is not true. It may be that one or two of the examination methods described in this module are not those that you routinely use, even that 'Dr Brilliant, who is a fantastic doctor, and an MRCP PACES examiner to boot' does not have exactly the same way of doing things. This does not matter. The important thing is that the method for examining a system progresses in a logical and fluent manner that seems second nature to the candidate, and that recognized methods are used to perform particular manoeuvres. Eccentricities are to be avoided since they will cause the examiner to think 'that looks a bit odd . . . they might have got away with it this time . . . but I'm not sure . . . down a grade, I think'. But there is no single rigidly prescribed method for many aspects of technique; for instance, examination of the carotid pulse. The candidate must not appear to strangle the patient, which both 'fails to maintain patient welfare' and is ineffective, since tension in the neck muscles induced by the threat will prevent useful palpation of the vessel, but it does not matter at all whether the fingers or thumb are used to feel the pulse itself. I prefer to use my thumb, but of the two best clinical cardiologists that I have come across, one used her thumb and one his fingers.

> Ask the examiner if they want you to explain your findings as you go.

Examiners will usually tell the candidate whether they want them to comment on their findings as they go, or if they want them to proceed without comment aside from the necessary enquiries and instructions to the patient. But some examiners do not do this, or forget to do so sometimes, in which case it is sensible for the candidate to ask 'do you want me to comment on my findings as I go?' It is always best to be clear from the beginning, and asking the question gives the impression (hopefully not dispelled by subsequent performance on the station) that 'this candidate is in control, they are master (or mistress) of the situation'.

> If a thing is clear-cut, then say so; but do not box yourself into corners if you are not sure.

In discussing your examination findings, there is a sensible balance to be struck. In one camp is the candidate that is terrified of getting anything wrong, who when confronted by an enormously obese, blue and bloated man, scarcely able to breathe, and whose wheeze can be heard from the corridor outside the examination room, says very tentatively that the patient 'seems a little breathless at rest' and only plucks up the courage to admit that they are deeply cyanosed when the examiner has asked for the third time 'do you notice anything else?' In the other camp is the candidate who wants to impress upon the examiners that they are decisive and will immediately cut to the heart to

the matter. After vigorously rolling the legs a few times they conclude that the tone is increased, almost undoubtedly because the candidate's technique was not conducive to relaxation, and before the examiner can blink or indeed any other signs have been considered, the patient has been diagnosed as having a spastic paraparesis and sent off for an MRI scan. Go for the middle ground: if the man is blue and wheezing, then say so; if the tone in the legs might be increased but isn't clearly grossly abnormal, then say 'the tone in the legs might be increased . . . I will look for other evidence of an upper motor neuron lesion as I proceed'.

> Prepare your thoughts in the ten seconds before you finish your examination.
> - What would you like to do to complete your examination?
> - What have you found?
> - What are the possible diagnoses?

As soon as you have finished your examination of the patient the examiner is going to ask you to comment, most probably by saying something along the lines of 'please tell me what you have found'. This may occur just as you complete your beautifully paced and thorough examination of the relevant system in precisely six minutes and zero seconds, but is also likely to happen at certain obvious 'break points' in the process of a complete examination. For instance, in the cardiovascular station the examiner is likely to stop you as soon as you have finished auscultation of the heart, or perhaps of the lung bases. They are unlikely to be able to allow you the time to progress to palpation of the liver and for an abdominal aortic aneurysm, to check for ascites (if relevant), and then to move on to the peripheral pulses and oedema in the legs – although the latter may be obvious from the foot of the bed and should always be looked for. You should be aware of when the examiner is likely to stop you and have ready the list of things you would like to do to complete your examination. Spend the last few seconds before you finish or know that you are going to be asked to stop considering how you will respond to 'what have you found?' and 'what is the diagnosis?' The simplest and shortest questions are always the most deadly.

> Present your findings clearly.

Candidates who know what is wrong with a case rarely have difficulty in presenting their findings to the examiners. But if they are not sure, then candidates very often fail

to do themselves justice. Consider two candidates examining the same difficult case. The examiners have agreed that the case is difficult, that the physical signs are not absolutely obvious, and that their interpretation is not straightforward.

As they are examining the case the first candidate thinks 'it isn't obvious to me what the problem is here . . . I can't be sure of any of these physical signs . . . this is bad . . . this is terrible . . . this is worse than terrible . . . I'm going to fail'. And they go on to present their findings in a hesitant manner, speaking so quietly that the examiners have great difficulty in hearing what they are saying at all, and looking for all the world as though they want a hole to open in the floor and swallow them up. It is impossible for the examiners to score them better than unsatisfactory for any of the clinical skills.

By contrast, as they are examining the case the second candidate thinks

'it isn't obvious to me what the problem is here . . . I can't be sure of any of these physical signs . . . it's a difficult case . . . let me think . . . the abnormality that seems most clear cut is x . . . I will talk about that . . . let me remind myself, what are the commonest causes of x?' They then present the case as follows: 'I found this a difficult case', and they then go on to present the findings in the logical order in which they elicited them, concluding with something along the lines 'I thought the most obvious abnormality was x . . . the commonest causes of which are . . .' This candidate has had the same difficulty with the case as had the first, but they have not panicked, they've worked their way through to a sensible analysis, which is what you need to do when confronted with something that isn't clear cut in the medical admissions unit, ward or clinic. Score satisfactory, or borderline at worst.

Details from the marksheet that the examiner will be looking at as you examine the patient are shown in Table 8.

From the foot of the bed

- Well or ill?
- Correctly positioned and exposed.
- General inspection.
- Respiratory rate.
- Cough.
- Open mouth, deep breath in and out – wheeze or stridor?

Does the patient look well or not? If they are unwell, then why? Severe respiratory disease may make the patient look sweaty, pale, breathless or cyanosed. Are they using their accessory muscles to breathe?

Is the patient positioned correctly? Ideally they should be lying on the

bed or couch with their torso propped up at 45° and undressed to the waist. However, if it is cool and to maintain decorum it is common practice to allow patients, particularly women, to keep some of their clothes on. This can pose a dilemma for the candidate: should they expose the patient fully to be seen to be thorough, but perhaps thought uncaring? Or should they allow the patient to keep their clothing on and be seen to be kind, but perhaps thought slapdash? The best solution is for the candidate to ask the examiner 'would you like me to ask Mrs Jones to remove her night dress?' But if the pyjama jacket or nightie is not removed, take great care when inspecting the chest to lift up the clothing to look all over.

Are there any clues around to indicate what sort of respiratory problem the patient might have? The salbutamol inhaler on the bedside

locker suggests asthma or chronic obstructive pulmonary disease and the sputum pot chronic bronchitis or bronchiectasis. The cylinder of oxygen probably implies chronic respiratory failure in the context of a PACES exam. If the patient has lots of bruises, then long-standing steroid treatment must be the likely cause. Bilateral ankle oedema could indicate cor pulmonale in a respiratory case. The candidate that observes and interprets these obvious things correctly is well on the way to scoring a four.

Uncommon in real life, but less so in PACES exams, look out for the patient who has a general appearance that can be associated with a respiratory abnormality. In particular, could the patient have scleroderma or another auto-immune rheumatic disorder that can be associated with interstitial lung disease? Don't

TABLE 8 KEY FEATURES OF EXAMINER'S MARKSHEET FOR RESPIRATORY SYSTEM EXAMINATION

Clinical skill	To score satisfactory	To score unsatisfactory
Physical examination	Technique must be correct, thorough, systematic and fluent. Specific requirement for professional methods of palpation, percussion and auscultation are noted.	Techniques are incorrect. Significant or important tests are omitted. Approach is unsystematic, hesitant, lacking confidence or unprofessional.
Identifying physical signs	Identifies correct signs. Signs that are not present are not found.	Important signs are missed. Signs that are not present are found.
Differential diagnosis	Sensible, and includes the correct diagnosis.	Poor, and fails to consider the correct diagnosis
Clinical judgement	Offers a sensible and appropriate management plan.	Offers an inappropriate management plan.
Maintaining patient welfare	Treats the patient in an appropriate manner.	Causes the patient physical or emotional discomfort, or treats them in an unsafe manner.

15

try to be too clever and invent these findings if they aren't there, but if you really think they might be, then say so – without boxing yourself completely into a corner at this early stage in proceedings – 'I notice that Mrs Jones has waxy fingers . . . this makes me think of scleroderma, which . . . although I know it's not very common in routine clinical practice . . . can be associated with respiratory problems'.

Before moving on to start examining the hands, count the respiratory rate (over 30 seconds, also noting the unlikely event in PACES that the patient has an unusual respiratory pattern), and then ask the patient to do two things: give a cough, and open their mouth and to take one big breath in and out as fast as they can. If the patient coughs up a large dollop of green sputum, then you have almost certainly made the diagnosis (bronchiectasis) before you have even laid hands on the patient, which is a very good start to the station. If you elicit wheeze or (even more precise diagnostically)

stridor, then again you are well on the way to the diagnosis.

Hands

Look in particular for clubbing (Table 9), nicotine staining of the fingers and peripheral cyanosis. Quickly feel the pulse: approximate rate, and sinus rhythm or atrial fibrillation? Ask the patient to cock their wrists back to see if they have a metabolic flap. Report your findings in a brisk manner: 'the hands are normal', if they are.

Face and neck

You will have noticed any obvious features on inspection from the foot of the bed, but look in particular for anaemia and for central cyanosis. If the patient is clearly cyanosed, then say so.

Note if the JVP is grossly elevated, and swiftly palpate the cervical and supraclavicular lymph nodes. Do not linger over these aspects, which do not appear on the PACES mark sheet for the respiratory station, although most physicians would regard them as a proper part of the examination of the respiratory system.

Trachea

Practise palpating the trachea.

- **Neck supported and slightly flexed.**
- **Approach from below.**
- **Don't appear to strangle the patient.**

To feel the trachea requires practice and a gentle touch. As with attempts to palpate the carotid arteries, the problem is that a less than subtle approach can lead the patient to think that they are about to be throttled, which naturally leads them to lower their chin and tense up, making access difficult. Palpation is easiest if the patient's head is supported on pillows and slightly flexed such that tension in the anterior muscles of the neck is not required to support the head. Let the patient know that you are going to feel their windpipe and bring your finger(s) over the top of the sternal manubrium from below, avoiding the presentation of a visual threat. Diagnose tracheal deviation only if the trachea is very clearly displaced from the midline.

Inspection of chest and assessment of expansion

Note the general shape of the chest, in particular look for pes carinatum, pectus excervatum, kyphosis and scoliosis. Look carefully for surgical scars at the front, sides and back. If there is a tunneled central line, then in the context of a respiratory case in PACES, it probably means that the patient has bronchiectasis (likely caused by cystic fibrosis): almost a 'hole in one' as far as you are concerned.

Ask the patient to take a deep breath in and out, looking at how well the chest expands and whether there is any asymmetry of movement. Then

TABLE 9 CAUSES OF CLUBBING	
Cause	**Diagnoses to consider**
Respiratory	Interstitial lung disease Bronchiectasis (including Cystic Fibrosis) Lung cancer/mesothelioma* Lung abscess/empyema*
Cardiac	Congenital cyanotic heart disease Infective endocarditis*
Abdominal	Liver cirrhosis Chronic active hepatitis Coeliac disease Ulcerative colitis Crohn's disease
Other	Idiopathic, sometimes hereditary

Notes
* Uncommon in PACES.

estimate expansion using your hands. For the upper lobes, place your hands on either side of the chest, fingers pointing up and with the tips just touching the clavicles, and ask the patient to take a second deep breath. Do your hands rise normally and symmetrically? For the lower lobes, clamp the sides of the chest between your hands, extending your thumbs towards the midline until they nearly meet, but keeping them just above the chest wall so that they are free to move. Ask the patient to take a third deep breath: the thumbs should move symmetrically apart by at least 5cm. There is no point in assessing expansion from the back of the chest: the spine is always fixed and you never find anything that is not clearer from the front.

Percussion and auscultation

Percuss the front of the chest, ensuring that you adequately cover all areas, but without going to the extreme of striking every square centimeter in an effort to be seen to be thorough. Begin over the clavicles, comparing right with left, and then percuss moving down the chest in (say) three positions in the mid-clavicular line, comparing right and left sides in each. Then progress to (say) three positions between the anterior and mid-axillary lines, moving down the chest and again comparing the two sides in each position.

Continue your examination by auscultating in the same places that you have percussed, again comparing right and left sides of the chest.

If you have detected any abnormalities on percussion or auscultation of the front of the chest, then proceed to check for abnormalities of vocal (tactile) fremitus or vocal resonance. The

former should be elicited by pressing symmetrically and firmly on the two sides of the chest, most physicians using the ulnar borders of their hands, and asking the patient (typically) to 'say 99'. The latter is determined by listening over the chest and asking the patient to 'whisper 99': if the words are intelligible, then whispering pectoriloquy is demonstrated and vocal resonance is said to be increased. If percussion and auscultation of the anterior chest are normal, then it is not necessary to check for abnormalities of vocal fremitus or resonance.

Finally, before you leave the anterior surface of the chest, ensure that you have located the mediastinum: palpate for the apex and, if you cannot easily feel it, swiftly percuss in a line between the two nipples to demonstrate the area of cardiac dullness.

After finishing with the front of the chest, proceed to examine the back, percussing in half a dozen places from the top to the bottom in the mid-clavicular line, comparing the two sides in each position, and then proceed to auscultate in the same way. Again check for vocal fremitus and vocal resonance if you have detected any abnormalities, but not if you have not.

Expect to be asked 'what else would you like to do?' and 'what are your findings?' as soon as you appear to have finished auscultating the chest.

Completing the respiratory examination

It is almost certain that the examiner will stop you when you have finished auscultation of the back of the chest, but if not, check

for ankle oedema, which might suggest cor pulmonale in this context. Then say that you would like to see a sputum pot, if there is one, and to check peak flow/ spirometry.

Check list – respiratory examination

1. Well or ill?
   (a) Correctly positioned and exposed.
   (b) General inspection.
   (c) Respiratory rate, accessory muscles.
2. Cough.
3. Open mouth, deep breath in and out – wheeze or stridor?
4. Hands – clubbing, metabolic flap.
5. Face – conjunctival pallor, central cyanosis.
6. Neck – lymph nodes (swiftly), JVP.
7. Trachea.
8. Inspection of chest.
9. Front of chest – expansion, percussion, auscultation (vocal fremitus and vocal resonance if appropriate).
10. Back of chest – percussion, auscultation (vocal fremitus and vocal resonance if appropriate).
11. Ankle oedema.
12. Sputum pot.
13. Peak flow.

Presenting your findings to the examiners

The examiner is most likely to start off by asking you to summarise your findings, which you should do in the same logical and systematic manner in which you have hopefully examined the patient. This is by far the best way of giving a sensible account that does not miss anything out, but – by the time you get to PACES – you should be able to do better than trot out an exhaustive stream of negative findings in the manner of an automaton. Present briskly and clearly. For instance, if you are presenting a case of interstitial lung disease, which is one of the commonest respiratory cases in PACES:

- 'From the foot of the bed I notice that Mrs Jones is rather breathless at rest and is using some of her accessory muscles to breath. I also notice the oxygen cylinder by the bedside . . .'

- 'She is clubbed (assuming she is), but there is no metabolic flap' . . .

- 'The pulse is about x beats/minute and in sinus rhythm (if it is), and the respiratory rate is x breaths/minute' . . .

- 'I find it difficult to be sure in this light (it's often difficult to tell, but assuming Mrs Jones is not dark blue), but Mrs Jones does not seem to be cyanosed' . . .

- 'The venous pressure in the neck is normal (assuming it is) and there is no lymphadenopathy (assuming there isn't)' . . .

- 'The trachea is normal (assuming it is) and the mediastinum is not displaced (assuming it isn't)' . . .

- 'There are no scars on the chest (unless there are), but chest

TABLE 10 PHYSICAL FINDINGS IN COMMON RESPIRATORY PACES CASES

Diagnosis	General inspection	Clubbing	Movement of chest	Percussion/auscultation	Other features to look for
Bronchiectasis	Cough produces sputum	Probably	Probably normal	Coarse crackles, often widespread but likely to be more prominent in some zones than others; may be wheeze.	Tunneled line or scars of previous central venous access, suggesting cystic fibrosis in this context. Evidence of cor pulmonale.
Chronic obstructive pulmonary disease	Cough may lead to wheezing (sometimes sputum). 'Over-inflated' chest. Nicotine staining of fingers.	No	Globally reduced	Wheeze; often a few widespread crackles, but not as prominent as in bronchiectasis or interstitial lung disease.	Evidence of cor pulmonale.
Interstitial lung disease	May be signs of autoimmune rheumatic disorder, particularly rheumatoid arthritis or scleroderma.	Probably	Globally reduced	Fine crackles, particularly at bases.	Evidence of cor pulmonale.
Pleural effusion		No (1)	Normal, or focally reduced (if large)	Stony dullness to percussion at base. Reduced vocal (tactile) fremitus (2). Reduced breath sounds, but sometimes increased vocal resonance (whispering pectoriloquy) (2).	Marks from previous insertion of chest drain.
Pneumonectomy/ lobectomy	Scar Deformity of chest	No	Focally reduced	Dullness to percussion and reduced breath sounds where lung has been resected.	Mediastinum may be shifted (tracheal deviation, displaced apex/cardiac dullness). Horner's syndrome.
Upper airway obstruction	Stidor Tracheostomy scar	No	Normal	Normal	

Notes
All cases may be breathless, using accessory muscles and cyanosed.
(1) Unlikely to be clubbed in the context of PACES.
(2) Why the disparity between vocal fremitus and resonance? An effusion reduces transmission of low frequency sounds (100–200Hz) to the chest wall, hence vocal (tactile) fremitus is reduced, but it increases transmission of high frequency sounds (300–400Hz), hence vocal resonance can be increased.

expansion seems generally reduced (assuming it is)' . . .

• 'Percussion is normal in all areas (assuming it is), but on auscultation I can hear fine inspiratory crackles in both bases extending up into the midzones bilaterally' . . .

And you can go on directly to give your interpretation of the findings, or wait for the examiner to inevitably ask 'what do you think the diagnosis is?'

. . . 'I think these findings suggest that Mrs Jones has interstitial lung disease . . . but I would also want to consider bronchiectasis'.

The examiner is then likely to proceed with questioning along very obvious lines: 'how would you establish the diagnosis?' The way to approach this is to think, 'what would I actually order if I was seeing this woman as a new patient in clinic?' Which would lead you to say sensible things like 'I would start off by checking lung function tests, expecting to find a restrictive picture, and a chest X-ray, expecting to see interstitial shadowing' . . . 'other tests that would be of particular interest would be a CT scan of the chest, also blood gases' . . . and then you are on a roll.

This is all very easy if you are confident that you know the diagnosis, but much harder if you are not sure. As suggested earlier, if confronted with a difficult case, you must get into the mindset 'this is a difficult case' and not 'Oh, this is awful . . . I'm going to fail'. Practise your method of presenting a respiratory case (and all other sorts of case) so that it becomes a question of 'filling in the blanks as relevant'. This will stand you in good stead when, as is likely on at least one of the PACES examination stations, you run into something tricky. You won't go to pieces, you will get the information out in a logical order, and you will pick up more marks than you otherwise would. In the respiratory station, consider the diagnoses and physical findings listed in Table 10.

Details from the marksheet that the examiner will be looking at as you examine the patient are shown in Table 11.

From the foot of the bed

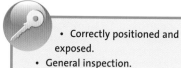

- Correctly positioned and exposed.
- General inspection.

Is the patient positioned correctly? Ideally they should be lying flat on the bed or couch and undressed to the waist. However, as discussed in the introduction to the section on respiratory examination, it is common practice to allow women to keep some of their clothes on. Again, ask the examiner what they would like you to do, but make sure that you inspect both arms and the torso properly by temporarily lifting up

the garments. Ask the patient if they can lie absolutely flat: some cannot do so, in which case ask them to let you know the flattest position in which they are comfortable.

Does the patient look well nourished or are they wasted? Some features of abdominal disease may be apparent from the foot of the bed, in particular some of the more dramatic signs of chronic liver disease such as obvious jaundice and a very swollen abdomen full of ascites. Look at this stage, and as you proceed with the abdominal examination, for all of the many signs of chronic liver disease (Table 12).

Remember that an abdominal case in PACES could have a gastroenterological/hepatological diagnosis, but is perhaps equally likely to have a haemato-oncological or renal condition. From the foot of

the bed, and as you proceed, look for any of the features in Table 13: these would be very useful clues.

Hands

Aside from clubbing (Table 9) and the other features of chronic liver disease listed in Table 12, look for koilonychia (spoon-shaped nails) suggesting iron deficiency. Ask the patient to extend their arms and spread their fingers out, looking for the fine tremor that is likely to indicate alcohol withdrawal, but bearing in mind that it might be caused by calcineurin inhibitors (ciclosporin or tacrolimus) in a patient with a transplant. Then ask the patient to cock their wrists back, as in the respiratory examination, to look for a metabolic flap, which in an abdominal case in PACES would almost certainly indicate decompensation in a case of chronic liver disease.

TABLE 11 KEY FEATURES OF THE EXAMINER'S MARKSHEET FOR ABDOMINAL SYSTEM EXAMINATION

Clinical skill	To score satisfactory	To score unsatisfactory
Physical examination	Technique must be correct, thorough, systematic and fluent. Specific requirements for professional method of palpation and percussion for masses, organomegaly and ascites are noted.	Techniques are incorrect. Significant or important tests are omitted. Approach is unsystematic, hesitant, lacking confidence or unprofessional.
Identifying physical signs	Identifies correct signs. Signs that are not present are not found.	Important signs are missed. Signs that are not present are found.
Differential diagnosis	Sensible, and includes the correct diagnosis	Poor, and fails to consider the correct diagnosis
Clinical judgement	Offers a sensible and appropriate management plan.	Offers an inappropriate management plan.
Maintaining patient welfare	Treats the patient in an appropriate manner.	Causes the patient physical or emotional discomfort, or treats them in an unsafe manner.

TABLE 12 SIGNS OF CHRONIC LIVER DISEASE

System	Sign
Skin	Jaundice Spider naevi Scratch marks Purpura 'Tissue paper' (especially on shins) Hyperpigmentation (rare – haemochromatosis – 'bronzed diabetes')
Hands	Leuconychia Clubbing Palmar eythema Dupuyten's contracture (some association with alcoholic liver disease)
Abdomen	Splenomegaly Ascites Hepatomegaly (rare – liver usually normal/small in size) Caput medusa (very rare)
General	Feminisation in men – gynaecomastia, loss of secondary sexual hair, testicular atrophy

TABLE 13 IS THE CASE GASTROENTEROLOGICAL/HEPATOLOGICAL, OR HAEMATO-ONCOLOGICAL, OR RENAL? – CLUES TO LOOK FOR OUTSIDE THE ABDOMEN

Cause	Look for
Gastroenterological or hepatological	Loss of body weight/cachexia. Signs of chronic liver disease (Table 12). Fine tremor (alcohol – but could just be ciclosporin in renal transplant patient)
Haemato-oncological	Loss of body weight/cachexia. Indwelling single-lumen tunneled line (Hickman, or similar) or portacath (subcutaneous chamber for injection of drugs, usually on upper left chest). Scars in neck from previous insertion of tunneled lines.
Renal	Indwelling double-lumen tunneled line (for dialysis). Scars in neck from previous insertion of dialysis lines. Fistula in arm: left or right; radiocephalic (at wrist) or brachiocephalic (at elbow). Scars from previous dialysis access surgery at wrists or elbows.

Note
All causes can be associated with pallor and purpura, but haemato-oncological diagnosis most likely if very prominent.
You MUST look carefully at the arms: if there is a fistula, or a lot of appropriate scars, then the case is renal (or most unlikely dual pathology).

Face and neck

Aside from looking carefully at the sclerae and conjunctivae for the obvious but extremely important features of jaundice and anaemia, look in the mouth for evidence of iron deficiency, namely angular cheilitis (painful cracks at the corners of the lips) and atrophic glossitis (pale, smooth tongue), also for the raw, beefy tongue of folate or B12 deficiency. Look and feel for parotid swelling, particularly common in malnourished alcoholics.

Give a moments thought to whether or not there are a lot of telangiectasiae on the face: cases of hereditary haemorrhagic telangiectasiae still sometimes appear in PACES.

After finishing with the face, proceed to feel for lymphadenopathy in the neck in a systematic manner. It does not matter if you palpate for glands from the front or the back of the patient, the key thing is that you cover all of the relevant areas in a businesslike manner, looking as though you have done it many times before. It is not uncommon for a candidate to palpate very carefully and then declare that there is lymphadenopathy, when what they have felt is a transverse process of one of the cervical vertebrae or a rather hard bit of thyroid cartilage. This sort of mistake only happens to those who have not felt many necks with due care and attention, so practise.

Inspection of the abdomen

Ask the patient to pull down their pyjama bottoms until the groins, but not the genitals, are exposed. Look carefully for any surgical scars. Incisions in the groins (often hernia repairs) or in the suprapubic region (typically for Caesarean section or other gynaecological procedures) often heal very well and are easy to miss, as are scars in the flanks from renal surgery. And on the renal theme, hockey-stick shaped scars in the right or left iliac fossae are usually if not always associated with kidney transplants. The examiners will expect you to note all scars and be particularly impressed if you spot something that they missed in the short time that they were able to see the case before the exam started. Note if the abdomen looks distended and if the superficial veins are prominent. Ask the patient to take a deep breath in and out: sometimes the movement of an enlarged organ will be visible from the foot of the bed. Ask them to give a cough, looking for bulges/herniae.

Palpation

Begin by asking the patient if they have any pain or tenderness before you start. If they say that they do, then reassure them that you will start off by feeling in a place that isn't painful or tender, and ask them to tell you if you hurt them at any time. This is important. The examiner can see if the patient is in distress and, as stated in the introduction to this section, the candidate who (literally) presses on when they are causing pain will not pass the exam. If this means that you are not able to palpate as thoroughly as you would like to do so, then you can and should explain this when reporting to the examiner – 'I was not able to palpate deeply in the right upper quadrant because this caused the patient pain' (or similar).

Palpation – as you know – can only properly be done if you get down to the level of the abdomen, hence the need for you to wear clothing that allows this without undue difficulty. Begin with light palpation around the four quadrants, then firmer, looking at the patient's face from time to time for evidence of discomfort rather than fixedly on the abdomen.

Next proceed to systematic palpation for organomegaly. You will almost certainly know if there is any gross enlargement of organs from your preliminary palpation. As in your routine clinical practice, you must be thorough, but do not overdo this by starting in the right groin crease, advancing your hand one centimetre nearer to the right costal margin with every breath. The patient will be dizzy with hyperventilation by the time you get half way up the

abdomen and the examiner will be irritated ('this candidate is performing for show . . . I don't like that . . . the liver obviously isn't very big . . . any sensible doctor would know that already'). Start in the right iliac fossa, moving up to the right costal margin in five or six breaths, unless you think that you feel something, in which case you will naturally home in to confirm. If the liver is enlarged, then remember that you will need to report not just on its size, but on whether it is tender, soft/hard, smooth/irregular, or pulsatile.

Feel for splenomegaly, again without inducing hypocapnia. If there is none, ask the patient to roll 45 degrees towards you and feel again at the left costal margin, most physicians placing their left hand behind the patients left posterior rib cage as they do so.

Palpate bimanually for enlargement of the kidneys. Many candidates do this very badly indeed, so it is not surprising that they fail to feel kidneys that are very obvious when proper technique is applied. The idea is to apply pressure to the retroperitoneum, thereby moving any retroperitoneal structure forward (almost inevitably the kidney), and to detect such movement anteriorly. Palpate using your right hand to apply firm and constant pressure to the abdomen half way between the midline and the edge of the flank, just above the level of the umbilicus. Use the flat palmar aspect of the fingers of your left hand to apply firm pressure for a few seconds in the renal angle, release the pressure, and then reapply it. Can you feel anything coming up towards the fingers of your right hand? Apply the pressure again and ask the patient to take a deep breath in. Can you feel anything moving beneath the right hand? Repeat in the other flank.

> ⚠ Palpation for the kidneys is often done very badly: common errors are –
>
> - Left (posterior) hand – incorrect location of renal angle (will not move kidney); 'flapping' hand up and down too quickly (no time to perceive change in feeling anteriorly).
> - Right (anterior hand) – incorrect location (usually too far lateral); not keeping hand still (cannot perceive change in feeling caused by posterior pressure).

Remember the five ways in which the left kidney can be distinguished from the spleen on physical examination (Table 14).

> 🔑 You must be able to explain clearly how you distinguish an enlarged kidney from an enlarged liver or spleen by physical examination.

Although not specifically mentioned on the PACES mark sheet, examination of the abdomen in routine clinical practice should include palpation for an abdominal aortic aneurysm. The initial manoeuvre for this involves nothing more than palpating deeply for two seconds just above the umbilicus. If the aortic pulsation cannot be felt, the patient does not have an abdominal aortic aneurysm; if it can, then further palpation is required.

Percussion

Some physicians prefer to leave percussion of any part of the abdomen until they have finished palpation; others prefer to percuss for the liver immediately after they have palpated for it, then percussing for the spleen after they have palpated for splenomegaly. Both approaches are entirely reasonable.

TABLE 14 DIFFERENCES BETWEEN THE SPLEEN AND THE LEFT KIDNEY ON PHYSICAL EXAMINATION

Finding	Spleen	Left kidney
Can you get above it?	No	Yes (usually)
Movement on inspiration	Towards right iliac fossa	Towards left iliac fossa
Can you feel it bimanually?	No	Yes
Percussion note	Dull	Resonant (usually)
Has a notch?	Sometimes	No

It is difficult to confuse a mildly enlarged spleen with a mildly enlarged kidney, but it can be hard to distinguish these organs if they are grossly enlarged. The very big polycystic kidney may be jammed under the ribs, so you cannot get above it; it may scarcely move with respiration; it may be dull to percussion. In such circumstances look carefully for clues listed in Table 7, and always consider 'is there a renal transplant?': the well-healed hockey-stick scar in one or other iliac fossa with the relatively unimpressive feeling mass beneath it could be just the thing you are looking for.

Check list – abdominal examination

1. Correctly positioned and exposed.
2. General inspection.
3. Are there signs of chronic liver disease?
4. Are there clues to tell you the case is gastroenterological/ hepatological, haemato-oncological or renal?
5. Hands – clubbing, koilonychia, metabolic flap.
6. Face – jaundice, conjunctival pallor, angular cheilitis, glossitis, mouth ulcers (telangiectasiae).
7. Neck – lymph nodes.
8. Inspection of abdomen – including flanks and groins ('give a cough', scars, herniae).
9. Palpation of abdomen – general; systematic for organomegaly.
10. Percussion of abdomen – to confirm organomegaly; for ascites if appropriate.
11. Auscultation of abdomen.
12. (External genitalia).
13. (Rectal examination).
14. Ankle oedema.
15. Urine – dipstick.

As usual the examiner is looking for an acceptable technique that seems second nature to you.

In addition to confirming the lower border of the liver, percussion can also define the upper border and vertical extent of the organ. Move downwards from the chest to the abdomen in the mid-clavicular line. The upper border to percussion is usually around the sixth rib and the vertical extent of the liver is about 8–10 cm, although this is very variable depending on the heaviness of percussion technique.

If the abdomen is swollen, but also if it isn't, you need to demonstrate percussion for ascites. If there is none, the examiner is very likely to stop you at this point and ask you 'what else would you like to do to complete your examination?' However, if allowed to proceed, you need to demonstrate solid technique. Many clinical methods for trying to detect ascites are described, some involving the requirement for a 'third hand' (fluid thrill), others involving drawing on the patient's skin. To me these seem difficult or inelegant. My preferred technique is as follows: percuss from the centre of the abdomen towards the flank; if it becomes dull in the flank, keep the finger that you strike (usually the middle finger of the left hand) absolutely still on the skin, just at the point where you think 'this is definitely dull'; ask the patient to roll away from the hand; wait 5 seconds or so; repeat percussion. If 'definitely dull' has become 'definitely resonant', shifting dullness has been demonstrated.

Expect to be asked 'what else would you like to do?' and 'what are your findings?' as soon as you seem to have finished palpating the abdomen.

Completing the abdominal examination

To complete your examination you would wish to 'listen for bruits over the liver and the rest of the abdomen, check the hernial orifices with the patient standing up, examine the external genitalia, perform a rectal examination, check for ankle oedema and stick test a urine specimen'.

Presenting your findings to the examiners

As usual, the examiner will almost certainly start off by asking you to summarise your findings, which you should again do in the same logical and systematic manner in which you have performed the examination. For instance, if you are presenting a case of chronic liver disease, which is one of the commonest abdominal cases in PACES:

- 'From the foot of the bed I notice that Mrs Smith seems comfortable at rest and well nourished, but I also see that she looks slightly jaundiced and has some scratch marks and bruises on her skin . . .' (if this is so, you have already demonstrated to the examiner that you are on the right track)

- 'The palms of her hands look a bit reddened, but there are no other stigmata of chronic liver disease and no metabolic flap . . .'

- 'Looking at her face and neck, the sclerae confirm that she is jaundiced and there are a few spider naevi on the cheeks, but she is not anaemic . . .'

- 'Moving on to the abdomen itself, I notice that there is a scar in the right iliac fossa that is almost certainly that of an appendicectomy, also a feint suprapubic scar that is likely to be due to gynaecological or obstetric surgery . . .' (all clocking up plus points in the examiners' minds)

- 'On palpation the most obvious finding is that the spleen is enlarged about 8 cm below the left costal margin . . .'

- 'The liver edge is also palpable about 2 cm below the right costal margin, the edge feeling smooth, firm and non-tender . . .'

- 'There is no ascites . . .'

- 'The diagnoses that I would like to consider in this case include . . .'

This should not be too difficult if the case is straightforward and you are confident of the physical signs, but if there are no very obvious stigmata of chronic liver disease, you can feel masses below both costal margins extending down into the flanks, you are 90% sure that these are due to hepatosplenomegaly but are worried that there might be two big kidneys, then how do you present?

- 'From the foot of the bed I notice that Mrs Smith seems comfortable at rest and well nourished . . .' (you have not panicked; you are starting to say sensible things in a logical order)

- 'The hands are normal, with no stigmata of abdominal disease, and there is no metabolic flap . . .'

- 'The face and neck are normal, with no jaundice, anaemia or other significant findings . . .'

- 'Moving on to the abdomen itself, I notice that there is a scar in the right iliac fossa that is almost certainly that of an appendicectomy, also a feint suprapubic scar that is likely to be due to gynaecological or obstetric surgery . . .' (always get these points in, even though they are most unlikely to be relevant to the main diagnosis: they say 'I am the sort of doctor who notices things', which the best doctors always do)

- 'On palpation the most obvious finding is that there are masses below both costal margins extending into the flanks . . .'

And recalling Table 14:

- 'The mass on the right side extends about 15 cm below the costal margin . . . it feels smooth, firm and non-tender . . . it is dull to percussion, I cannot get above it, and I cannot palpate it bimanually . . .' (you are not quite confident enough just to say 'it's a liver' . . . so you are giving sensible data that explains why, later on, you will say you think it's a liver)

- 'The mass on the left side also extends about 15 cm below the costal margin . . . it feels smooth, firm and non-tender . . . it is dull to percussion, I cannot get above it, I cannot palpate it bimanually, and I cannot feel a notch . . .' (again you aren't confident enough just to say 'spleen', but you are giving the examiner information that says 'I know how to try to do this')

- 'There is no ascites . . .'

- 'I think that this is a case of hepatosplenomegaly . . .'

See Table 15 for causes of hepatomegaly, splenomegaly, hepatomegaly and big kidneys to consider in PACES.

TABLE 15 CAUSES OF ABDOMINAL ORGANOMEGALY IN PACES

Finding		Cause	Comments
Hepatomegaly	Common	Alcoholic liver disease Autoimmune hepatitis Primary biliary cirrhosis	Cirrhosis often associated with normal or small liver. Carcinomatous secondaries are a very common cause of hepatomegaly in routine clinical practice, but unlikely in PACES.
	Unlikely	Congestive cardiac failure Polycystic liver Other rarities – amyloid, storage disorders	Hepatomegaly due to cardiac failure common at cardiovascular station, but is JVP grossly elevated? Polycystic liver likely if kidneys palpable or other clue that patient has renal condition (arteriovenous fistula, renal transplant).
Splenomegaly	Common	Myeloproliferative disorder – chronic myeloid leukaemia*, myelofibrosis*, primary polycythaemia. Lymphoproliferative disorder – lymphoma, chronic lymphatic leukaemia. Portal hypertension	
	Unlikely	Infective – malaria (chronic)*, leishmaniasis (kala-azar)*. Autoimmune/rheumatological – rheumatoid arthritis (Felty's syndrome), SLE. Other rarities – amyloid, storage disorders	Infective causes common if taking PACES in centre where malaria or leishmania endemic.
Hepatosplenomegaly	Common	Myeloproliferative disorder – chronic myeloid leukaemia, myelofibrosis, primary polycythaemia. Lymphoproliferative disorder – lymphoma, chronic lymphatic leukaemia. Portal hypertension	
	Unlikely	Other rarities – amyloid, storage disorders	
Big kidneys	Common	Adult polycystic kidney disease	May be associated with palpable polycystic liver, especially in women
	Unlikely	Tuberous sclerosis	Can have large angiomyolipomatous kidneys

Notes
* The most likely causes of a very large spleen (>10cm below costal margin).
Many acute or subacute infections can cause hepatomegaly or splenomegaly, but it is not common for such cases to appear in PACES.

Details from the marksheet that the examiner will be looking at as you examine the patient are shown in Table 16.

From the foot of the bed

- Well or ill?
- Correctly positioned and exposed.
- General inspection.

Does the patient look well or not? If they are unwell, then why? Severe cardiac disease may make the patient look sweaty, pale, breathless or cyanosed.

Is the patient positioned correctly? Ideally they should be lying on the bed or couch with their torso propped up at 45° and undressed to the waist. However, if it is cool and to maintain decorum it is common practice to allow patients, particularly women, to keep some of their clothes on. This can pose a dilemma for the candidate: should they expose the patient fully to be seen to be thorough, but perhaps thought uncaring? Or should they allow the patient to keep their clothing on and be seen to be kind, but perhaps thought slapdash? The best solution is for the candidate to ask the examiner 'would you like me to ask Mrs Jones to remove her night dress?' But if the pyjama jacket or nightie is not removed, take great care when inspecting the chest to lift up the clothing to look all over. The lateral thoracotomy scar from a mitral valvotomy may be not at all obvious, particularly if obscured by a pendulous breast, and you certainly don't want to miss it.

Are there any signs that might indicate what sort of cardiac problem they have? The GTN spray on the bedside locker suggests ischaemic heart disease. The median sternotomy scar clearly indicates cardiac surgery, the scar visible on their calf below their pyjamas most likely due to vein harvesting meaning that they have had coronary artery by-pass grafts. Bilateral ankle oedema suggests right-sided cardiac failure. The candidate that observes and interprets these obvious things correctly is well on the way to scoring a four.

Uncommon in real life, but less so in PACES exams, look out for the patient who has a general appearance that can be associated with a cardiac abnormality. In particular, is the patient Marfanoid? Could they have ankylosing spondylitis? Don't try to be too clever and invent these findings if they aren't there, but if you really think they might be, then say something along the lines of 'I notice that Mr Brown is very tall

---

TABLE 16 KEY FEATURES OF THE EXAMINER'S MARKSHEET FOR CARDIOVASCULAR SYSTEM EXAMINATION

Clinical skill	To score satisfactory	To score unsatisfactory
Physical examination	Technique must be correct, thorough, systematic and fluent. Specific requirements for professional method of assessment of arterial and venous pulses, and palpation and auscultation of the praecordium are noted.	Techniques are incorrect. Significant or important tests are omitted. Approach is unsystematic, hesitant, lacking confidence or unprofessional.
Identifying physical signs	Identifies correct signs. Signs that are not present are not found.	Important signs are missed. Signs that are not present are found.
Differential diagnosis	Sensible, and includes the correct diagnosis	Poor, and fails to consider the correct diagnosis
Clinical judgement	Offers a sensible and appropriate management plan.	Offers an inappropriate management plan.
Maintaining patient welfare	Treats the patient in an appropriate manner.	Causes the patient physical or emotional discomfort, or treats them in an unsafe manner.

and thin, with very long fingers . . . this makes me think of Marfan's syndrome, which . . . although I know it's not very common in routine clinical practice . . . can be associated with a number of cardiovascular problems'.

Hands

Look in a business-like manner for clubbing and splinter haemorrhages, but do not spend a minute gazing at the hands in the manner of a fortune teller. Note also their temperature: low cardiac output can cause cool hands and peripheral cyanosis. Report your findings in a brisk manner: 'the hands are warm and well perfused with no stigmata of endocarditis'. This suggests that you are operating at a level above that of the candidate who laboriously lists a string of negatives: 'the hands are not cool or

cyanosed; there is no clubbing; there are no splinter haemorrhages'.

Radial pulse

Start off by briefly feeling both radial pulses, then feel the right radial pulse for fifteen seconds and comment on its rate and rhythm.

In routine clinical practice pulse rate is of vital importance in assessing any patient, with tachycardia (pulse >100/min) commonly associated with pain, fear, hypovolaemia, fever/sepsis and a host of other acute conditions. These are not likely to be relevant in a patient examined in PACES, poorly controlled atrial fibrillation being the likeliest cause of a tachycardia. Bradycardia (pulse <60/min) is most probably due to a β blocker in the exam situation, as it is in the medical admissions unit.

By far the commonest abnormality of rhythm is the irregularly irregular pulse of atrial fibrillation, but see Table 17 for other causes of an irregular pulse.

> If the patient is obviously in atrial fibrillation, then say so.

After assessing the pulse rate and rhythm at the wrist, ask the patient if their arm or shoulder is painful or stiff, and – if not – raise the arm whilst feeling for a 'collapsing pulse' suggestive of aortic incompetence. But remember, the odds of getting a case of aortic incompetence in Station 3 must be about 25 to 1 against, and not all patients with aortic incompetence will have this physical sign, so don't overinterpret unless the finding is truly dramatic. And do not forget that, aside from a collapsing pulse, the character of the pulse cannot be assessed reliably from palpation of the radial artery.

Brachial pulse and blood pressure

After examining the radial pulses, move on to assess the brachial pulses, from which you can comment on any abnormality in pulse character. The default position must be to say that this is normal, because it usually is. If the pulse is difficult to feel and seems to be of low volume, then say something along the lines of 'the pulse is of low volume, perhaps slow rising, which means that I will obviously look carefully for signs of aortic stenosis as I proceed'. This indicates to the examiners that you are thinking as you go along, which is as it should always be, and it does not box you into a corner in the way that baldly declaring 'the pulse is slow rising, this is aortic stenosis' does.

There are many bits of the cardiovascular examination where

Likelihood in PACES	Cause	Radial pulse is
Common	Atrial fibrillation	Irregularly irregular
	Sinus arrhythmia	Cyclically variable with respiration: rate increases on inspiration and decreases on expiration
Less common	Atrial extrasystole	Regular, with weak (or impalpable) pulse followed by incomplete compensatory pause and strong subsequent beat, but at the bedside it can often be impossible to say that the compensatory pause is incomplete rather than complete
	Ventricular extrasystole	Regular, with weak (or impalpable) pulse followed by complete compensatory pause and strong subsequent beat
Rare	Atrial flutter with variable ventricular response	Irregularly irregular
	Second degree heart block	Regular with (fairly) regular missed beats

TABLE 17 CAUSES OF AN IRREGULAR PULSE

There are physical signs that can be used to distinguish between the causes of an irregular pulse. For instance, the appearance of a cannon A wave in the neck during a pause in the radial pulse indicates that the pause is due to a ventricular extrasystole, when the right atrium beats against a tricuspid valve that has been closed by the premature ventricular contraction. But DO NOT spend time looking for such things in the PACES exam because (1) you don't have time to do so, (2) >90% of examiners will not know what you are talking about and think you are showing off, and (3) in real life you'd check an ECG, as would the examiner.

the examiner can pretty well only judge you by what you say: for instance, if you appear to be looking at the hands then it is just about impossible for the examiner to conclude that you are not, unless you fail to describe some very obvious feature. Feeling the brachial pulse is different: the examiner knows that it lies just medial to the biceps tendon, that you are unlikely to be able to feel it well unless you support the elbow in slight flexion, and that it is easiest to feel the patient's right brachial pulse with your right thumb and their left brachial pulse with your left thumb. You are unlikely to be able to do all this smoothly if you first attempt it in the PACES examination, and the examiner will be able to see you failing to do so. Moral of the story: practise palpating the brachial arteries.

After finishing the palpation of the brachial arteries tell the examiner that you would like to know the patient's blood pressure before swiftly moving on to examine the face.

Face

You will have noticed if the face is very abnormal during your general inspection from the foot of the bed, but now look in particular for generalized pallor or a 'mitral facies', conjunctival pallor and/or (most unlikely) petichiae, central cyanosis and/or (not quite so unlikely) a high arched palate.

Jugular venous pressure

> **Finding the JVP is crucial in clinical practice and in PACES**
> The examiner can see things as well as you can (or better).
>
> • Neck slightly flexed and supported.
> • No tension in sternocleidomastoid muscles.
> • Practise, Practise, Practise.

Finding the jugular venous pressure is a key part of the cardiovascular examination because determining the filling pressure of the right side of the heart is important diagnostically. In PACES it assumes even greater importance because the examiners can see exactly what you are doing and themselves determine where the JVP is, that is if you have got the patient into a position where it is visible. It is quite clear that many candidates are unable to do this and after ten seconds of staring hopefully at the neck, which seems to be an eternity for all concerned, they then – usually after an appropriate comment to the patient – press the abdomen in the hope that this will reveal something useful. It will not do so unless the patient has been positioned correctly.

The single most important issue in finding the JVP is to ensure that the neck is adequately supported and that there is no tension in the sternocleidomastoid or other muscles. There is very little pressure in the jugular veins, literally only a few centimeters of blood, which is not enough to cause any visible movement of the skin of the neck if the muscles are tense. If the sternocleidomastoids are taut to support the head when the candidate is looking for the JVP, then the examiner knows for certain that any statement about the height of the pulse can be nothing more than a guess, and guesses don't score well. So, both to see the JVP in your routine clinical practice and (just as important in PACES) to demonstrate to the examiner that you can see it, make sure that the patient's head is supported by the pillow and that the sternocleidomastoids are relaxed. It is standard practice to look for the JVP on the right side, when sometimes it is easier to see if the patient's chin is tilted a little to the left, which serves to shorten the right

sternocleidomastoid, but excessive rotation will lead to tension in the neck and obscure things. Remember the following basic points:

• The external jugular venous pulse is easier to see than the internal and can be used to judge the height of the JVP if the vein is pulsating, but not if it is distended without pulsation, which indicates that it is not freely connected to the intrathoracic pressure.

• The JVP cannot be judged from the internal jugular vein low down in the neck where it runs deep to the sternocleidomastoid muscle, through which any venous pressure wave cannot be seen. The JVP in the internal jugular vein can be seen from the mid part of the neck upwards.

• With a patient lying at 45°, the upper limit of normal for the JVP is 3cm in vertical height above the angle of Louis.

If, after positioning the patient correctly, you can see the JVP, then proceed directly with the rest of the cardiovascular examination. But if you cannot, then you need to find out why. Is it too high to be seen easily, or is it too low?

If a cardiac patient looks breathless, plethoric or unwell, then it is a reasonable bet that their JVP will be elevated, so look very carefully anterior to the ear. Can you see a pulsation? If so, you've got it. A pulsation anterior to the ear is not arterial and must be venous: it is a constant source of surprise to examiners who have seen this from the end of the bed that candidates frequently declare that 'the JVP is not raised'. Norway: null points.

By contrast, if the patient looks well, then it is more than likely that their JVP is normal and to be found in the root of the neck. The application of abdominal pressure may be of help in demonstrating this, which is sometimes loosely called a hepatojugular or abdominojugular test (because it is not what the test of this name was described for). After appropriate explanation to the patient, positioned in a manner such that their JVP could be seen, put your hand on the middle of the abdomen, look at the neck, and then apply reasonably firm sustained pressure for five seconds or so. This causes a temporary increase in venous return to the heart that, for literally a few seconds only – which is why you must be looking at the base of the neck as you press – leads to a temporary elevation of the JVP such that it can be seen. But enough to establish with certainty that the JVP is not elevated.

Table 18 shows the ways in which the JVP can be distinguished from the carotid pulse.

Palpation of the carotid arteries

Practise palpating the carotid arteries.

- Neck supported and slightly flexed.
- Approach from the side.
- Don't appear to strangle the patient.

Although the examiners cannot feel through your fingertips (or thumb) as you palpate the carotid arteries, this is another aspect of the cardiovascular examination that is very revealing, simply because the vessels can be difficult to feel and doctors who have not felt a lot of them are unlikely to have developed a good technique for doing so. As with looking for the JVP, the essential requirement is to make sure that the anterior neck muscles are relaxed. If your technique involves approaching the patient in the manner of someone bent on strangulation, then the inevitable and natural response of the patient will be to tense up. Ensure that the head and neck have remained comfortably supported on the pillow, bring your fingers or thumb up to the sternocleidmastoid muscle from below to avoid any sensation of visual threat, and palpate in the middle of the neck just medial to the sternocleidmastoid. The pulse character will usually be normal, but think to yourself 'is it slow rising?' (could be aortic stenosis), 'is it jerky?' (likely to be normal, but could just be hypertrophic cardiomyopathy) and 'is there a thrill?' (almost certainly aortic stenosis).

Inspection of the chest

Note any deformity of the chest and, as stated before, look carefully for surgical scars, also for implanted pacemakers/cardioverter-defibrillators. The latter are frequently apparent to the examiners, even as they stand at the foot of the bed, and a candidate who fails to spot them is likely to be in difficulties.

Palpation of the apex beat and praecordium

Locate the apex and note its character, feel for a left parasternal heave and for thrills in the pulmonary and aortic areas (Table 19). If you cannot feel the apex beat, then percuss in a line between the two nipples, which will demonstrate the area of cardiac dullness. Dextrocardia or other causes of mediastinal shift are exceptionally rare in routine clinical practice, but less so in PACES.

Auscultation

The examiner cannot hear what you are (or aren't) hearing, but they can tell whether or not you are listening in a systematic manner, and whether or not the business seems second-nature to you. It is usual to begin at the apex before moving on to the left sternal edge, pulmonary area, aortic area and (for radiating murmurs or carotid bruits) the neck. It is debatable whether in routine clinical practice it is necessary to listen in all areas with both the bell and the diaphragm (I don't do so), but it is absolutely essential to do so at the apex, the diaphragm picking up the usually high pitched sound of mitral regurgitation and the bell the low pitched sound of mitral stenosis. For PACES, the advice must be to listen to all areas with both, in which case some will systematically listen in all areas with the diaphragm and then repeat the circuit with the bell,

Feature	JVP	Carotid
Present anterior to ear	Yes	No
Character of movement	Descending most prominent	Ascending most prominent
Number of pulsations	Usually two per heart beat	One
Is pulse palpable?	No	Yes
Change with inspiration	Drops lower in neck	No change
Change if patient sits up	Drops lower in neck	No change
Change if light pressure applied to base of neck	Less prominent or abolished	No change
Change with abdominal pressure	Temporary rise in neck	No change

TABLE 18 WAYS OF DISTINGUISHING THE JVP FROM THE CAROTID PULSE

TABLE 19 PALPATION OF THE PRAECORDIUM

Finding	Interpretation
Non-displaced heaving apex	Left ventricular hypertophy – a common sign, most likely due to hypertension, also aortic stenosis
Non-displaced tapping apex	Tapping apex beat is due to palpable first heart sound of mitral stenosis – a relatively rare sign nowadays
Double apical impulse	Said to be typical of hypertrophic obstructive cardiomyopathy – but a very rare sign and not to be over-diagnosed
Palpable left parasternal heave	Right ventricular hypertrophy and/or dilatation – due to any cause of pulmonary hypertension, including cor pulmonale
Palpable thrill	Most likely due to aortic stenosis, when can be felt in neck, aortic area, over the sternum, or at the apex. Much less likely to be due to a ventricular septal defect, when typically felt at left sternal edge (consider in cases that seem likely to have congenital heart disease)

whereas others will listen in each area with both diaphragm and bell before moving on to the next area. Both are acceptable.

When listening to the heart it is essential that you simultaneously feel the carotid pulse to allow you to establish the timing of the sounds that you hear. We all know that this is scarcely necessary in the patient with a normal or slow heart rate and with no murmur or a very obvious abnormality, but it is an entirely different matter if you are trying to make a diagnosis in a patient that is unwell with a tachycardia. Such patients are not likely to feature in PACES, but it is vital that you demonstrate to the examiner that you have a method that might stand up to the difficulties presented by the breathless woman with fast atrial fibrillation who will probably pitch up on your next medical take. It is not acceptable to time the sounds by palpating the radial pulse: this would not mislead in the patient with a normal pulse rate, but could do so with tachycardia, and it's no good having a method that might break down in this circumstance.

After listening to all areas with the patient resting in the standard position, proceed to perform the standard manoeuvres to accentuate the sounds. Ask the patient to roll onto their left side, breathe quietly, and then listen at the apex with both diaphragm and bell. Ask the patient to sit forward, place the diaphragm of your stethoscope in the fourth intercostal space just to the left of the sternum, and give clear instructions 'breathe in . . . breathe out . . . and hold it'. This gives the best chance of hearing the diastolic murmur of aortic incompetence.

As suggested in the preliminary comments to this section, it is very likely that the examiner will tell you to stop examining the patient at this point. They may ask 'what else would you like to do to complete your examination?', in which case reply as in Table 20.

Expect to be asked 'what else would you like to do?' and 'what are your findings?' as soon as you stop listening to the heart.

Completing the cardiovascular examination

If the examiner does not stop you after you have finished listening to the heart, then continue with the examination in the systematic manner given in Table 20.

Check list – cardiovascular examination

1. Well or ill?
2. Correctly positioned and exposed.
3. General inspection.
4. Hands – clubbing, splinters.
5. Radial pulses – rate, rhythm.
6. Brachial pulse – character.
7. Face – conjunctival pallor, central cyanosis.
8. Jugular venous pressure.
9. Palpation of carotid arteries.
10. Inspection of chest.
11. Palpation of apex/praecordium.
12. Auscultation of the heart – apex, left sternal edge, pulmonary area, aortic area, neck; then with standard manoeuvres to accentuate particular murmurs.
13. Chest – auscultate lung bases.
14. Abdomen – palpate for hepatomegaly and abdominal aortic aneurysm, listen for bruits.
15. Legs – peripheral pulses, ankle oedema.
16. Blood pressure.
17. Urine – dipstick.

Presenting your findings to the examiners

The examiner is most likely to start off by asking you to summarise your findings, which you should do in the same logical and systematic manner in which you have hopefully examined the patient. This is by far the best way of giving a sensible account that does not miss anything out, but – by the time you get to PACES – you should be able to do better than trot out an exhaustive stream of negative findings in the manner of an automaton. Present briskly and clearly.

TABLE 20 'WHAT ELSE WOULD YOU LIKE TO DO TO COMPLETE YOUR EXAMINATION?'

Chest	Percuss for pleural effusions Listen for basal crepitations Check for sacral oedema
Abdomen	Palpate for the liver – if it is enlarged, then is it pulsatile? Feel for abdominal aortic aneurysm Listen for bruits over aorta and femorals Examine for ascites (if relevant)
Legs	Feel for peripheral pulses Check for oedema
Other	Check blood pressure Dipstick test of urine for blood and protein

- 'From the foot of the bed I notice that Mr Brown is/has . . .'

- 'There are no stigmata of cardiac disease in the hands'

- 'The pulse is whatever rate it is in whatever rhythm it is and of normal character (unless it is clearly abnormal)'

- 'Mr Brown is not pale or cyanosed (unless he clearly is)'

- 'The JVP is normal (assuming it is)'

- 'On inspection of the chest there are no scars (unless there are)'

- 'The apex beat is normal (assuming it is) and there are no palpable heaves or thrills (unless there are)'

'On auscultation . . .', and here comes a bit that very often sorts those that pass from those that fail. Candidates who are in difficulty nearly always hit the buffers at this point, speaking more and more indistinctly, and often able to whisper little more than that 'there was a murmur'. This will not do. Even if you really don't know what the murmur is, it is still possible to score a 3, certainly a 2, if you present your findings in a sensible manner and follow that up with a reasonable discussion. Two types of presentation can lead to success. First, not available to you if you don't know what the diagnosis is: 'I found signs consistent with aortic stenosis (or whatever is appropriate) . . . there was a . . .' and go on to say what you heard. Secondly, a logical presentation of the auscultatory findings, aided perhaps by a bit of presentational technique. Supposing that (as is likely) the patient is not cyanosed or clubbed, which would probably suggest some form of congenital cardiac disease in this context. You have heard a loud murmur that radiates widely over the chest, but you cannot decide where it is coming from, and there doesn't seem to be any part of the cardiac cycle that is quiet, but you don't really think there is anything that sounds like mitral stenosis. It would be easy for you to land up saying something along the lines of 'there was a lot of noise' and going red in the face. How about:

- 'I found the findings on auscultation difficult' (you are not the sort of doctor who is going to pretend that you are sure when you are not – and you shouldn't be in your routine practice or you'll get into trouble)

- 'I thought the first heart sound was normal' (it nearly always is)

- 'I thought the second heart sound was normal' (it nearly always is)

- 'In systole I could hear a loud murmur that radiated widely over the praecordium' (loud murmurs are inevitably systolic)

- 'There was a sound in diastole which I think was a third heart sound' (the commonest cause of a sound in diastole)

This approach of analyzing each element of the findings on auscultation is both the correct way to try to work out the diagnosis in routine clinical practice, and also the best way of demonstrating that this what you do to the PACES examiner. If the case above was mixed mitral valve disease and the diastolic sound was not due to a third heart sound, then all would not be lost with the presentation given if you had examined in a fluent manner and discussed the case sensibly.

If you have not given the diagnosis earlier, then when you have finished presenting your findings you should say how you interpret them; if not, the examiner will certainly ask you to do so. If you know the answer, simply say 'these findings indicate that the diagnosis is . . .' If you aren't sure, then say 'these findings might be explained by x or y' . . . and go on to explain what aspects are for and against x, and what for and against y. Even if you haven't elicited all of the physical signs correctly, a reasonable technique for performing the physical examination, with a logical method of presenting the findings, followed by a sensible discussion of their implications, is likely to score 3 marks in a case where the physical signs aren't blindingly obvious.

TABLE 21 DIFFERENTIAL DIAGNOSIS OF A SYSTOLIC MURMUR

Cause	Findings on auscultation		Other features to look for
	Common	Less common	
Aortic stenosis	Ejection systolic murmur – usually louder in aortic than in mitral area; may radiate to neck; unlikely to radiate to axilla	Ejection click Second heart sound may be quiet (usually declared after diagnosis established)	Pulse pressure low Pulse slow rising Thrill palpable in neck Apex heaving but not displaced
Aortic sclerosis	Ejection systolic murmur – usually louder in aortic than in mitral area; may radiate to neck; unlikely to radiate to axilla		No features to suggest aortic stenosis (heaving apex may be due to concurrent hypertension)
Mixed aortic valve disease/aortic regurgitation	Ejection systolic murmur – usually louder in aortic than in mitral area; may radiate to neck; unlikely to radiate to axilla Early diastolic murmur – loudest at lower left sternal edge	Ejection click	Apex likely to be displaced
Aortic flow murmur associated with aortic regurgitation	Ejection systolic murmur – usually louder in aortic than in mitral area; may radiate to neck; unlikely to radiate to axilla Early diastolic murmur – loudest at lower left sternal edge		Pulse pressure wide Pulse character collapsing Apex likely to be displaced Other features of aortic incompetence
Mitral regurgitation	Pansystolic murmur – loudest in mitral area; may radiate to axilla; unlikely to radiate to neck 3rd heart sound		Apex displaced Thrill palpable at apex (rare)
Mitral valve prolapse (1)	Mid- or late- systolic murmur – loudest in mitral area; may radiate to axilla; unlikely to radiate to neck Mid-systolic click	3rd heart sound	
Mixed mitral valve disease	Pansystolic murmur – loudest in mitral area; may radiate to axilla; unlikely to radiate to neck Mid-diastolic murmur at apex	Opening snap	Mitral facies Atrial fibrillation very common
Hypertrophic obstructive cardiomyopathy (2)	Ejection systolic murmur – usually louder in aortic than in mitral area; may radiate to neck; unlikely to radiate to axilla		Pulse character jerky Apex – double impulse (rare)

Notes
(1) Purely on auscultation, it can be difficult to distinguish between mitral valve prolapse (mid-systolic click, mid/late-systolic murmur that extends to S2, followed by an S3) from aortic stenosis (ejection click, ejection systolic murmur, followed by an S2). If the murmur is loudest in the aortic area, then aortic stenosis is most likely; if it is loudest in the mitral area, then mitral valve prolapse. Are other features of aortic stenosis present?
(2) Hypertrophic obstructive cardiomyopathy is a less common diagnosis than aortic or mitral valve disease, but suspect in younger patient;
(3) Tricuspid regurgitation is rare as an isolated diagnosis but produces a pansystolic murmur best heard at the lower left sternal edge. The physical signs that establish the diagnosis are a grossly elevated JVP with prominent V waves and a pulsatile liver;
(4) Ventricular septal defect – see Table 23;
(5) In any patient who has had cardiac surgery, ALWAYS consider the possibility of valve replacement(s), which may be associated with flow or (if leaking) regurgitant murmurs. Does S1, indicating a mitral valve replacement, or S2, indicating an aortic valve replacement, sound mechanical?

Many cardiac cases will have a systolic murmur, when in a middle aged or elderly patient the most common diagnoses to consider are shown in Table 21. The differential diagnosis of a diastolic murmur is generally straightforward, as shown in Table 22. If the patient is young (or even middle aged), particularly with features such as clubbing, cyanosis or scars of cardiac surgery, then consider the possibility of congenital heart disease. With improvements in paediatric care, more and more children with congenital heart disease are surviving into adulthood, but the examiners all know that such cases are not common, and most (myself and 99% of others at a guess) would not be at all confident if they were

TABLE 22 DIFFERENTIAL DIAGNOSIS OF A DIASTOLIC MURMUR

| Cause | Findings on auscultation | | Other features to look for |
	Common	Less common	
Aortic regurgitation	Early diastolic murmur – loudest at lower left sternal edge Ejection systolic flow murmur – aortic area 3rd heart sound	Mid-diastolic murmur (Austin Flint) – apex; caused by regurgitant aortic jet hitting mitral valve	Pulse pressure wide Pulse character collapsing Apex displaced Other features of aortic incompetence related to wide pulse pressure, e.g. Corrigan's pulse
Pulmonary regurgitation	Early diastolic murmur – loudest in pulmonary area	Features of mitral stenosis/mixed mitral valve disease	Raised JVP Palpable right ventricular heave No features of aortic incompetence
Mitral stenosis	Mid-diastolic murmur at apex	S1 loud Opening snap Early diastolic murmur (Graham Steell) – pulmonary area; caused by pulmonary hypertension secondary to mitral disease	Mitral facies Atrial fibrillation very common Apex tapping but not displaced Features of pulmonary hypertension and/or tricuspid incompetence

asked to say what the diagnosis was before reading their briefing notes. They will allow for this in their marking. So don't panic: a fluent physical examination and description of your findings together with very limited knowledge of the commonest congenital cardiac conditions (Table 23) should get you through, even though you haven't really got a clue what might be wrong with the heart.

TABLE 23 DIFFERENTIAL DIAGNOSIS OF CONGENITAL CARDIAC CONDITIONS

Cause	Pathology	Cyanosis	Findings on auscultation		Other features to look for
			Common	Less common	
Tetralogy of Fallot	Large VSD Over-riding aorta RV outflow tract obstruction Right ventricular hypertrophy – leading to right-to-left shunting	Yes	P2 absent (1) Ejection systolic murmur – pulmonary area		Scars from cardiac surgery (systemic to pulmonary artery shunt or complete correction) Clubbing Palpable right ventricular heave Palpable thrill in pulmonary area
Eisenmenger's	Large left-to-right shunt causes increased pulmonary blood flow, pulmonary hypertension and right ventricular hypertrophy. Pressures in systemic and pulmonary circulations equalize such that murmur of original shunt (ASD, VSD, PDA) disappears	Yes	P2 loud (1) S4 at left sternal edge	Pulmonary ejection click Early diastolic murmur in pulmonary area (pulmonary regurgitation, Graham Steell) Pansystolic murmur at left sternal edge (tricuspid regurgitation)	Scars from cardiac surgery Clubbing JVP very high Giant V waves in JVP (tricuspid regurgitation) Palpable right ventricular heave Palpable P2
Atrial septal defect	Ostium primum or ostium secundum. Blood shunts from left-to-right across ASD because the right ventricle is more compliant than the left	No (2)	S2 – wide fixed splitting throughout respiratory cycle	Ejection systolic murmur – pulmonary area, due to increased flow across pulmonary valve (not the ASD itself) if large shunt. RV heave	None Signs of pulmonary hypertension can develop (as pulmonary pressure rises, flow falls, and murmur from pulmonary valve decreases)
Ventricular septal defect	Left-to-right shunt from LV to RV	No (2)	Pansystolic murmur – lower left sternal edge (can radiate widely)		Palpable thrill at left sternal edge Apex – thrusting Palpable pulmonary artery
Patent ductus arteriosus	Persistence of normal part of the foetal circulation that connects the descending aorta to the left pulmonary artery. Left-to-right shunt from aorta to pulmonary artery	No (2)	Continuous machinery murmur – loudest in second left intercostal space (3)		Signs of pulmonary hypertension can develop (as pulmonary pressure rises, flow falls, and murmur from VSD decreases)
Coarctation of the aorta	Narrowing of aorta at site of fetal ductus arteriosus	No	Systolic murmur at left sternal edge and/or interscapular		Signs of pulmonary hypertension can develop (as pulmonary pressure rises, flow falls, and murmur from PDA decreases) Radiofemoral delay

Notes

(1) In a cyanosed patient, if P2 is loud, the working diagnosis is Eisenmenger's; if you cannot hear P2, the working diagnosis is Fallot's;
(2) Unless complicated by Eisenmenger's; (3) BEWARE the renal patient with a large arteriovenous fistula in the left arm, which can make a continuous sound (bruit): if you think you hear a PDA, listen to the arm and examine it if you can hear the sound there.
There are an enormous number of other congenital heart conditions, but these are not likely to appear in PACES, and if they do the examiners – who will most certainly not be experts in the field – will simply expect you to identify the physical signs correctly and make logical comments about them.

Details from the mark sheet that the examiner will be looking at as you examine the patient are shown in Table 24.

From the foot of the bed

- Correctly exposed.
- General inspection.

The written instructions for the case will direct you towards the part of the nervous system that needs to be examined – cranial nerves, arms or legs – but from the foot of the bed take stock of the whole patient and not just the part specified. Table 25 lists common neurological diagnoses in patients seen in PACES and clues to look for: if you spot one or more of these and recognize their significance, then you are probably already more than half way to a good performance.

Assessment of higher cortical function

It is very uncommon for this to be the subject of the central nervous system examination in PACES, but it is possible for the station instructions to say something along the lines of 'this man has difficulty communicating, please ask him some questions'. The most likely diagnoses in such a case are dysarthria or dysphasia, with disturbance of higher mental functions very much less likely.

After introducing yourself to the patient you will obviously begin your assessment by getting them to talk: 'what is your name?', 'what is your address?' Simply listening to the way that they do so may give the answer to the case. To further demonstrate and analyse dysarthria or dysphasia, proceed as described in Table 26.

In the unlikely event that the patient's problem is not a dysphasia or dysarthria, then proceed to test higher cortical function using an abbreviated mental test score by asking the following questions.

- What is your age?
- What is the time (to nearest hour)?
- Address for recall at end of test – 42 West Street (ask patient to repeat to ensure that they have heard it correctly)
- What year is it?
- What is the name of this place?
- Recognition of two persons (can the patient identify your job and that of a nurse?)
- Date of birth (date and month)
- Year of First World War
- Name of present monarch
- Count backwards from 20 to 1
- What was the address given earlier in the test?

TABLE 24 KEY FEATURES OF THE EXAMINER'S MARKSHEET FOR CENTRAL NERVOUS SYSTEM EXAMINATION

Clinical skill	To score satisfactory	To score unsatisfactory
Physical examination	Technique must be correct, thorough, systematic and fluent. Specific requirements for professional method (as appropriate) of assessment of tone, power, reflexes, sensation, coordination and cranial nerve function are noted.	Techniques are incorrect. Significant or important tests are omitted. Approach is unsystematic, hesitant, lacking confidence or unprofessional.
Identifying physical signs	Identifies correct signs. Signs that are not present are not found.	Important signs are missed. Signs that are not present are found.
Differential diagnosis	Sensible, and includes the correct diagnosis.	Poor, and fails to consider the correct diagnosis.
Clinical judgement	Offers a sensible and appropriate management plan.	Offers an inappropriate management plan.
Maintaining patient welfare	Treats the patient in an appropriate manner.	Causes the patient physical or emotional discomfort, or treats them in an unsafe manner.

TABLE 25 COMMON NEUROLOGICAL DIAGNOSES IN PACES – CLUES FROM THE FOOT OF THE BED

Condition	Features to consider as patient speaks or moves spontaneously
Multiple sclerosis	Speech – pseudobulbar or cerebellar Eyes – nystagmus Coordination – cerebellar Bladder – convene/urinary catheter/leg bag
Hemiplegia	Speech – dysphasia or dysarthria Face – asymmetry Posture – asymmetry
Spinal cord lesion	Legs – spastic: face looks normal and arms may look muscular (from wheelchair use) if, as is likely, lesion below cervical cord level Bladder – convene/urinary catheter/leg bag
Motor neuron disease	Speech – bulbar or pseudobulbar Muscles – global wasting, fasciculation (if prominent)
Huntington's disease	Choreoathetoid movements
Muscular dystrophy	Muscles – wasting
Myotonic dystrophy	'Myotonic facies' – frontal balding, ptosis
Peripheral neuropathy	Muscle wasting – particularly distal legs Feet/ankles – ulcers/amputated toes/Charcot joints
Parkinson's disease	Facies – immobile, unblinking Posture – 'Parkinsonian' Movement – tremor, general paucity
Neurofibromatosis	Skin – neurofibromata, café-au-lait spots

Examination of the cranial nerves

There are few areas in which your examination technique is more visible to external scrutiny than when you are examining the cranial nerves. The experienced practitioner has a method that enables them to move smoothly and reasonably quickly through the complex series of maneuvers required, guiding the patient simply but firmly and unambiguously as they do so. Many candidates cannot do this, frequently halting to think 'what do I do next?', and further betray their lack of skill by giving instructions that confuse the patient and lead to yet more interruptions in the process.

It is vital that any neurological examination is performed in a reasonably brisk manner – more so than the examination of any other system. This is not just because in PACES and in routine clinical practice you do not have the luxury of unlimited time, but because the tests that you are doing require the patient's effort or concentration. Although it may be an irritation to the examiners if you spend a long time listening to the heart, the heart sounds are exceedingly unlikely to change with the passage of time during a PACES station. By contrast, if you are too slow with the neurological examination it is more than likely that the patient will become tired or their concentration waver, in which case your findings are prone to become unreliable.

I nerve (olfactory)

'Do you have any problem with your sense of smell?' Unless the patient says that they do, which is most unlikely, then you are not expected

TABLE 26 ANALYSIS OF DYSARTHRIA AND DYSPHASIA

Problem	Tests	Comments
Dysphasia	Obeying simple commands – build up in complexity, starting with the most simple: 'open your mouth', 'touch your nose', 'put your left hand on your right ear' (deficient in receptive dysphasia). Quality of speech – if the patient's speech does not have a normal pattern, listen carefully for features suggesting an expressive dysphasia (circumlocutions, word substitutions, word salads etc). Ability to name objects – present your tie, pen, stethoscope to the patient and ask them to say what it is (deficiency indicates nominal dysphasia).	Indicates a cortical lesion in the dominant hemisphere, usually the left. Look for other evidence, eg. right-sided visual defect/inattention, weakness (facial droop, pronator drift), sensory deficit/inattention.
Dysarthria	Repetition of phrases that are difficult to articulate – 'British constitution', 'west register street', 'biblical criticism'.	Consider bulbar or pseudobulbar palsy – test lower cranial nerves. Consider cerebellar problem – test for nystagmus, cerebellar signs in the limbs, truncal ataxia.

to test this. If testing is required, get the patient to sniff through one nostril after blocking the other by pressing on the side of the nose with their finger. Assuming the nostril is clear, present whatever odour is available and ask the patient if they can smell it; then repeat on the other side. Olfaction is preserved if the patient can smell anything at all: they are not required to name the odour correctly, although they may do so.

II nerve (optic) – visual acuity and visual fields

Begin by asking the patient if they have any problem with their vision. If they say that they wear spectacles, ask them to put them on before you

test acuity. Get the patient to cover each eye in turn and test ability to read from the Snellen's chart or, if none is available, any printed matter at the bedside. If print cannot be read, check the ability to count fingers, and failing that, perceive hand movements or see light. The patient with a glass eye will usually have broken out into a smile by this stage and told you.

Assuming that the patient has the necessary acuity, now proceed to examine the visual fields by confrontation. The standard method (Table 27) requires a lot of assistance from the patient: it is suitable for 'outpatient practice' that forms the bulk of neurologists' work,

also for most patients that are likely to appear in PACES. A variation of technique that needs less assistance must be employed whenever the patient cannot comply with instructions such as 'cover one of your eyes' for any reason: it is frequently the only method that can be applied in the context of an acute medical take.

Again assuming the necessary acuity, test for visual inattention – a feature of parietal lobe lesions – by asking the patient to look directly at your face whilst you raise a finger just inside the outer limits of each of their temporal fields. Tell them not to move their eyes from your face, but to say 'yes' or point if they see

	TABLE 27 **EXAMINING THE VISUAL FIELDS BY CONFRONTATION**	
	Standard method	**Variation**
Technique	1) Directly face the patient, about 1m away 2) Ask the patient to cover their right eye and look with their left eye into your right eye, whilst you cover your own left eye 3) Tell the patient to keep looking directly into your eye and not to look anywhere else 4) Confirm that the patient can see your finger by placing it midway between you and waggling it 5) Move your waggling finger in the vertical plane midway between you and the patient from outside of one quadrant of your vision towards the centre of the visual field, asking the patient to 'tell me as soon as you see my finger out of the corner of your eye'. Patients will often be unable to stop themselves glancing towards the finger as it appears, but this also tells you that they've seen it 6) Repeat the process bringing your finger into the visual field from the patient's superotemporal, nasotemporal, inferonasal and inferotemporal directions 7) Repeat the whole process with the patient covering their left eye and looking into your left eye	1) Directly face the patient, an arm's length away 2) Cover the patient's right eye with your left hand 3) Tell the patient to keep looking directly at your face and not to look anywhere else 4–6) As standard method 7) Repeat the whole process covering the patient's left eye with your right hand
Advantages	Standard technique. Allows comparison of patient's visual fields with examiner's visual fields	Requires lesser degree of compliance from patient
Disadvantages	Requires high degree of compliance from patient	Does not allow comparison of patient's visual fields with examiner's visual fields unless examiner can comfortably close their left and right eyes separately – but this is not critical: significant visual field defects are obvious without confirmation by comparison with your own visual fields
Common errors of technique	Lack of clarity in giving instructions leads to poor method and unreliable findings Moving waggling finger in vertical plane that is not equidistant from patient and examiner means that visual fields cannot be compared	Also requires clear instructions to patient

one of your fingers moving. Waggle the finger on one side of the patient and then the finger on the other side, checking that they can identify when each moves. Then waggle both fingers together. Visual inattention is present if the patient indicates that only one finger moves when both have done.

The next step in a complete examination of the visual fields is to examine for a central scotoma and the size of the blind spot using a red hat pin. You must know how to do this, but it is unlikely that you will be asked to do so in the PACES exam because it would require two or three minutes, and if – as is likely – there are abnormal physical signs elsewhere, the examiner will ask you to move on. So ask the examiner 'would you like me to examine for a central scotoma and the size of the blind spot?' (all clocking up points, 'this doctor knows what they are looking for'). If (bad luck) they say yes, then remember the following:

1. It is absolutely vital that the patient's eye remains fixed upon yours throughout testing: any movement at all will mean that it is very difficult it not impossible to demonstrate a small central scotoma, or indeed find the blind spot at all.

2. Examine for a central scotoma in the right eye by asking the patient to cover their left eye (whilst you cover your right) and look directly at your eye. Put the head of the pin directly in the line of sight between you and ask the patient 'can you see the head of the pin?' Move the head of the pin about over a range of 10cm or so around the line of fixation and ask 'does the head of the pin disappear at any time?' If there is a defect, map out the area of the

scotoma. Then proceed to check if there is a more subtle defect of central vision, namely that colour perception is altered. Clear instructions to the patient are paramount: whilst moving the pin head around the line of fixation say 'does the colour of the pin head change as I move it around?' (if yes, then ask how – optic nerve lesions typically lead to the pin head to look paler or pinker at the point of fixation than a few centimeters away from that point); or hold the pin head directly in the line of fixation and say to the patient 'remember the colour of the pin head . . . keep looking straight at my eye . . . I am going to move the pin . . . there, and there, and there, and there (presenting the pin head 5–10cm above, below, to left and to right of the fixation point) . . . did it look the same colour in the middle as in the other places?'

3. Remember that the blind spot is located about 15° to the temporal side of the point of visual fixation. As with

examining for a central scotoma, it is vital that you give the patient very clear directions. Rather than saying something along the lines of 'tell me if you notice anything', or (in a rather vague way) 'tell me if the pin disappears', say 'keep looking straight at my eye . . . I am going to move the pin around to find your blind spot . . . the red head of the pin will disappear . . . (you haven't gone mad, it will disappear) . . . tell me when it does . . . (and when it has done) . . . tell me when it comes back'.

Common visual field defects are shown in Table 28.

Pupillary responses

Note the size and shape of the pupils, then examine with a bright pen torch, looking at both direct and consensual responses and their symmetry. The pathway of the pupillary response to light is shown in figure 1.

Examine for a relative afferent pupillary defect as follows:

1. Shine the light into the right eye for 5 seconds

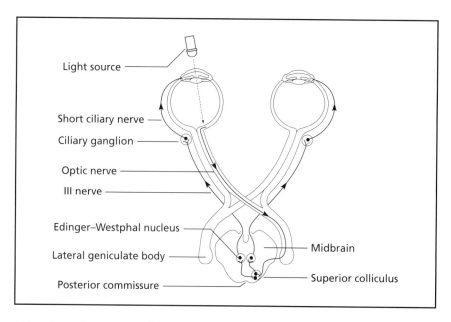

▲ **Fig. 1** The pupillary response to light.

TABLE 28 ABNORMALITIES OF VISUAL ACUITY AND VISUAL FIELDS

One eye or both eyes?	Defect	Interpretation	Common causes
Monocular	Reduced acuity	Cataract Macula disease Optic nerve disease	Optic neuritis – demyelination* Optic neuritis – ischaemia Compression
	Altitudinal	Retinal disease Optic nerve disease	Glaucoma Vascular occlusion
	Central scotoma	Retinal disease Optic nerve disease	Macular disease Optic neuritis – demyelination* Optic neuritis – ischaemia Compression
Both eyes	Reduced acuity	Cataract Macula disease Optic nerve disease	Hereditary optic atrophy (Leber's) Toxins/drugs
	Homonymous hemianopia	Lesion of optic tract behind chiasm	Cerebrovascular accident* Tumour
	Bitemporal hemianopia	Lesion at optic chiasm	Pituitary tumour* Craniopharyngioma Suprasellar meningioma
	Central scotoma	Retinal disease Optic nerve disease	Macular disease Hereditary optic atrophy (Leber's) Toxins/drugs
	Tunnel vision	Retinal disease	Retinitis pigmentosa* Choroidoretinitis
One or both eyes	Enlarged blind spot(s)	Papilloedema	Brain tumour Accelerated phase hypertension Benign intracranial hypertension*

Notes: * most likely causes in PACES.

2. Observe the pupil of the left eye

3. Move the light swiftly to shine in the left eye

4. Does the left pupil dilate? – if so there is a relative afferent pupillary defect on the left side

5. Now observe the pupil of the right eye

6. Move the light swiftly back to shine on the right eye

7. Does the right pupil dilate? – if so there is a relative afferent pupillary defect on the right side

This test compares the afferent pathway (comprising the retina and optic nerve anterior to the chiasm) of the light reflex of one eye with that of the other. If there is a problem with the afferent pathway on one side, that pupil dilates when the light is shone directly into it.

Examine the near response by asking the patient to look at the wall on the far side of the room and then focus on your finger tip, held about 30 cm away from their face just above their line of vision. A common error is for candidates to hold their finger below the patient's line of vision so that it is difficult to see their pupils as they focus on the near object.

The pupil's near response is normally the same as its response to light, but there are a few unusual conditions – very uncommon in routine clinical practice, but more likely to appear in PACES – where the response to light is sluggish, with the response to near better preserved. These include Adie's pupil, Argyll Robertson pupil, Parinaud's midbrain syndrome, and aberrant regeneration of the third nerve.

Table 29 lists causes of pupillary abnormalities.

Eye movements

First look at the general appearance of the eyes: in particular, is there ptosis, indicating a third nerve palsy

TABLE 29 COMMON CAUSES OF UNEQUAL OR IRREGULAR PUPILS			
Condition	**Pupil features**	**Light reaction**	**Near reaction**
Simple anisocoria	Round and regular	Normal	Normal
Horner's syndrome	Small and regular	Normal	Normal
Third nerve palsy*	Dilated	Absent	Absent
Pharmacological	Dilated or small	Absent	Absent
Traumatic	May be irregular or oval	Reduced	Reduced
Adie's pupil	Dilated and irregular	Poor/absent	Sustained (tonic)
Argyll Robertson pupil	Small and irregular	Absent	Present
Iritis (synechiae)	Irregular	Normal	Normal

Notes: * there are likely to be other obvious clues to a third nerve palsy: ptosis, down and out position of eye, abnormalities of eye movement.

(if ptosis complete, eye position abnormal and pupil sometimes large) or Horner's syndrome (if ptosis partial, eye position normal and pupil small)?

Examine pursuit movements by gently putting one of your hands on the patient's forehead to prevent them from turning it when you ask them to follow your finger as you move it smoothly but reasonably briskly up and down and then from side to side. Most patients are unable to suppress the natural tendency to turn their head in pursuit of an object if you simply say 'keep your head still as you follow my finger'. Ask the patient to tell you 'if they see double at any point', but remember that vision becomes indistinct at the far peripheries of the visual fields, particularly when the eyes are at the extremes of their movement. Many patients will declare that they have 'a bit of double vision (or similar)' at this point, analysis of which is never revealing, excepting to demonstrate that the PACES candidate lacks experience. Do not move your finger such that viewing it requires deviation of more than about 45° from the neutral position when testing eye movements. Significant diplopia will always be detectable within this range and sense will not

be achieved beyond it. If the patient does say that they see double, then usually it will be obvious which eye is to blame and you should say so directly: 'the left eye is failing to abduct properly (or as appropriate)'. Further examination of the problem is not required if this is the case, but in the unlikely event that there is doubt as to which eye is not moving properly, then ask clear questions and give clear instructions to analyse

the defect. 'Are the two images side by side and parallel (sixth nerve lesion)?' . . . 'or does one of the images seem to be tilted and below the other (likely to be a fourth nerve lesion)?' Then, 'keep your head still . . . I am going to cover one of your eyes . . . (and taking your hand off their forehead, cover one of their eyes) . . . is it the inner or outer image that goes away when I cover this eye . . . (and then repeat when covering the other eye)?' The eye responsible for the outer image is the one that is not moving properly.

Test saccadic movements in the horizontal plane by holding your hands to left and right of the patient's field of vision and asking them to look at 'which hand moves?' as you waggle one and then the other alternately a few times: then repeat the test in the vertical plane, holding one hand in the upper and one in the lower visual field. Brainstem or cerebellar disorders can impair saccadic movements.

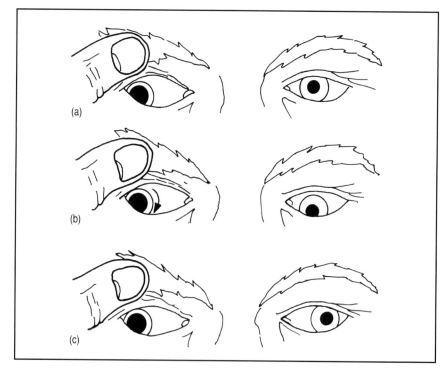

▲ **Fig. 2** Right third nerve palsy. (**a**) At rest, when the eyelid is lifted up it can be seen that the eye is looking down and out, and the pupil is fixed and dilated. (**b**) On attempted down-gaze the right eye rotates inwards. (**c**) On attempted gaze to the left, the right eye does not move.

TABLE 30 COMMON ABNORMAL EYE MOVEMENTS AND THEIR CAUSES

Abnormality	Cause	Comment
Ptosis, eye is 'down and out', pupil dilated (sometimes), no movement possible excepting abduction (sixth nerve action) and intorsion of eye on downgaze (fourth nerve action when third nerve paralysed)	Third nerve palsy	See figure 2
Diplopia on looking downwards and away from the side of the affected eye	Fourth nerve palsy	Uncommon; difficult to spot; patient likely to tilt head to overcome diplopia (defective eye uppermost)
Eye fails to abduct on lateral gaze	Sixth nerve palsy	See figures 3 and 4
On attempting to gaze to the left the right eye does not adduct; the left eye does abduct, but shows nystagmus (or vice versa)	Classical internuclear ophthalmoplegia (3)	Lesion in right medial longitudinal fasciculus; may be bilateral; usually due to multiple sclerosis. See figure 4
Nystagmus – horizontal or rotatory	Peripheral lesion (labyrinth or vestibular nerve) Cerebellar lesion	
Nystagmus – vertical	Central lesion	Vestibular nuclei in brainstem
Non-stop pendular 'wobble' of the eyes, without fast and slow phase	Congenital nystagmus	

Notes
(1) Local disease of the eye/orbit can impair eye movement and cause diplopia.
(2) A few nystagmoid jerks are normal when the eyes are deviated to the extremes, hence – as with examining for diplopia – do not ask the patient to track an object beyond about 45° from the neutral position.
(3) It is also possible to have a form of internuclear ophthalmoplegia where on attempting to gaze to the side there is a failure of abduction of one eye, with adduction preserved in the other (nystagmus is absent/minimal).

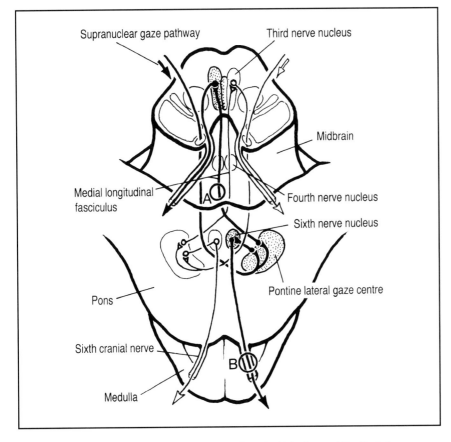

▲**Fig. 3** Nerve pathways for lateral gaze. The pathways shown in thicker lines and the stippled areas are responsible for gaze to the left. For the significance of 'A' and 'B', see Fig. 4.

Table 30 lists causes of abnormal eye movements.

Fundoscopy

Ask the examiner if they would like you to perform fundoscopy. It is unlikely that they will want you to do this on station 3, fundoscopy typically being tested in station 5.

V nerve (trigeminal)

Practise testing sensation.

- Give clear instructions.
- Move at a reasonable pace.
- Light touch should be light touch, not stroking.
- 'Does the pin feel sharp?', not 'can you feel it?'.

Assess light touch and pin prick in the territories of V_1, V_2 and V_3 (Figure 5). Testing sensation can be difficult and it is very easy to obtain equivocal findings. Many

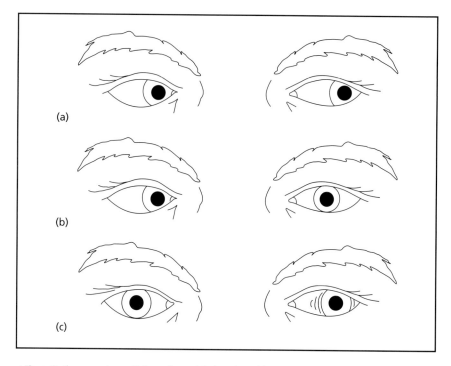

▲ **Fig. 4** Sixth nerve palsy and internuclear ophthalmoplegia. (**a**) Normal gaze to the left. (**b**) A patient with a left sixth nerve palsy attempting to look to the left. The left eye fails to abduct. Lesion at 'B' in Fig. 3. (**c**) A patient with left internuclear ophthalmoplegia attempting to look to the left. The right eye does not adduct; the left eye tries to abduct but shows nystagmus. Lesion at 'A' in Fig. 3.

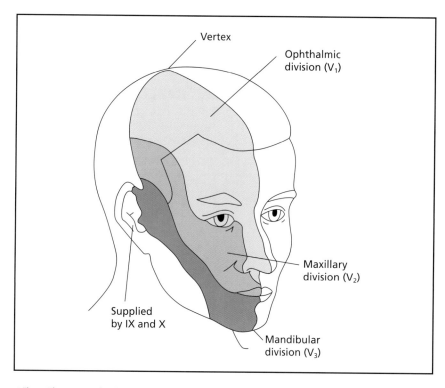

▲ **Fig. 5** The sensory distribution of the trigeminal nerve.

such as 'it feels a little bit lighter on that side (or similar)'. The pursuit of marginal sensory abnormalities is not likely to be useful, indeed it will almost certainly lead only to confusion.

Test light touch using either cotton wool or your finger tip (the best neurologist I ever worked for used his finger tips, saying 'that's what they're for . . . touching things'). Do not apply a stroking motion, which is a more complex stimulus than light touch. Say 'please close your eyes . . . I am going to touch you very gently on the face . . . say 'yes' if you feel anything at all'. The trigeminal nerve also mediates touch sensation on the anterior two-thirds of the tongue, but I have never seen a neurologist test this and it would not be expected by any examiner that I have met in PACES.

Use a Neurotips™ to test for pin prick/pain sensation. There are two well recognized ways of doing this, both of which are acceptable. The first simply tests whether or not the patient can perceive the sharpness of the pin. The key is that they must be clear that you are testing for pain, not simply awareness of touch. Say 'does this feel sharp?' and then test each of the trigeminal subdivisions. If the patient says that they can feel it, but that it isn't sharp, then they have a defect of pin prick/pain sensation. The second method tests the patient's ability to distinguish between the sharp and the blunt end of the Neurotips™. Having established that they can perceive the sharpness and can tell the difference between the two ends with their eyes open – 'this is sharp . . . and this is blunt' – ask them to close their eyes and say sharp or blunt as appropriate when they feel anything touch them on the face.

candidates display very poor technique: those that can do it stand out a mile. The keys are to be clear in your own mind what you

are testing for, to give clear instructions to the patient, to move at a reasonable pace, and not to pay too much attention to comments

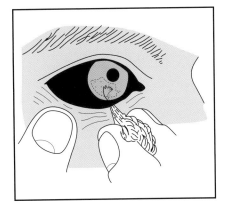

▲**Fig. 6** Testing the corneal reflex.

TABLE 31 COMMON ABNORMALITIES OF THE TRIGEMINAL NERVE

Abnormality	Causes
Unilateral loss of sensation in one or more branches	Following herpes zoster. Direct injury following facial fracture (V_2 especially).
Loss of corneal reflex, sensation in V_1, accompanied by dysfunction of nerves III, IV and VI	Lesion in cavernous sinus
Brisk jaw jerk	Bilateral upper motor neurone lesions above the level of the pons, but also with anxiety

Abnormality of the V nerve with other cranial nerve lesions suggests a cerebellopontine angle lesion (see Table 34).

Look at the face for wasting of the muscles of mastication and then feel the masseters after asking the patient to clench their teeth. Get the patient to open their mouth against resistance, noting any deviation to a weaker side. Test the jaw jerk by asking the patient to let their mouth hang loosely open, putting your forefinger between lower lip and chin and then striking the finger with a tendon hammer.

Finally, test the corneal reflex as shown in figure 6.

Common abnormalities of the trigeminal nerve are shown in Table 31.

VII nerve (facial)

Look carefully for any asymmetry. Ask the patient to wrinkle their forehead and then show you their teeth. Demonstrating what you want them to do can be helpful. Explain to the patient that you want them to 'screw their eyes tightly shut, and don't let me open them'. Look to see how deeply the eyelashes are buried on the two sides before trying with reasonable (but not excessive) firmness to prize the eyelids apart. Then ask the patient to 'blow out your cheeks with your lips closed' and demonstrate what you want them to do. Feel both cheeks simultaneously to assess the

TABLE 32 COMMON ABNORMALITIES OF THE FACIAL NERVE

Abnormality	Explanation	Causes
Weakness of upper and lower facial muscles	Lower motor neurone lesion	Bell's palsy (1) Surgical injury – look for scar over parotid. Ramsay Hunt syndrome (2)
Weakness of lower facial muscles, with upper facial muscles relatively preserved/intact	Upper motor neurone lesion	Stroke. Other upper motor neurone lesion.

Notes
(1) The commonest cause of a lower motor neurone facial lesion.
(2) A rare condition caused by herpes zoster of the facial (geniculate) ganglion, which also leads to a painful vesicular eruption in the external auditory meatus.
(3) Abnormality of the VII nerve with other cranial nerve lesions suggests a cerebellopontine angle lesion (see Table 34).

tension generated in the muscles, also note if air escapes through the nose, which would indicate palatal weakness (see below).

The facial nerve also supplies taste sensation to the anterior two-thirds of the tongue, but I have never seen a neurologist test this and it would not be expected by any examiner that I have met in PACES.

Common abnormalities of the facial nerve are shown in Table 32.

VIII nerve (vestibulocochlear)

Occlude one ear by gently pressing on the tragus and whisper 'seven, eight, nine' (or similar) into the other; repeat the test, whispering 'ten, eleven, twelve' (or similar) into the other. If hearing is abnormal (Table 33) proceed to perform Weber's and Rinne's tests. If hearing is normal, ask the examiner if they would like you to do so.

Rinne's test – hold a 512Hz tuning fork on the mastoid until it is no longer audible. If it is then held by the external auditory meatus it will still be audible to the normal ear, meaning that air conduction is better than bone conduction. If a patient has sensorineural deafness then, although their hearing is (by definition) impaired, air conduction will remain better than bone. By

---

TABLE 33 COMMON CAUSES OF DEAFNESS

Conductive deafness	External ear canal – wax Tympanic membrane – damage Inner ear – fluid Ossicle damage – head injury Otosclerosis – degenerative
Sensorineural deafness	Cochlear nerve/organ of Corti – acoustic neuroma, fracture of petrous temporal bone Degenerative

Abnormality of the VIII nerve with other cranial nerve lesions suggests a cerebellopontine angle lesion (see Table 34).

TABLE 34 CEREBELLOPONTINE ANGLE LESIONS

Neurological deficit	Causes
Tinnitus and deafness (VIII) Loss of corneal reflex (V) Vertigo, ataxia (cerebellum) Facial weakness (VII, a late sign)	Acoustic neuroma Other masses

Notes
(1) Always consider neurofibromatosis in a patient with an acoustic neuroma.
(2) Involvement of VII nerve is rare in acoustic neuroma: if present, consider another diagnosis.

---

contrast, in conductive deafness bone conduction is better than air because air conducted sound, but not that conducted through bone, depends on proper function of the auditory ossicles.

Weber's test – place the tuning fork on the vertex. It should normally be heard equally in both ears. In sensorineural deafness the sound will not be heard in the affected ear, whereas in conductive deafness it will be heard in both.

IX and X nerves (glossopharyngeal and vagus)

The glossopharyngeal nerve carries sensation from the oropharynx and sensation and taste from the posterior third of the tongue; the vagus nerve carries motor fibres to the palate and vocal cords.

In your interaction with the patient you will already have noticed if they have dysarthria or dysphonia, but ask them to repeat 'yellow lorry' as a test of lingual sounds and 'baby hippopotamus' as a test of labial sounds. You will also have found if air escaped through the nose when the patient puffed out their cheeks as a test of facial nerve function: if it did so, then this indicates weakness of palatal movement. Whilst they say 'Aaah' look at the movements of palate and uvula using a torch: normally both sides elevate symmetrically and the uvula remains in the midline. Ask the patient to give a cough, listening particularly for the bovine sound of recurrent laryngeal nerve palsy.

If these tests are normal then it is not necessary to proceed to test pharyngeal sensation and the gag reflex, which are unpleasant for the patient. But if there are abnormalities then explain to the patient exactly what you are going to do and be gentle, very gentle. Taking an orange stick and a tongue depressor say 'I am going to touch the inside of your mouth very gently . . . (depress the tongue and touch the palate gently on each side with the orange stick) . . . now say Aaah . . . (touch the posterior pharyngeal wall very gently on both sides) . . . (and after taking the tongue depressor out) . . . could you feel the stick touching you in all those places? . . . did it feel the same on both sides?' Finding out whether the patient wretches if the posterior pharyngeal wall is stabbed with the orange stick is both deeply unpleasant and of no diagnostic utility.

Common causes of lower cranial nerve lesions are shown in Table 35.

XI nerve (spinal accessory)

Look at and palpate the sternocleidomastoid muscles: are they symmetrical; is one or both wasted? Test strength by asking the patient to twist their neck to the right side as you resist the movement by placing the flat of your hand against that side of their face. Make sure that you can see the muscle belly of the left sternocleidomastoid and palpate to determine that it is contracting. Repeat as the patient turns to the left side.

From behind the patient, inspect the trapezius muscle for wasting or asymmetry before testing power by asking the patient to shrug their shoulders and then telling them to 'keep them up' as you press down to elicit weakness.

It is very uncommon to get an isolated lesion of the XI nerve, but it can sometimes be damaged by surgery, penetrating injury or tumour in the posterior triangle of

TABLE 35 COMMON CAUSES OF LESIONS OF THE LOWER CRANIAL NERVES

Neurological deficit	Site of lesion	Cause
Unilateral IX and X	Skull base	Tumour Fracture
	Brain stem	Lateral medullary syndrome
Bilateral X	Lower motor neurone (progressive bulbar palsy)	Motor neurone disease
	Upper motor neurone (pseudobulbar palsy)	Multiple sclerosis Cerebrovascular disease
Recurrent laryngeal	Mediastinum	Lung cancer Other mediastinal mass
	Neck	Thyroid (esp after surgery – look for scar)
Unilateral IX, X and XI	Jugular foramen (1)	Tumour within skull Lateral brain stem lesion (usually vascular accident)
Unilateral IX, X, XI and XII	Lesion at jugular foramen and hypoglossal canal (2)	Tumour outside skull
Unilateral IX, X, XI, XII and Horner's syndrome	As above (3)	Tumour outside skull

Notes
(1) The IX, X and XI nerves exit the skull through the jugular foramen. Deficit of these three nerves is called Vernet's syndrome.
(2) The XII nerve exits the skull through the anterior condylar canal, just above condyle of the occipital bone. Deficit of these four nerves is called Collet-Sicard syndrome.
(3) This deficit called Villaret's syndrome.
(4) It is not necessary to know the names of these syndromes for PACES.

against the inside of each cheek in turn while you press from the outside with your finger.

Check list – examination of the cranial nerves

1. General inspection.
2. 'Any problem with sense of smell?' (I: Olfactory).
3. Visual acuity, visual fields, (blind spot and fundoscopy if examiner affirms) (II: Optic).
4. Pupillary responses.
5. Eye movements (III, IV, VI: Oculomotor, Trochlear, Abducens. Also cerebellum/brain stem).
6. Sensation on face, corneal reflex, muscles of mastication (V: Trigeminal).
7. Facial muscles (VII: Facial).
8. Hearing; Rinne's and Weber's tests (if appropriate) (VIII: Vestibulocochlear).
9. 'Yellow lorry', 'baby hippopotamus', puff out cheeks, palatal movement ('say Aaah') (IX and X: Glossopharyngeal and Vagus).
10. Sternocleidomastoid and Trapezius muscles (XI: Accessory).
11. Tongue (XII: Hypoglossal).

the neck. Wasting and weakness of the sternocleidomastoids is often seen in dystrophia myotonica.

XII nerve (hypoglossal)

Tell the patient to open their mouth and look carefully at the tongue for wasting, fasciculation or involuntary movement as it lies in the floor of the mouth. Remember that the normal tongue often shows flickering movements when protruded: these are not pathological. Ask the patient to stick their tongue out and waggle it from side to side: look for asymmetry of protrusion (deviation is towards the weak side) and slowness/incoordination. Test power by asking them to press their tongue

TABLE 36 COMMON CAUSES OF TREMOR AND INVOLUNTARY MOVEMENTS IN PACES

Tremor/movement	Cause
Resting tremor	Parkinson's disease
Intention tremor	Cerebellar disease
Postural tremor	Benign essential tremor (sporadic or familial) Physiological (exacerbated by anxiety)
Chorea	Huntington's
Athetosis	Cerebral palsy Cerebral anoxia Wilson's disease
Dystonia	Phenothiazines/butyraphenones

Note
(1) Other causes of chorea include Sydenham's (rheumatic fever), thalamic lesions, oral contraceptive pill/pregnancy, thyrotoxicosis, SLE, polycythaemia rubra vera and senility.

TABLE 37 MOTOR POWER IN THE ARM

Movement	Nerve root	Peripheral nerve
Shoulder abduction	C5	Suprascapular (first 90°) Axillary (second 90°)
Shoulder adduction	C7	Nerves to latissimus dorsi and pectoralis major
Elbow flexion	C5,6	Musculocutaneous
Elbow extension	C7	Radial
Wrist extension	C7	Radial
Wrist flexion	C7	Median
Finger extension	C8	Radial
Finger flexion (squeeze my two fingers)	C8,T1	Median (thumb, index and middle fingers) Ulnar (ring and little fingers)
Finger abduction (spread your fingers apart)	T1	Ulnar (dorsal interossei)
Finger adduction (hold this piece of paper between your fingers and stop me pulling it out)	T1	Ulnar (palmar interossei)
Abduction of thumb away from the palm (holding palm horizontal and facing upwards, put thumb pointing toward ceiling at 45° to palm, and ask the patient to keep it there whilst you press it down)	T1	Median (abductor pollicis brevis)

Neurological examination of the arms

After inspection from the end of the bed for the features described in Table 25, look closely at the posture of the arms/hands, for tremor or other involuntary movements (Table 36), for wasting (and the pattern of any wasting), and for fasciculation.

Ask the patient to 'put their arms out in front of them (with the palms facing upwards) . . . and then close their eyes'. This is an excellent screening test, in particular for pyramidal weakness, when the arm drifts down, and for sensory abnormality, when (if power is normal) the arm tends to wander upwards. After observing for a few seconds ask the patient to 'keep their eyes closed . . . and touch their nose with this finger (examiner touches the index finger of the patient's right hand) . . . put the arm out again . . . and now touch your nose with this finger (examiner touches index

finger of the patient's left hand). A patient with any significant weakness, sensory deficit or problem with coordination will not be able to perform this test normally. Now with the arms still outstretched, but with the palms facing downwards, ask the patient to 'play the piano with their fingers' and demonstrate what you mean. This simple maneuver will often elegantly demonstrate the presence of any unilateral motor problem.

Test tone at the wrists and at the elbows: is there a 'catch' with quick movements, particularly on extension, suggestive of an upper motor neurone lesion, or a lead-pipe feeling, perhaps with cogwheeling, indicating parkinsonism?

Examine power by systematically moving from shoulder abduction as shown in Table 37. The correct method is to get the patient to place the relevant joint in the position that you want to be maintained and then ask them to try to keep that position as you attempt to move the joint by overcoming the relevant muscle group. For instance 'put your arms out at the side . . . (demonstrate arms abducted to 90° at the shoulder, with elbows flexed) . . . keep them there . . . stop me pushing them down'. When reporting power, use the MRC grading scale correctly (Table 38).

Test the biceps (C5,6), supinator (C6), triceps (C7) and finger (C8) jerks, using reinforcement ('clench your teeth') if needed.

Test coordination, in particular looking for cerebellar problems, by performing the finger-nose test, also by asking the patient to perform rapidly alternating movements of their hands/fingers. Two are commonly used: tapping the palm of one hand with the front and then

TABLE 38 MRC SCALE FOR GRADING MUSCULAR POWER

Grade	Description
0	No flicker of movement
1	Flicker of movement in muscle, but not enough to move joint at all
2	Joint can be moved, but not against gravity
3	Joint can move against gravity, but not against any other resistance
4	Movement against resistance, but weaker than normal
5	Normal power

Note – The MRC grading system was developed in the context of trying to find out if it was worthwhile suturing nerves that had been transected, when any flicker of movement that moved the assessment from grade 0 to grade 1 indicated a degree of re-innervation. Movement of grade 3 or less is of no functional use.

the back of the fingers of the other hand as fast as possible, and opening and closing a pinch of fingers and thumb together as fast as possible. Common causes of cerebellar signs are shown in Table 39.

Test sensation to light touch and then pin prick, using clear instructions as described for testing sensation on the face. It is essential to move at a reasonable pace to prevent the patient from getting fatigued, when responses become unreliable, also to prevent the examiner from becoming bored and irritable. Begin with one touch to the tip of the middle finger (C7, median nerve or peripheral neuropathy), then to the tip of the thumb (C6, median nerve, peripheral neuropathy), then the tip of the little finger (C8, ulnar nerve, peripheral neuropathy), and then proceed proximally testing the medial and lateral surfaces of forearm and upper arm, remembering the dermatomes as shown in figure 7.

If you detect any loss of light touch or pin prick, you then need to analyse the deficit to determine its cause. Tell the patient 'I just want to check this out a bit more . . . (and starting to apply the stimulus within the area in which it is not perceived and then progressively moving towards an area of normal sensation) . . . tell me as soon as you feel this . . . (and then return to the starting point and explore in another direction)'.

> Expect to be asked 'what else would you like to do?' and 'what are your findings?' as soon as you appear to have finished testing light touch/pin prick sensation in the arms

If there is no deficit to light touch, check for sensory inattention by telling the patient that you are going

TABLE 39 COMMON CAUSES OF CEREBELLAR SIGNS	
Condition	**Other neurological signs to look for**
Multiple sclerosis	Nystagmus Internuclear ophthalmoplegia Optic atrophy Spastic paraparesis
Brain stem vascular lesion	Other evidence of focal brain stem lesion
Alcoholic cerebellar degeneration	Nystagmus Peripheral neuropathy
Friedreich's ataxia (1)	Scoliosis Pes cavus Dysarthria Absent tendon jerks (ankle especially) Absent vibration sense and joint position sense (feet especially) Upgoing plantars
Posterior fossa space-occupying lesion (2)	Papilloedema
Paraneoplastic syndrome (2)	Cachexia Clubbing

Notes: (1) More common in PACES than in routine clinical practice; (2) Not likely in PACES. Alcohol and phenytoin intoxications are common acute causes of cerebellar dysfunction, but uncommon in PACES.

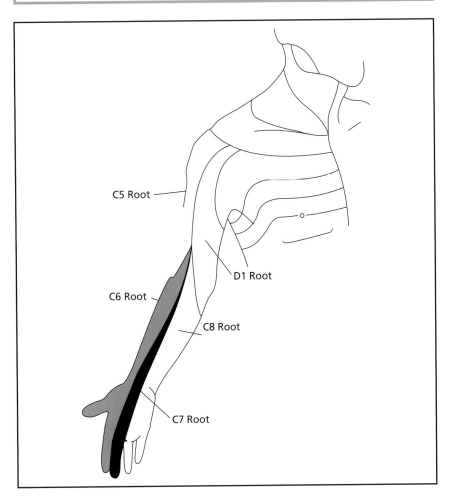

▲ **Fig. 7** The dermatomes of the arm.

TABLE 40 SENSORY AND MOTOR DEFICITS OF ROOT OR NERVE LESIONS IN THE ARM

Lesion	Sensory deficit	Motor deficit
C5	Lateral border upper arm	Shoulder abduction
C6	Lateral forearm/thumb	Elbow flexion
C7	Middle finger	Elbow extension
		Wrist extension/flexion
C8	Medial forearm/little finger	Finger extension
T1	Axilla down to elbow	All small muscles of hand
Axillary nerve	Small area over deltoid	Shoulder abduction
Radial nerve*	Dorsum of thumb and index finger	Elbow extension
		Wrist extension
		Finger extension
Median nerve	Lateral palm and lateral fingers and thumb	Wrist flexion
		Long finger flexors
Ulnar nerve*	Medial palm, little finger and medial half ring finger	All small muscles of hand, excluding abductor pollicis brevis

Notes
(1) * sensory loss may not be prominent.
(2) Causes of root and nerve lesions in the arm are shown in Table 41.

to touch them on their left, right or both hands and ask them to say 'left, right or both' when they feel anything. Then touch them gently on both hands at the same time. They will almost certainly say 'both', but if they say 'left', then they have demonstrated right-sided sensory inattention (or vice versa if they say 'right') suggestive of a parietal lesion.

Test joint position sense in the middle finger of each hand. Again, clear instructions to the patient are paramount. Begin by grasping the sides of the middle and distal phalanges, asking the patient to look, and demonstrating 'this is up . . . and this is down'. Then, with the patient's eyes closed, make small but precise movements, saying 'tell me which

way I move the joint, up or down . . . now . . . and now'. If the patient cannot perceive movements at the distal interphalangeal joint, proceed to move the whole finger up and down at the metacarpophalyngeal joint (then the wrist, then the elbow if necessary).

Test vibration sense at the tip of the middle finger of each hand using a 128 Hz tuning fork, having first established that the patient can feel it buzzing on their sternum. If it is not perceived in the finger, proceed proximally to the metacarpophalyngeal joint, radial styloid and olecranon as appropriate.

If you demonstrate any sensory abnormality, then the first question in your mind should be 'is this a peripheral neuropathy?', which would be most likely if the problem affects both hands/arms in a glove distribution. By contrast, a clearly unilateral sensory problem is extremely unlikely to be due to peripheral neuropathy, in which case does it fit best with a root or nerve lesion (Table 40)?

TABLE 41 CAUSES OF ROOT AND NERVE LESIONS IN THE ARM

Lesion	Common cause
Any root	Cervical spondylosis
	Disc lesion
	Cervical cord lesion (syringomyelia)
Axillary nerve	Fractured neck of humerus
	Deep IM injection
Radial nerve	Crutch palsy
	Saturday night palsy
	Fractured humerus
Median nerve	Carpal tunnel syndrome
	Trauma to wrist
Ulnar nerve	Lesion at elbow
	Lesion at wrist

Notes
(1) Lesions of suprascapular and musculocutaneous nerves are extremely rare.
(2) Syringomyelia associated with dissociated sensory loss over one or both of the arms and often with upper motor neurone signs in the legs.

Check list – neurological examination of the arms

1. General inspection.
2. Appearance of arms – posture, tremor, spontaneous movements, wasting, fasciculation.
3. Screen for problem – 'arms out in front, palms facing up, with eyes closed'; 'touch your nose'; play the piano.
4. Tone.
5. Power – shoulder abduction, shoulder adduction, then systematically move peripherally.
6. Tendon jerks – biceps, supinator, triceps, finger.
7. Coordination – finger-nose, rapidly alternating movements.
8. Sensation – light touch, pin prick, sensory inattention, joint position, vibration.

TABLE 42 PATTERNS OF MUSCLE WASTING IN THE LEGS

Pattern of wasting	Likely diagnosis	Other neurological features in legs
Unilateral, global	Polio	No sensory signs
Bilateral, distal (inverted champagne bottle)	Hereditary Motor Sensory Neuropathy (Charcot-Marie-Tooth disease) (1)	Pes cavus Clawing of toes Absent ankle jerks Peripheral neuropathy (sometimes)
Bilateral, proximal, with calf hypertrophy	Muscular dystrophy (Duchenne or Becker) (2)	No sensory signs

Notes
(1) Predictable PACES question – 'supposing the patient presented with a short history of peripheral neuropathy, what diagnoses would you consider?'
(2) Another predictable PACES question – 'supposing the patient presented with a short history of proximal muscle weakness, what diagnoses would you consider?'

Neurological examination of the legs

After inspection from the end of the bed for the features described in Table 25, look closely at the posture, for involuntary movements, wasting (and the pattern of any wasting, Table 42) and for fasciculation, which almost always indicates motor neurone disease.

Ask the patient if they are able to get off the bed/couch and walk. If they say 'no', proceed with the examination, but if they say 'yes', then get them to do so (unless the examiner tells you not to), providing any assistance that is necessary and offering them their stick/walking aid if they have one. Depending on their speed, ask them to walk 5 or 10 metres and then return, looking for any typical pattern of abnormality (Table 43). Ask them to walk 'heel-toe', demonstrating what you mean by this, and before getting them back on the couch ask them to stand facing you with their feet together, and then maintain this posture with their eyes closed (Romberg's test: Table 43).

TABLE 43 COMMON ABNORMALITIES OF GAIT AND THEIR FREQUENT CAUSES

Abnormality of gait	Gait	Frequent cause	Heel-toe	Romberg's test
Slow initiation Small steps	Festinant	Parkinson's disease	Appropriate (1)	Negative (2)
Small steps Body sways from side to side	Waddling	Proximal myopathy	Appropriate	Negative
Unilateral Stiff-legged Dragging foot	Hemiplegic	Stroke	Appropriate	Negative
Bilateral Stiff-legged Dragging feet	Paraplegic	Spinal cord lesion	Appropriate	Negative
Wide-based stance Unsteady Reels to one side or to both sides	Cerebellar	See Table 39	Significantly impaired	Negative
Bilateral Wide-based stance High-stepping Flapping feet	Sensory ataxic	Peripheral neuropathy	Significantly impaired	Positive
Unilateral High step Flapping foot	Steppage/Equine	Foot drop	Appropriate	Negative
Affected by pain	Antalgic	Painful condition of back, hip, knee, ankle or foot	Appropriate	Negative

Notes
(1) An 'appropriate' heel-toe test means that the patient's performance is not significantly impaired in the context of their overall motor difficulty.
(2) A negative Romberg's test means that the patient is not more unsteady with their eyes closed than they are with their eyes open.

Ask the patient to relax their legs and test tone. Rock the right leg such that it rotates to and fro at the hip joint, placing one hand behind the knee as you do so. After a few seconds, flip the knee joint up from below. If tone is normal, the heel will stay on the bed: if it is increased, the heel will flip up off the bed. Repeat with the left leg. Test, with the knee flexed to 45–90°, for clonus at each ankle: after a few small but unpredictable movements, moving the foot up and down and from side to side to encourage relaxation, push it into dorsiflexion and hold it there with reasonably firm pressure. Failure to sustain the pressure is a common reason for candidates to fail to elicit clonus that is very obvious when the examination is performed correctly. If clonus is present at the ankle, but not if it is absent, test for clonus at the knee: with the leg relaxed and the knee extended, push the patella firmly down towards the foot and hold it there.

Practise your technique for eliciting ankle clonus

- Knee flexed to 45–90°.
- Get the ankle loose.
- Push ankle firmly into dorsiflexion and hold it there.

Examine power by systematically moving from hip flexion as shown in Table 44. As stated previously, the correct method is to get the patient to place the relevant joint in the position that you want to be maintained and then ask them to try to keep that position as you attempt to move the joint by overcoming the relevant muscle group. For instance 'lift your leg straight up off the bed . . . keep it there . . . stop me pushing it down'.

Test the knee (L3, 4) and ankle (S1) jerks, using reinforcement ('clench your teeth') if needed. Check the plantar responses by drawing an orange stick or similar blunt object up the lateral aspect of foot towards the little toe.

Practise your technique for eliciting the ankle jerks.

- Get the ankle loose.
- Take a good swing.

Test coordination, in particular looking for cerebellar problems, by performing the heel-shin test. This is often done badly, with the patient simply asked to rub their heel up and down their shin. The correct method, which will demonstrate abnormalities not found by the simple rubbing method, is as

follows. Ask the patient to put their right heel on the top of their left shin and run it down the shin towards the foot, pointing to demonstrate exactly what you want them to do. Then ask them to lift their heel off the bottom of the shin and replace it at the top. Repeat the cycle once more, and then do so on the other side. Patients with significant weakness will not be able to perform the test in a normal manner and this needs to be recognized in your interpretation of their performance. However, if their difficulty is out of proportion to any weakness, remember the common causes of cerebellar signs (Table 39) and anticipate the question from the examiner 'what else would you look for if you think the patient might have a cerebellar problem?' (nystagmus; cerebellar signs in the arms; truncal ataxia).

Test sensation to light touch and then pin prick, using clear instructions and a brisk approach as described previously. Since a peripheral neuropathy if by far and away the commonest cause of sensory deficit in the leg in both general clinical practice and PACES, begin by touching the feet and then progressing proximally, as shown in figure 8. If you detect any loss of light touch or pin prick, then – if it is not obviously in the stocking pattern of a peripheral neuropathy – you need to analyse the deficit in the manner described previously.

Expect to be asked 'what else would you like to do?' and 'what are your findings?' as soon as you appear to have finished testing light touch/pin prick sensation in the legs.

Test joint position sense in the big toe of each foot, using instructions

TABLE 44 MOTOR POWER IN THE LEG		
Movement	**Nerve root**	**Peripheral nerve**
Hip flexion	L2	–
Hip extension	L4,5	Sciatic
Knee flexion	S1	Sciatic
Knee extension	L3, L4	Femoral
Foot dorsiflexion	L5	Peroneal (lateral popliteal)
Foot plantarflexion	S1	Tibial (medial popliteal)
Toe dorsiflexion	L5	Peroneal (lateral popliteal)
Ankle eversion	L5, S1	Peroneal (lateral popliteal)
Ankle inversion	L4, L5	Tibial (medial popliteal)

Note – The main nerve root(s) for each movement are shown: other roots may play a lesser role.

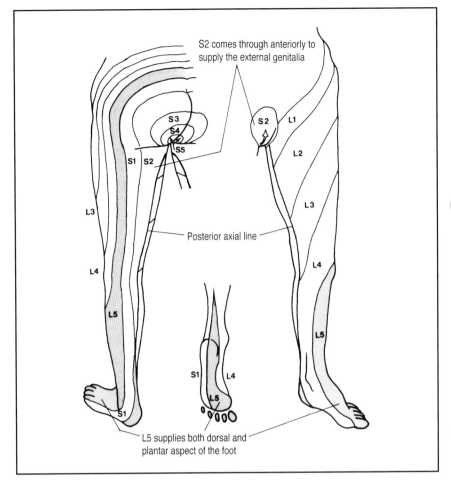

S2 comes through anteriorly to supply the external genitalia

Posterior axial line

L5 supplies both dorsal and plantar aspect of the foot

▲ **Fig. 8** The dermatomes of the leg.

and technique as explained for the finger (and proceeding to move the foot up and down at the ankle joint if required).

Test vibration sense at the tip of the big toe of each foot using a 128 Hz tuning fork, having first established that the patient can feel it buzzing

on their sternum. If it is not perceived, proceed proximally to the medial malleolus, patella and iliac crest as appropriate.

A clearly unilateral sensory problem is extremely unlikely to be due to peripheral neuropathy, in which case does it fit best with a root or nerve lesion (Table 45)?

> **Check list – neurological examination of the legs**
>
> 1. General inspection.
> 2. Appearance of legs – posture, spontaneous movements, wasting, fasciculation.
> 3. Walk – is there a characteristic gait abnormality?, heel toe.
> 4. Romberg's test.
> 5. Tone, including ankle clonus.
> 6. Power – hip flexion, hip extension, then systematically move peripherally.
> 7. Tendon jerks – knee, ankle.
> 8. Plantar response.
> 9. Coordination – heel-shin.
> 10. Sensation – light touch, pin prick, joint position, vibration.

Presenting neurological findings to the examiners

More so than with examination of any other system, the examiner can see exactly what physical signs you are able to elicit as you perform a neurological examination. A lengthy list of all the (likely very many) negative findings is not required, and if you embark on giving a litany of unremarkable findings – perhaps in an attempt to cut down the length of time that the examiner can ask you questions – then this is likely to cause irritation, and irritated examiners are unlikely to score you highly. Your strategy must be to present only the significant findings in a crisp and logical manner.

It may be that this is straightforward: 'from the foot of the bed I notice that Mr X has

TABLE 45 SENSORY AND MOTOR DEFICITS OF ROOT OR NERVE LESIONS IN THE LEG

Lesion	Sensory deficit	Motor deficit
L2	Often none (across upper thigh)	Hip flexion
L3	Often none (across lower thigh)	Knee extension
L4	Medial leg	Foot inversion
L5	Dorsum of foot	Toe dorsiflexion
S1	Behind lateral malleolus	Foot plantarflexion and eversion
Femoral nerve	Anterior thigh and medial knee	Knee extension
Peroneal nerve	Lateral aspect lower leg and dorsum of foot	Foot dorsiflexion, inversion and eversion
Tibial nerve	Sole of foot	Foot plantarflexion and eversion

Note: Causes of root and nerve lesions in the leg are shown in Table 46.

TABLE 46 CAUSES OF ROOT AND NERVE LESIONS IN THE LEG

Lesion	Common causes/comments
Roots L2,3,4	Neurofibroma Meningioma Neoplastic disease (1)
Roots L5, S1	Disc lesions (2)
Femoral nerve	Diabetes Lesion in posterior abdomen/psoas/femoral canal
Peroneal nerve	Pressure palsy at fibula neck Hip fracture/dislocation
Tibial nerve	Very uncommon as isolated lesion

Notes
(1) Uncommon in PACES; disc lesions a rare cause of compression of L2,3,4.
(2) Neurofibroma, meningioma and neoplastic disease also possible.

a pair of elbow crutches (as appropriate) . . . on examination of the cranial nerves the abnormalities are that visual acuity is reduced to counting fingers in the right eye, but is normal in the left eye . . . eye movements are grossly abnormal . . . on attempting to gaze to the right the left eye does not adduct . . . the right eye abducts but shows nystagmus . . . which indicate an internuclear ophthalmoplegia . . . there are no other abnormalities'. In which case you can go on to say 'these findings are most likely to be explained by multiple sclerosis causing optic atrophy . . . which I would want to confirm by fundoscopy . . . a lesion in the median longitudinal fasciculus . . . and either spasticity or cerebellar problems in the legs'.

However, if the signs are not so clear cut, then it remains important to describe them well. The examiner is as likely to have found them as difficult as you have done, if not more so. Very few **PACES** examiners are neurologists and most will be mightily impressed by a candidate who appears to be able to make some sense of a less than straightforward neurological case. Description of ocular movements often causes difficulty. If the patient's gaze does not seem normal in any direction and there is nystagmus when the patient looks anywhere, then it is easy in the heat of the moment to end up saying little more than 'the eye movements are abnormal . . . and there's a lot of nystagmus', which is not going to impress. Try something along the

lines of 'I found the eye movements difficult to analyse, but they were clearly abnormal . . . the patient was unable to direct their gaze in any direction in a normal manner . . . the most marked abnormality was on attempted gaze to the right (or wherever it was), when the right eye did whatever it did and the left eye did whatever it did . . . in all directions of gaze, but particularly to wherever, there was complex nystagmus with horizontal/rotatory (as appropriate) as well as a vertical component . . . (all you've said so far is that the eye movements are abnormal, and there's a lot of nystagmus, although you have added the key point about the nystagmus having a vertical component) . . . all these findings suggest a central lesion in the brain stem'.

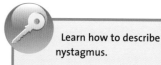

Learn how to describe nystagmus.

Above all, keep a firm grasp of the basics. It is very unlikely that the PACES examiner will know more. If the knee jerks are brisk, but tone is otherwise normal and the plantars are flexor, then don't say that the patient might have an upper motor neurone lesion or a spastic paraparesis: most likely they haven't relaxed. If there are sensory abnormalities, then don't say that the diagnosis might be a myopathy: it isn't.

The brief clinical consultations are designed to replicate professional behavior that is frequently required of specialty registrars and consultants, when in a limited period of time they need to make a focused assessment of a patient, explain the plan for investigation and management, before moving on to the next case in the clinic or the Emergency Department. They are challenging in the PACES exam, and of great importance because station 5 carries a lot of marks (56/172; 32.5%).

The format of Station 5 is shown in Table 47, and details from the marksheet that the examiner will be looking at as you conduct the consultations are shown in Table 48.

General approach

Time is short in Station 5, hence the key word is 'focus'.

Two sorts of cases are typical: the patient presenting with a common discrete medical presentation, and the patient with a spot diagnosis, most often dermatological, rheumatological or endocrinological. The instructions to the candidate will give unambiguous direction, and it is very important that these are followed: there is simply no time for going 'off track'.

The common medical presentation
The scenario may be set in the Emergency Department or on

a ward, and the problem to be addressed will be clear cut. For instance, the patient 'complains of a sharp pain in the chest'. The good candidate will immediately think of the common causes of pleuritic-type chest pain – pulmonary embolism, pneumonia, pneumothorax, musculoskeletal – and the history that they take will immediately focus on sorting out this differential diagnosis: what were you doing when the pain came on? has it affected your breathing? is the pain worse if you twist or turn? have you had any other chest symptoms (cough, haemoptysis etc)? have you felt unwell over the last few days (feverish etc)? have you had any problems in your legs (pain, swelling) etc? have you ever had anything like this before (and what was the diagnosis)? have you have had any other illnesses recently? have you been on any long coach trips or aeroplane flights?

There is no time for beating about the bush. The information above could be obtained in not much more time than it took you to read the paragraph, following which matters should proceed to relevant examination of the heart, lungs and legs. It would not be appropriate to spend time looking for clubbing or a metabolic flap: after briefly feeling the pulse and saying that you'd like to know the blood pressure, the next step would be to have a quick look for cyanosis and at the JVP, perform rapid palpation, percussion and

TABLE 47 BRIEF CLINICAL CONSULTATIONS – FORMAT OF STATION 5	
Time	
5 minutes before starting station	Read the two scenarios very carefully. What are the main tasks? – working out the diagnosis?; sorting out and explaining a plan for investigation or management?; often both of these are required. Write down any points that you want to be sure of covering.
0–8 minutes	Take a focused history from the patient and perform an appropriate focused examination. Examiner reminds 'two minutes to go' at 6 minutes – this will act as a prompt to the patient to ask the question(s) that they have been briefed to ask (if these haven't already come up naturally in the course of the consultation).
8–10 minutes	Examiner asks candidate to give relevant findings on history and examination and to suggest appropriate diagnosis and/or plan for investigation and/or plan for treatment.

TABLE 48 KEY FEATURES OF THE EXAMINER'S MARKSHEET FOR A BRIEF CLINICAL CONSULTATION

Clinical skill	To score satisfactory	To score unsatisfactory
Clinical communication skills	Elicits history relevant to the complaint and explains information to the patient in a focused, fluent and professional manner.	Omits important areas of the history and/or appears unpractised or unprofessional. Explains things poorly to the patient.
Physical examination	Techniques must be correct, appropriate practised and professional.	Techniques are incorrect; significant or important tests are omitted; approach is inappropriately focused, hesitant, lacking confidence or unprofessional.
Clinical judgement	Offers a sensible and appropriate plan for investigations and treatment.	Offers an inappropriate plan for investigations and treatment.
Managing patient's concerns	Listens and is empathetic. Seeks, detects and attempts to address the patient's concerns.	Does not listen well and/or is not empathetic. Overlooks patient's concerns.
Identifying physical signs	Identifies correct signs. Signs that are not present are not found.	Important signs are missed. Signs that are not present are found.
Differential diagnosis	Sensible, and includes the correct diagnosis.	Poor, and fails to consider the correct diagnosis.
Maintaining patient welfare	Treats the patient in an appropriate manner.	Causes the patient physical or emotional discomfort, or treats them in an unsafe manner.

auscultation of the heart and lungs, and look at the legs to see if one was swollen.

The patient will have been primed to ask one or two straightforward questions, for instance 'is this serious?' and 'can I have a painkiller and go home?' These are not devastatingly difficult questions to answer: all that's required is that the candidate says something sensible and reasonably reassuring, and doesn't allow themselves to be talked into an unwise cause of action. 'It probably isn't serious . . . but there is a chance it could be and we should check things out . . . we need to get a scan of your lungs to check that there isn't a blood clot'. 'No, I will give you a painkiller to try to get rid of the pain, but I would not be happy with you just going home afterwards . . . there might be a clot of blood in the lungs . . . and if there is then it will heal up . . . but we would need to thin the blood to stop more clots causing trouble . . . they can cause serious trouble, and sometimes even kill people'.

The 'spot diagnosis'

Many of the patients seen in Station 5 will have 'spot' dermatological, rheumatological, endocrinological or (probably less likely) ophthalmological diagnoses, not least because all centres hosting PACES exams will have many such patients on their books who used to participate in station 5 of the previous format of the exam (which comprised one case from each of these four categories).

In preparing for Station 5 it is worthwhile thinking of the obvious questions a patient with one of the common spot diagnoses might be primed to ask: dermatological – 'will the rash go away?'; 'can the rash be treated?'; rheumatological – 'do I need any tests for the arthritis?'; 'what is the treatment for the arthritis?'; endocrinological – 'will my eyes always look like this?'; 'how can (the particular condition) be treated?'; ophthalmological – 'will I go blind?' Details regarding particular dermatological, rheumatological, endocrinological and ophthalmological conditions can be found in the appropriate modules of Medical Masterclass: further description here will be confined to matters of dermatological, rheumatological, endocrinological and ophthalmological examination routine.

Examination of the skin

The patient will typically be presented in such a way that the relevant abnormality is visible, but it is important to recognize that a proper examination of a difficult case means looking at all of the skin, and making the correct diagnosis often depends on knowing which areas are or are not involved. It is sensible to ask the patient 'are any other areas affected?' – which is what you would do in routine clinical practice – and go on to look at any parts suggested by them unless the examiner indicates that you should not do so. It is very unlikely that the examiner will let you strip a patient to look all over their skin because there is only a limited amount of time, buy they are likely to say 'what would you be looking for in particular?', so be prepared for this question and remember the typical locations of common dermatological conditions (Table 49).

TABLE 49 LOCATION OF COMMON DERMATOLOGICAL CONDITIONS

Location	Common in routine clinical practice	Also consider in PACES
Scalp	Psoriasis Alopecia	
Face	Xanthelasma Rosacea Basal cell carcinoma	Systemic sclerosis Discoid lupus erythematosus Dermatomyositis Sturge-Weber
Mouth	Candidiasis Herpes simplex Lichen planus	Osler-Weber-Rendu Peutz-Jeghers
Neck	Contact dermatitis (nickel)	Pseudoxanthoma elasticum
Trunk	Herpes zoster (1) Pityriasis	Dermatitis herpetiformis
Axillae		Pseudoxanthoma elasticum Acanthosis nigricans
Elbows	Psoriasis (extensor) Atopic dermatitis (flexor) Rheumatoid nodules (extensor) Gouty tophi (extensor) Olecranon bursitis	Pseudoxanthoma elasticum (flexor) Xanthomata (extensor)
Hands	Contact dermatitis Scabies	Systemic sclerosis Addison's disease Dermatomyositis
Nails	Psoriasis Fungal infection Leuconychia Koilonychia	Tuberous sclerosis
Legs	Venous ulcer Varicose eczema Necrobiosis lipoidica diabetorum Erythema nodosum Henoch-Schonlein purpura	Pyoderma gangrenosum
Feet	Diabetic ulcer	Keratoderma blenorrhagica
Any	Vitilgo Purpura Erythema multiforme	Neurofibromatosis Pemphigus Pemphigoid

Note
(1) Shingles can affect any dermatome, but particularly common on trunk.

1. Do all the lesions look the same (monomorphic rash), or are there lesions of different sorts (pleiomorphic rash)?

2. What part(s) of the body is/are affected?

3. What type of rash is it? – macular (flat, discrete lesions that are not palpable), papular (raised, discrete lesions up to 1cm in diameter that are palpable), nodular (like papular, but bigger), vesicular (small well-defined fluid-filled lesions), bullous (like vesicular, but larger) or pustular (contain purulent – but sometimes sterile – fluid). Is there ulceration?

4. What is the colour (eg. erythematous, pigmented, purpuric), size (approximately) and shape of a typical lesion; what is the surface of the lesion like (eg. smooth, scaling, crusted, eroded); is there evidence of scarring where lesions have healed?

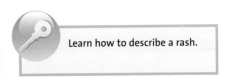

Learn how to describe a rash.

Examination of the locomotor system

The commonest rheumatological diagnoses in PACES are rheumatoid arthritis, psoriatic arthropathy, systemic sclerosis, gout or Charcot's joints, but aside from giving the obvious 'spot' diagnosis you should be able complete a standard GALS (Gait, Arms, Legs, Spine) examination in a smooth and efficient manner to demonstrate the functional impact of any musculoskeletal problem (Table 50 and Figure 9).

Very few PACES examiners are dermatologists and most will feel insecure when dealing with anything other than common dermatological conditions, hence – unless the diagnosis is both common and obvious – they will almost certainly not mark you down too heavily if you do not recognize something that is rare, as long as you demonstrate an ability to describe the lesions accurately and make one or two other sensible comments. But saying 'there's a rash . . . and I don't know what it is' will not impress, and yet some candidates to come up with little more than this in the heat of the moment. Remember and use the correct vocabulary to describe any lesions accurately in a systematic manner.

TABLE 50 THE GAIT, ARMS, LEGS AND SPINE (GALS) EXAMINATION

GALS	Manoeuvre	Figure 9, panel	Tests
Gait	Walk a few steps away from you, turn and come back		Is the gait normal? If not, then how is it abnormal (table 43)?
Arms	Stand in front of the patient and press on the midpoint of each supraspinatus	1	Detect hyperalgaesia, suggesting fibromyalgia
	Hands behind the head, with elbows back	2	Abduction and external rotation of glenohumeral joint
	Bend the arms up to touch shoulders	3	Elbow flexion
	Arms straight out in front of body	4	Elbow extension
	Elbows by the side, flexed to 90°, turning palms up and down	5	Pronation and supination at elbow and wrist
	Make a 'prayer sign', bending wrists back as far as possible; repeat with backs of hands together	6	Wrist extension and flexion
	Clench the fists and then open the hands out flat	7	Wrists and hands; make sure you check for full extension of fingers – if not, then which joints fail to extend?
	Squeeze my fingers (index and middle)	8	Grip strength
	Touch each finger tip onto thumb in turn	9	Precision and coordination
	Gently squeeze metacarpal heads	10	Tenderness suggests an inflammatory condition
Legs	Thomas' test (1)	11	For fixed flexion deformity of hips
	Flex and extend each hip and knee with your hand on the knee	12	Hip and knee extension; crepitus in patellofemoral joint
	Flex hip and knee to 90° and passively rotate each hip internally and externally	13	Pain and limitation of movement of hip rotation
	Palpate each knee for warmth and swelling; check patella tap	14	For inflammation and effusions
	Look at feet		For any abnormality; calluses or ulcers may suggest abnormal load bearing
	Gently squeeze metatarsal heads	15	Tenderness suggests an inflammatory condition
Spine	Stand behind patient and assess straightness of spine and symmetry of trunk/legs. Are the iliac crests level? Are the muscles of the back of the legs and the Achilles' tendons normal?		Scoliosis, kyphosis, gibbus, abnormal lumbar lordosis (increased or decreased); leg length
	Touch your toes (watching from side)	16	Abnormal spinal curvature; limited hip movement
	Turn from side to side (standing behind and holding pelvis to prevent rotation)	17	Thoracolumbar rotation
	Slide hand down leg towards knee (repeat on other side)	18	Lateral lumbar flexion
	Put ear on shoulder (repeat on other side)	19	Lateral cervical flexion
	Look up at ceiling then down at the floor	20	Cervical flexion and extension
	Let jaw drop open and move it from side to side	21	Temporomandibular joints

Tests

(1) Thomas' test should not be performed if the patient has a hip replacement because forced flexion can cause dislocation. Patient lies face up on firm couch. Place your left palm under the patient's lumbar spine. Passively flex both legs (hips and knees) as far as possible. Keep the non-test hip maximally flexed such that spine remains flat (lumbar lordosis remains eliminated). Ask patient to extend non-test hip. Incomplete extension indicates a fixed flexion deformity. Then test other hip.

Examination of the endocrine system

The most likely spot diagnoses are exophthalmos/Graves' disease, acromegaly, goitre, hypothyroidism, Cushing's syndrome and Addison's disease.

The only part of the patient that you are likely to have to examine systematically in the endocrine section of station 5 is the neck, so practise your method for doing this. Make sure that the neck is fully exposed, and after initial inspection (aside from the neck take note of the general appearance, and in particular the eyes) ask the patient to take a sip of water (it is more than likely that one will be to hand) and hold it in their mouth. Then, whilst you look carefully at the neck, ask them to swallow. Watch for movement of any goitre, also for the appearance of a nodule that had previously been obscured beneath sternocleidomastoid.

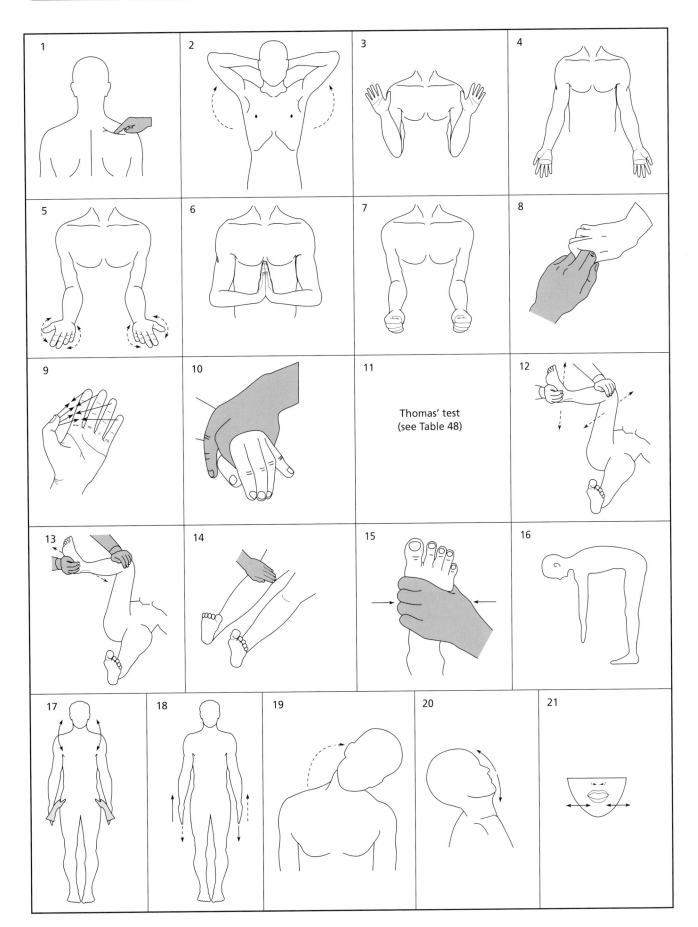

Thomas' test
(see Table 48)

▲ **Fig. 9** The Gait, Arms, Legs and Spine (GALS) examination. See Table 50 for further details.

With appropriate comments to the patient, move behind them and proceed to palpate the thyroid in a systematic manner. With the neck slightly flexed feel below the thyroid cartilage for the isthmus, then palpate for the two lobes that extend laterally below the sternocleidomastoid muscles. If the gland is enlarged, then aside from its size note whether it is soft/firm and nodular/diffusely swollen.

After palpating for the thyroid, examine for lymphadenopathy in a systematic manner, proceeding through the groups – submental, submandibular, preauricular, postauricular, suboccipital, anterior and posterior triangles, and supaclavicular. If you feel nodes, are they separate/matted together, mobile/fixed, fleshy/rubbery/hard?

Percuss over the upper sternum for retrosternal extension of any goitre, and auscultate over the thyroid for a bruit, but if you hear something listen in the aortic area to check that this is not a murmur radiating to the neck.

If there is anatomical abnormality of the thyroid, remember and examine for the eye signs of thyrotoxicosis (Table 51), and proceed to ask questions to discern whether the patient could be hypo- or hyper-thyroid, or has been in the past (and if so, about treatment).

Examination of the eyes

External examination of the eyes will most commonly be required in a patient with thyroid disorder (Table 51). Fundoscopy is rarely tested in PACES, because to perform it adequately requires that the patient be in a darkened room and with one or both pupils dilated, which tends to render the history taking and discussion elements of the station artificial and difficult. Furthermore, when a candidate is using an ophthalmoscope, all that the examiner can see during this time is the bobbing and weaving of their head, and whether or not the light from the ophthalmoscope is falling on the pupil. As always, a good method of examination will stand a better chance of achieving a correct diagnosis, and also incline the examiner to generosity in marking. Proceed as follows:

1. Select the large aperture if the pupil is dilated, the small one if not. Stand about 1m from the patient and rotate the lens dial to provide the sharpest image.

2. Look at the pupils to look for the normal red reflex from the retina. Any opacity such as a cataract or vitreous haemorrhage will darken the red reflex, and subluxation of the lens may be seen (rarely).

3. Ask the patient to 'keep your eyes on that (object) on the wall on the far side of the room . . . it's OK to blink, but please keep the eyes still'.

4. Examine each eye in turn using a systematic approach. Initially approach from a slightly temporal direction to see the optic disc, then follow the four main vascular arcades peripherally, then ask the patient to 'look at the light' for you to see the macula, and finally examine the peripheral retina in all quadrants by asking the patient to look up and down, right and left.

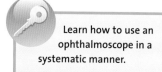 **Learn how to use an ophthalmoscope in a systematic manner.**

Describe your findings in the logical manner in which you examined them, and remember that common things are common: 'the red reflex was normal in both eyes indicating that there are no opacities in the lens or the vitreous . . . the optic discs looked normal . . . the arterioles and venules looked normal . . . there were dot haemorrhages and hard exudates in all quadrants . . . and photocoagulation scars in the peripheries . . . these are features of diabetic retinopathy'. The most likely diagnosis in PACES is diabetic retinopathy, with optic atrophy and retinitis pigmentosa commonly appearing (much more commonly than in routine clinical practice).

Acknowledgement

Many of the neurological drawings in *Clinical Skills for PACES* were drawn by Dr John P Patten BSc FRCP, latterly Consultant Neurologist, King Edward VII Hospital, Midhurst, West Sussex.

TABLE 51 EYE SIGNS OF THYROTOXICOSIS	
Sign	**Comment**
Lid retraction	The sclera can be seen above the iris as the patient looks straight ahead. Common in thyrotoxicosis of any cause.
Lid lag	The sclera can be seen above the iris as the patient follows your finger as you move it from the upper to the lower part of the visual field. Common in thyrotoxicosis of any cause.
Proptosis Ophthalmoplegia Chemosis Periorbital oedema	Features of Graves' disease, not of other causes of thyrotoxicosis.

PAIN RELIEF AND PALLIATIVE CARE

Authors:

JR Ross and DC Traue

Editor:

DC Traue

Editor-in-Chief:

JD Firth

PACES STATIONS AND ACUTE SCENARIOS

1.1 History-taking

1.1.1 Pain

> ### Letter of referral to palliative medicine outpatient clinic
>
> Dear Doctor
>
> **Re: Mrs Fiona Woods, aged 45 years**
>
> Thank you for seeing this woman who was diagnosed with breast carcinoma 4 years ago. She was treated with neoadjuvant chemotherapy prior to surgery, mastectomy and axillary dissection, followed by a course of adjuvant Taxotere (docetaxel) chemotherapy. Two years later she presented with left lung collapse and a malignant pleural effusion, which was treated with drainage and pleurodesis. Her disease continued to progress despite two further chemotherapy regimens. Her recent CT scan shows not only a loculated pleural effusion and small-volume lung metastases but also widespread pleural disease.
>
> Her main problem now is increasing pain in the left side of her chest. She has been taking tramadol 100 mg qds, but this has been making her feel nauseous and does not seem to be controlling her pain. She is not sleeping well at night and is often woken by the pain. She is aware that her disease has progressed and that further options for treatment are now limited. Please would you see her and advise further regarding pain control.
>
> Yours sincerely,

Introduction

Pain is a common symptom in patients with cancer. In assessing pain it is important to consider its aetiology, remembering that in some cases it may not be related to the underlying malignancy. The principles of good pain management include a stepwise increase in the strength of the opioid analgesic prescribed (Fig. 1), which should be titrated individually for each patient, and appropriate use of non-opioid and adjuvant analgesics. Patients need to be encouraged to take regular analgesia (by the clock), via the oral route where possible. Predictable side effects of opioids need to be discussed with the patient: prophylactic laxatives should be prescribed and antiemetics may also be needed when treatment is started. You also need to consider how the pain is affecting the patient's quality of life and ability to perform activities of daily living. When treating pain it is important to remember the 'total pain model' and address other concerns, such as fear regarding disease progression or coexisting depression. Non-pharmacological interventions are a helpful adjunct to all drug therapies.

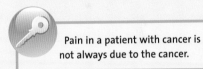

Pain in a patient with cancer is not always due to the cancer.

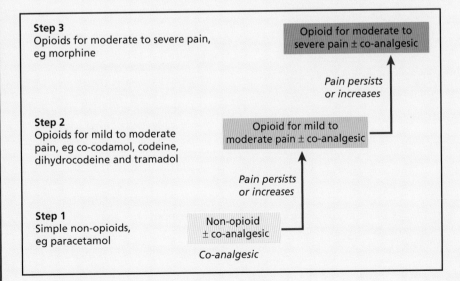

▲ **Fig. 1** WHO (World Health Organization) analgesic ladder.

Step 3
Opioids for moderate to severe pain, eg morphine

Step 2
Opioids for mild to moderate pain, eg co-codamol, codeine, dihydrocodeine and tramadol

Step 1
Simple non-opioids, eg paracetamol

Opioid for moderate to severe pain ± co-analgesic

Pain persists or increases

Opioid for mild to moderate pain ± co-analgesic

Pain persists or increases

Non-opioid ± co-analgesic

Co-analgesic

History of the presenting problem

An accurate history of the pain may give important clues to the aetiology. Ask the following questions.

- Where is the pain?

- Is it in more than one site?

- What is it like? Ask the patient to use descriptive terms, eg 'aching' or 'burning'.

- How severe is it? A score out of 10 can be helpful, particularly when gauging response to a treatment, eg before and after tramadol.

- When did it start and is it getting worse?

- Is it constant?

- Does it radiate anywhere?

- What precipitates or relieves it? Pain that is clearly related to movement is likely to be due to bony metastases in this context.

- Can she sleep at night? Does the pain wake her from sleep?

- How has the pain stopped her from continuing her usual routine?

- What does she think the pain is due to?

Other relevant history

Check for the following.

- Increasing shortness of breath and coughing, which might indicate infection, pulmonary emboli or pleural effusion.

- Side effects to current analgesics, eg constipation and nausea or vomiting: these may affect compliance with any prescription and adequate pain control.

- Anxiety or depression: these will affect both perception of pain and coping strategies.

Ask in particular if she has suffered in the past from asthma, peptic ulcer or renal failure, which would be a relative contraindication to use of an NSAID, or has a history of depression or anxiety, which may have recurred and benefit from treatment.

Take a full drug history (both prescribed and non-prescribed).

- Has she taken other analgesics in the past and, if so, did they help? Given a choice of pharmacologically acceptable medications, using one that the patient thinks has worked for her in the past is more likely to be effective than one that she is convinced is no good.

- Has she previously experienced side effects that might influence her compliance with future medication or your choice of drugs for her?

Remember that social history is crucial in this context.

- Is she living alone? Can she manage activities of daily living?

- Has she any dependants to care for?

- Has she either an informal or professional social support network, eg is she known to a community palliative care team?

> ⚠️ There is much more to pain control than prescribing analgesia: if the patient is very worried that no one is looking after the dog, then getting someone to sort this out may be more effective in relieving pain and distress than doubling the dose of morphine.

Plan for investigation and management

Investigations

- The CT scan performed by the oncology team suggests her pain may be due to pleural disease. However, if indicated by her history, investigations should be considered for bony metastases (bone scan) and pulmonary emboli (spiral CT scan as ventilation–perfusion scan will not be informative in this context).

- Blood tests: in particular check renal function and ensure her platelet count is not low. Alkaline phosphatase or calcium may be elevated with bony metastases.

Management

- Initially titrate with regular opioid analgesia, eg morphine sulphate immediate release (Oramorph) 10 mg 4-hourly (minimum starting dose as tramadol not effective). Give advice to patient not to drive until dose is stabilised: further details can be found on the medical issue pages of the UK Driver and Vehicle Licensing Agency (DVLA) website (http://www.dvla.gov.uk/).

- Commence regular laxative, eg co-danthramer 10 mL bd, and give antiemetics if necessary (eg metoclopramide hydrochloride 10 mg prn).

- Encourage her to keep a pain diary, including a record of breakthrough doses.

- Consider addition of NSAID (eg in the event of bony pain use diclofenac sodium SR 75 mg bd).

- Consider the use of a neuropathic agent if her history suggests neuropathic pain and the pain she is feeling is not responding to opioids. A sedating drug such as amitriptyline hydrochloride 25 mg nightly would be appropriate given difficulty sleeping at night.

This may need titration depending on response.

Follow-up
Notify primary care team and refer to or notify community palliative care team. Fix follow-up consultation with the palliative care team in the outpatients department and/or by community palliative care nurse.

Further discussion
Some patients are not comfortable with being started on strong opioids, often for reasons that are based on misunderstandings of one sort or another. The following issues should be discussed in case they are relevant:

- concern over the potential side effects that taking opioids might have;
- fear that there would not be any effective analgesics when pain gets really bad;
- fear that they might become addicted;
- fear that starting morphine means 'it's the end'.

Stepwise approach to using opioid analgesics
- Dose titration.
- Conversion of immediate-release to prolonged-release preparations.
- Calculation of a breakthrough dose.

Short-lived and continuing side effects
- Nausea and drowsiness are self-limiting and will disappear after a few days.
- Constipation and dry mouth will be present from when the patient starts the drug and will continue as long as it is taken.

Impact of other factors on the 'total pain' the patient is suffering
- Depression.
- Fear of disease progression.
- Social isolation.
- Spiritual distress.

1.1.2 Constipation/bowel obstruction

Letter of referral to palliative medicine outpatient clinic

Dear Doctor

Re: Mrs Claire Wilson, aged 76 years

Thank you for seeing this woman who was diagnosed with Dukes B/C carcinoma of the colon 2 years ago, treated with a hemicolectomy and chemotherapy. She developed liver metastases 9 months ago and had second-line chemotherapy, but her disease has progressed. Her main problem now is change in bowel pattern. She has previously had episodes of diarrhoea, but is now constipated despite a combination of laxatives. She has also had some abdominal pain, for which she uses prn morphine sulphate (Oramorph) and diclofenac sodium, and over the last few weeks has had some nausea for which she is using the anti-sickness medication that she had left over from her last course of chemotherapy.

There is nothing abnormal on examination. I would be grateful for your help with further symptom management.

Yours sincerely,

Introduction
Constipation is a common symptom in elderly patients and those with cancer (Table 1). Doctors may need to ask specifically about it when taking a history as patients often do not mention the problem. It is a predictable side effect of some drugs, eg opioids, and prophylactic laxatives should be prescribed when starting these, as it is better to prevent the problem than to treat it once established. If a patient does suffer from constipation, it is important to identify and treat it early because it can have significant complications, including overflow diarrhoea, urinary retention and bowel obstruction.

History of the presenting problem
Many patients describe the problem inaccurately, and hence a detailed history is necessary to establish the cause of constipation.

- What was her normal bowel frequency prior to having problems with constipation?
- When did she last open her bowels?
- What were the characteristics of her last stool (eg loose or formed; small, hard pellets or thin)?
- Did she need to strain to defecate?
- Was it painful to defecate?
- How typical of her recent bowel actions was the last stool?
- What is her current bowel frequency?
- Does she feel the need to defecate but is unable to? This would suggest hard stool or rectal obstruction.
- Is the urge to defecate largely absent? This could indicate colonic inertia.

TABLE 1 COMMON CAUSES OF CONSTIPATION IN PATIENTS WITH MALIGNANCY

Disease related	Tumour within bowel
	Extrinsic bowel compression by abdominal or pelvic disease
	Metabolic abnormalities (hypercalcaemia, hypokalaemia)
	Ascites resulting in bowel compression
	Neurological damage, eg spinal cord compression
Treatment related	Chemotherapy, eg vincristine
	Drugs, eg opioids, tricyclic antidepressants, diuretics, ondansetron
Debility	Dehydration
	Poor nutrition
	Weakness and inactivity
	Difficulties in use of bed pan and condition of lavatories
Concurrent problems	Haemorrhoids
	Anal fissures
	Hypothyroidism
	Diabetes

- Is there blood or mucus on/in her stool? This could be caused by tumour obstruction or haemorrhoids, or be a combination of both.

- Does she have abdominal pain or colic?

- Does she have abdominal bloating?

- Does she have nausea and/or vomiting?

- What treatments has she already tried (laxatives or rectal intervention) and what dose and combinations?

Other relevant history

General health

Establish if there are any broader issues in her day-to-day heath, such as debility, oral intake and mobility, which could be causing or influencing the constipation.

Other medical conditions

Check if the patient has any other serious medical problems that may have an effect on her bowel habit, eg hypothyroidism or diabetes.

Medications (prescribed and non-prescribed)

Many drugs can have a constipating effect, eg opioids. Check the *British National Formulary* or datasheets for any drugs the patient is taking to see if they might have caused her problem.

Plan for investigation and management

Investigations

- Blood tests: check for electrolyte abnormalities, eg hypercalcaemia or hypokalaemia, which can affect bowel function.

- Stool culture: if the patient has diarrhoea, it is important to rule out an infective cause, which is more common in immunocompromised patients, including those with cancer.

- Plain abdominal radiography: carry out only if you are concerned about proximal faecal impaction or bowel obstruction, *not* as routine.

Further investigation (CT scan and/or endoscopy) should only be considered if there are abnormal findings in other investigations that need to be explored, or if the patient's symptoms do not respond to treatment.

Management

Implement any simple lifestyle measures tolerable to the patient that will support the alleviation of her constipation, principally increases in fluid intake and physical exercise, as well as an improved diet.

- Treat reversible factors: rationalise any medication she is on, stopping constipating drugs if possible or switching to less constipating alternatives. Correct any metabolic abnormalities.

- Drug management: prescribe a combination of oral stimulant and softener laxatives, titrating up the dose if necessary. This can be accompanied by rectal intervention depending on the result of a rectal examination. An empty rectum would require no other prescription, but the presence of a hard stool would be best addressed with glycerol suppositories to soften and the presence of a soft stool by bisacodyl suppositories to stimulate.

Follow-up

To review the results of investigations and response to initial treatment. Aim to transfer the patient back to her primary care team and specialised community staff (such as Macmillan Nurses in the UK) once your investigations are complete.

Further discussion

Understanding the different classes of laxatives and the indications/side effects of these is essential to prescription of an effective course of treatment for the patient.

- Stimulant versus softeners: stimulants act mainly on the large bowel and may cause colic, so must be avoided in cases of bowel obstruction. Softeners are often used in combination with stimulants, but can be used alone to treat bowel obstruction.

- Polyethylene glycols (macrogols) such as Movicol: these are osmotic agents that need to be dissolved in water to be effective such that their use requires significant fluid intake by the patient.

- Combination preparations, eg co-danthramer: using a drug that is a combination of a stimulant and softener may help with compliance, but should be avoided in patients who are catheterised or have incontinence as it can cause skin burns.

There are a number of possible sequelae of untreated constipation, including urinary retention, overflow diarrhoea, faecal impaction and bowel obstruction.

Overflow diarrhoea

The history and examination should differentiate between true diarrhoea and faecal impaction with overflow, the latter being preceded by a varying period of constipation during which bacterial liquefaction of proximal faeces occurs. This directly results in offensive overflow diarrhoea and may be accompanied by faecal leakage, rectal discharge, distension and colic.

Simple constipation or bowel obstruction?

It is essential to differentiate between these to enable timely and appropriate management. Bowel obstruction is characterised by the presence of other symptoms (pain,

colic, nausea and vomiting, absence of flatus) as well as signs including distension, borborygmi or the absence of bowel sounds. When deciding on the management strategy for bowel obstruction the choice between medical or surgical treatment depends largely on the extent of the disease, including level(s) of obstruction, but must also consider the current performance status of the patient and his or her personal wishes.

1.2 Communication skills and ethics

1.2.1 Pain

Scenario

Role: you are a junior doctor working on an oncology ward.

Mrs Fiona Woods is a 45-year-old woman who was diagnosed with breast carcinoma 4 years ago, and treated with neoadjuvant chemotherapy prior to surgery, mastectomy and axillary dissection, followed by four cycles of adjuvant Taxotere (docetaxel) chemotherapy. Two years later she presented with left lung collapse and a malignant pleural effusion, which was treated with drainage and pleurodesis. Her disease continued to progress despite two further chemotherapy regimens. Her recent CT scan shows not only a loculated pleural effusion and small-volume lung metastases, but also widespread pleural disease.

Her main problem now is increasing pain in the left side

of her chest. She has been taking tramadol 100 mg qds, but this has been making her feel nauseous and does not seem to be controlling her pain. She is not sleeping well at night and is often woken by the pain. She is aware that her disease has progressed and that further options for treatment are limited, and wants to get home from hospital as soon as possible to be with her 5-year-old son.

Your task: to explain that you would like her to commence regular morphine analgesia and to discuss referral to the community palliative care team for ongoing support at home.

Key issues to explore

Try to identify as quickly as possible what the key problems are likely to be in the discussion of this scenario.

- What does the patient understand about her current disease status and prognosis?

- How does she feel about starting morphine and does she (and those who look after her) understand how to titrate and use it appropriately?

- Does she understand the role of the community palliative care team?

Key points to establish

It is very important to make certain points clear about yourself, the patient's condition and possible treatments from the start.

- Clarify what the patient understands regarding the results of the investigations and the cause of her pain. Also make sure that she understands that future treatments will be with palliative intent, focusing on symptom control.

- Explain about the introduction of morphine therapy. Make sure you discuss the common side effects (initial nausea, drowsiness and ongoing constipation), the role of 4-hourly dosing in the titration phase, the intention to convert to twice-daily preparation when stable, and use of breakthrough doses. With regards to breakthrough doses, explain that they will take approximately 20 minutes to work and can be repeated if ineffective. Encourage the patient to keep a record of how many breakthrough doses she takes, and whether or not they work.

- Establish if the patient has (unfounded) concerns over starting morphine treatment, eg fear of addiction or fear of tolerance.

- Discuss the role of the community palliative care team, emphasising the importance of specialist advice and input regarding symptom control.

Appropriate responses to likely questions

Patient: does this mean that there is nothing more that you can do for me?

Doctor: although we do not have any further treatment to reduce the cancer, we do have a number of ways to improve how you are feeling and particularly to make sure that you are not in pain. It is important that we focus now on helping you to feel as well as possible so that you can do the things that are most important for you.

Patient: if you give me morphine now, what will I do when the pain gets really bad?

Doctor: morphine is a drug that we use a lot and we know is effective at

controlling pain at all stages of an illness. There is scope to increase the dose slowly over time if we need to, and for most patients the morphine continues to help them. If for some reason morphine does not work for you, we have other drugs that we can use instead. The most important thing is to control and prevent your pain.

Patient: my friend's mum took morphine and she became really confused and muddled. I don't want that to happen to me.

Doctor: there are some side effects from morphine that people may experience. You may initially feel a little drowsy, but within a couple of days that will wear off as your body gets used to the medicine, although the benefit of controlling the pain will continue. In addition, for the first couple of days you may feel a little nauseous, and if so you can take some anti-sickness tablets, but this too will wear off quite quickly. Another reason we are going to increase the dose slowly is to help prevent any side effects.

Patient: can I go home as soon as possible?

Doctor: yes . . . we can start the medication here, and there are specialist nurses in the community who can continue to help you to adjust your dose until it is right for you. We will give them some information about you and they will offer you support and specialist advice at home. They have a lot of experience at helping people control their symptoms at home and will remain in contact with us in case they need any specific advice.

Patient: how much pain medication am I allowed to take?

Doctor: you can take breakthrough medication as often as you need it.

You should take one dose and then wait for 20–30 minutes to enable it to work. If the pain is still there, you can take another dose. If the pain is still not under control after a further 20 minutes, you should call the community team for advice. We always advise taking the extra pain medicine as soon as the pain starts rather than waiting for it to get more severe. If you regularly require more than one breakthrough dose a day, but this is helping your pain, then we may need to increase the background dose of medication that you are taking.

1.2.2 Breathlessness

Scenario

Role: you are a junior doctor working on an oncology ward.

Mr Will Bradbrook is a 70-year-old man with non-small-cell lung cancer. This was treated with a right upper lobectomy 18 months previously, followed by palliative chemotherapy 6 months ago for local recurrence with lung metastases. He had been referred to the Medical Assessment Unit (MAU) by his GP with worsening breathlessness. The latest investigations have been reviewed at the Lung Cancer multidisciplinary team meeting and show that his lung metastases have progressed despite the recently completed treatment with palliative chemotherapy, and also that he has developed a pleural effusion, although this is not large enough to be responsible for his problems breathing. He was transferred to the oncology ward from the MAU this morning for further management.

> **Your task:** to explain to Mr Bradbrook that there is no further disease-modifying treatment possible for his lung cancer and that the focus of future treatments will be on the palliative management of his breathlessness.

Key issues to explore

Establish what the key problems are likely to be in the discussion of this scenario.

- What does the patient already understand about the aims of treatment for his cancer to date, ie does he realise that his chemotherapy was palliative not curative?

- What does he understand about the current status of his disease and what the most recent investigations have shown?

- Does he understand the difference between active and palliative management?

- Does the patient understand the implications for his prognosis?

- What concerns does the patient have about his quality of life and symptom control?

Key points to establish

The patient will almost certainly be concerned and quite possibly distressed, hence it is important that you:

- use open questions appropriately;

- ask if the patient would like a member of his family to be present during the discussion;

- be clear that investigations have shown disease progression despite treatment;

- be explicit that the decision of the multidisciplinary team is that no

further disease-modifying treatment is possible, and would not be offered even at his request;

- explain that the focus from this point forward is on palliation (symptom control) and quality of life;

- explain what palliative care is and what services are available locally.

Appropriate responses to likely questions

Patient: was the wrong chemotherapy used this time and how do you know another won't work?

Doctor: the chemotherapy you were given was the one that is most successful in treating your type of cancer. Unfortunately, not all patients respond to treatment and that is what has happened in your case. There are many types of chemotherapy, but they are not proven to be helpful for your type of cancer and have significant side effects. This means there would be no benefit in using them and they could make you more unwell.

Patient: can you get rid of my breathlessness?

Doctor: we cannot promise to completely control it, but we can try a variety of different medications and approaches to see what helps you. There are a variety of things we can use to try and help you cope with the breathlessness and keep you functioning at the best possible level.

Patient: does this mean you're just leaving me to die?

Doctor: although there is nothing more we can offer to treat the cancer, we will work together with your GP and local palliative care team to monitor things regularly. There are many different treatments we can offer to help with any

symptoms you may have and the goal will be to ensure you have the best quality of life possible.

Patient: why don't you just drain the fluid from my lung?

Doctor: the X-ray shows that there isn't a lot of fluid there, so we don't think that draining it would do you any good. We don't want to go sticking needles and tubes into your chest if they really aren't going to help.

Patient: will I have to stay in hospital?

Doctor: no . . . the aim will be to get you home, supported by your GP and the community palliative care team as needed. What other help might you need at home?

Patient: can I stay in hospital if I want to?

Doctor: hospital is the best place for the management of some problems, but is not a good place for ongoing care. We can discuss with you and your family your needs and what help, if any, you will require when supporting yourself at home. If that isn't possible, then we can explore the alternatives, such as a nursing home, if they would better meet your needs. Is there anything that particularly worries you about going home?

1.2.3 Nausea and vomiting

Scenario

Role: you are a junior doctor working on an oncology ward.

Mrs Sharon Headley is a 52-year-old woman who was diagnosed with ovarian cancer 18 months ago, and was treated with a hysterectomy and bilateral salpingo-oophorectomy.

She was well with no evidence of recurrence at her last check-up 3 months ago. She presented to the Emergency Department earlier this week with abdominal pain, vomiting and abdominal distention. On examination she was found to have a palpable large pelvic mass and was admitted for further investigation.

Her symptoms are currently well controlled with regular analgesics and antiemetics. However, routine blood tests found that she was in renal failure, with a urea of 27 mmol/L (normal <7) and creatinine of 250 µmol/L (normal <120). A renal ultrasound scan has shown right-sided hydronephrosis. A staging CT scan confirmed the ultrasound findings, demonstrating ureteric compression due to recurrent ovarian cancer with widespread peritoneal seedlings. She has been referred for a ureteric stent.

Her case was discussed at the multidisciplinary team meeting and it was felt that surgery was not an option because of how widely the disease has spread. She would be suitable for palliative chemotherapy if her renal function improves with stenting.

Your task: to explain to the patient that she has developed recurrent cancer that is now incurable and that surgical intervention is not possible but palliative chemotherapy may be if her renal function improves.

Key issues to explore

Identify what the key problems are likely to be in the discussion of this scenario.

- Does the patient understand that she has a recurrent disease that is causing her symptoms?

- Does she understand the significance of a recurrent disseminated disease to her prognosis, ie that her cancer is now incurable?

- Does she understand that any treatment will be palliative not curative?

- Does she understand the implications to possible treatment options if her renal function does not improve with stenting?

Key points to establish

This is unquestionably going to be very hard for the patient, so your approach must be clear and leave absolutely no room for doubt over the points that you make.

- Establish who else the patient wishes to be present/involved in the discussions.

- Explain the results of the investigations, the most important point being that her illness has become recurrent disseminated cancer and that this has led to ureteric obstruction causing renal failure.

- Explain that because of its extent, the cancer cannot be cured.

- Explain that surgery to remove the cancer is not an option due to how widespread it has become.

- Explain that chemotherapy could only go ahead if renal function improved, because this determines whether the benefits outweigh the burdens of treatment.

Appropriate responses to likely questions

Patient: why didn't the doctors know something was wrong when I had my last check-up?

Doctor: it may be possible that the cancer wasn't present when you were last seen, or was so small that it wasn't possible to feel any sign of it when you were examined. Symptoms, such as the pain and vomiting, sometimes only start when the cancer is advanced.

Patient: the operation helped me last time, so why can't I have another one?

Doctor: when you had your last operation, the cancer was small and in one place, making it easier to remove. The scan has shown that the cancer is now spread widely throughout your abdomen, so it would be impossible to remove it all. Chemotherapy – that's treatment with drugs – might be the best option for future treatment because it will work through your whole body, but I'm afraid that I can't say that it will cure the cancer completely.

Patient: if the chemotherapy can't cure the cancer, what will it do?

Doctor: I'm sorry, but I'm afraid we haven't got any treatment that will cure the cancer. I'd like to say that we do, but we don't. Although the chemotherapy cannot cure the cancer, we hope that it will reduce the size of it and increase the time that you have left to live. It may also help with the symptoms that you are having, reducing the pain and swelling in your abdomen. It may also relieve the pressure from around the tube between your kidney and bladder and reduce the risk of further problems with your kidney function.

Patient: why can't I start the chemotherapy now?

Doctor: the chemotherapy will be excreted from the body by the kidneys. However, because of your renal problems, if we give it to you now it may cause further damage to the kidneys and give you more problems than benefits. We would only go ahead with the chemotherapy if you are well enough and it would be likely to improve things rather than make them worse. The last thing we want to do is to give you a treatment that makes you worse and not better.

Patient: *how long do I have to live?*

Doctor: it's difficult to say exactly, because everyone responds differently to the chemotherapy. If your cancer responds well, you may live for several years. Even if you do not respond to this course of chemotherapy, there may be the option to try another type. But if your kidney function does not improve and you are unable to have the chemotherapy, time may be much shorter.

Patient: *will I always need to be on the painkillers?*

Doctor: the pain is likely to be due to the mass in your abdomen. If the chemotherapy can shrink this mass, the pain may improve. We would hope to then either decrease or even stop the painkillers. However, if you do need to stay on them, we would try to find the dose that suits you best, causing the most benefits and the least side effects.

1.2.4 Bowel obstruction

Scenario

Role: you are a junior doctor working on an oncology ward.

Mrs Claire Wilson is a 76-year-old woman who was diagnosed with Dukes B/C carcinoma of the colon 2 years ago, and treated with a hemicolectomy and chemotherapy. She developed liver metastases 9 months ago and had second-line chemotherapy, but her disease has progressed. She has had constipation for some weeks and was under review in the palliative medicine clinic. When she attended the clinic today for her follow-up, she reported worsening abdominal pain and vomiting. She was admitted for investigation and was found to have bowel obstruction. A CT scan has shown a discrete single level of obstruction, and the surgical team feels that a bypass procedure could be performed. However, Mrs Wilson is relatively frail and there is concern about how she would tolerate surgery. At the multidisciplinary team meeting it was felt that her age and underlying diabetes would adversely affect her recovery, and that her low albumin (28 g/dL) might contribute to poor wound healing. However, as her performance status was good it was felt appropriate to offer surgery if she wanted to pursue this option.

Your task: to explain to the patient that she has developed bowel obstruction and that surgical intervention is possible, but that owing to her frailty there are significant risks attached to this. Help her to decide if she wants to pursue this or opt for medical management.

Key issues to explore

Determine what the main problems are likely to be before discussing the benefits and risks of a surgical versus a medical approach.

- What does the patient understand about the significance of her bowel obstruction with regard to the status of her disease and its prognosis?

- What are her goals? These will probably centre on prolongation of life, quality of life or a particular place of care.

- What does she understand about potential outcomes of surgery, eg colostomy?

- Does she understand that surgery would be a palliative and not a curative procedure?

Key points to establish

The patient is in a frail condition and this is pertinent to how she is treated. You must be explicit about the options available to her and leave no doubt over their possible consequences.

- Establish if she wishes anyone else to be present/involved in the decision-making process.

- Explain the results of the investigations clearly, ie that she has bowel obstruction.

- Explain all the treatment options available to her, including the risks and benefits of each.

- Explain that depending on the course of treatment chosen you will need to consider the benefits and burdens of continuing versus withdrawing some current treatments, eg intravenous fluids, and commencing or withholding others, eg artificial nutrition.

- Ensure that the decision-making process occurs correctly. You must first ensure that the patient is competent to make this decision and then provide all the

Station 4: Communication Skills and Ethics   **69**

information available so that fully informed consent can be given. It is important to respect her autonomy: a competent patient has a right to decide whether or not to accept a particular treatment.

Appropriate responses to likely questions
Patient: how will I eat and drink if I don't have the surgery?

Doctor: I know that you are vomiting at times and that makes it difficult, but if you are not able to take in enough fluids orally to keep you comfortable, then we can look at ways to give you extra fluids.

Patient: what sort of ways can you give me fluid?

Doctor: while you are deciding about whether or not you want the operation, we would provide fluids via a drip into one of your veins, but this can only be done in hospital and is a short-term option. If you decide not to go ahead with the surgery and are unable to drink enough to keep yourself comfortable, then we could give you extra fluid by a small needle that goes under the skin and this could be continued at home if necessary.

Patient: do I have to decide straight away?

Doctor: you do not have to decide immediately, but if you leave it too long and become less well then it may no longer be possible to go ahead with the surgery. If you want to think it over or discuss it with your family, I can come back tomorrow and we can talk again.

Patient: if I don't have the operation, will I always have the pain and vomiting?

Doctor: whether or not you have the operation, from now on we will

focus on controlling your symptoms using different drugs. We can give you painkillers and anti-sickness medicine via a small pump to try and get you feeling as well as possible.

Patient: if I don't have the operation, will I have to stay in hospital?

Doctor: no . . . all the medications can be given at home. If you are having medications by a syringe driver, then that can be done at home with help from your GP, district nurse and the community palliative care team, who have all the equipment if you need it.

Patient: will the operation mean that I live longer?

Doctor: that isn't certain. The aim of the operation is to help your symptoms by bypassing the blockage in your bowel. I'm afraid that an operation wouldn't be able to remove the cancer and cure it, but if it were successful it would enable you to eat and drink again, and that may mean that you lived longer.

Patient: doesn't that mean that I should have the operation?

Doctor: no, it doesn't mean that. There are risks attached to having the operation that could cause problems and even shorten your life, and there is the possibility that even if the operation were successful another blockage could occur in your bowel and we'd be back in the situation we're in now. So having the operation would not definitely prolong your life, but would hopefully help your symptoms.

Patient: so what's the right thing to do?

Doctor: there isn't a right and a wrong thing to do here. Having medical treatment with drugs to control the symptoms has advantages and disadvantages,

and having an operation has advantages and disadvantages. You need to decide which you'd feel most comfortable with, but no one is going to push you into having an operation that you don't want.

1.2.5 End of life

Scenario

Role: you are a junior doctor working on a care of the elderly ward.

Mrs Caroline Morgan is an 84-year-old woman with disseminated small-cell lung cancer. Her condition has slowly deteriorated over the past few months, resulting in her becoming less mobile and spending most of her days in bed. Investigations on admission showed no reversible cause for her deterioration and, 2 weeks later, she is no longer managing oral intake and is increasingly drowsy. At the request of her daughter you are called to see Mrs Morgan, who appears agitated and has audible respiratory secretions. Her daughter is very upset and wants to know what you are going to do to help her mother now that she is not drinking any fluids.

Your task: to explain to her daughter that Mrs Morgan is at the end of her life, and that the medical focus is on symptom control and patient comfort.

Key issues to explore
The condition of the patient is clear, but her daughter is deeply upset by the situation so you must identify the following points.

• What is the daughter's main concern?

- What does the daughter understand about her mother's illness to date, ie that her condition is incurable?

- Does the daughter understand that her mother is now in the end stage of her illness?

- What goals does the daughter expect for the management of her mother's illness?

Key points to establish

You will need to address several issues quickly and succinctly owing to the distress Mrs Morgan's daughter is in. Clearly establish that all treatment decisions will be based on what is in Mrs Morgan's best interests and not solely on her daughter's wishes. Ensure that you:

- explain that Mrs Morgan is in the terminal stage of her illness and that no treatment can reverse this;

- explain that no obligation exists to provide treatments that would be futile;

- outline the benefits and burdens of any treatment options that have been proposed and explain that the decision to withhold or withdraw treatments, such as artificial hydration and nutrition or cardiopulmonary resuscitation, will be based on the balance between these.

Appropriate responses to likely questions

Patient's daughter: *if you don't give my mother food and fluids she'll die.*

Doctor: I'm afraid that your mother is at the end stage of her illness and we cannot reverse this. People with advanced cancer often stop eating and drinking as the disease progresses and this has been the case with your mother. She only has a short time to live and giving her

fluid or nutrition artificially is unlikely to significantly change this. It is also unlikely to make her feel better or more comfortable, but may worsen some of her symptoms, such as the secretions causing the bubbling sound in her chest.

Patient's daughter: *does that mean that when her heart stops beating you won't try to start it again?*

Doctor: that's right. Doing heart massage and putting a breathing tube into her lungs is only sensible if something reversible has caused the heart to stop, for example a heart attack. Your mother is deteriorating because she has advanced cancer, and when her heart and breathing stop it will be because of this, which we cannot reverse. It simply wouldn't work if we tried to resuscitate her, so no, we wouldn't do it.

Patient's daughter: *are you just leaving her to die?*

Doctor: no . . . we need to make sure that she remains as comfortable as possible. Although we cannot reverse her illness, we want to make sure that we control any symptoms that she has to the best of our ability. You know her best; do you feel she is currently uncomfortable in any way?

Patient's daughter: *her breathing is very loud. What's causing that?*

Doctor: everyone produces secretions that they usually swallow. When people become weaker and less alert, these secretions may pool in the throat. Air moving through them makes a noise when your mother breathes in and out. Although it can sound distressing, it is unlikely that she is aware of this or troubled by it. We will try giving her some medication and simple things like changing her position to reduce this.

Patient's daughter: *she is very unsettled. Is she in pain?*

Doctor: as people come towards the end of life, it is not uncommon for them to be restless or agitated. I will examine your mother to make sure there is nothing simple that is making her uncomfortable, such as a full bladder, which we need to address. If I cannot find anything reversible disturbing her, then there are medicines that we can use to help her be more settled and relaxed. We will continue to keep a close eye on her, and if she suffers from any pain we will treat it.

1.3 Acute scenarios

1.3.1 Pain

Scenario

A 45-year-old woman presents to the Emergency Department with increasing breathlessness and pain in the left side of her chest. She was diagnosed with breast carcinoma 4 years ago and treated with mastectomy and chemotherapy. She tells you that she has had more chemotherapy, but that the disease has now spread to her lungs and she has been told there is now no more treatment to give. Two months ago she had a pleural effusion that was treated with drainage and pleurodesis. She has been taking regular morphine sulphate (modified release) 60 mg bd at home, which had helped with her pain, but over the past 48 hours she has had increasing pain in her left chest wall.

Introduction

The main aim is to establish the cause of the patient's sudden increase in pain and to re-establish good symptom control. Consider the following.

- What is the cause of her increase in pain? Has the pleural disease progressed, has she developed pulmonary emboli, or is it caused by bony metastasis or a fractured rib?

- Which drugs should she be given? To decide on the prescription you will need to know if the pain is opioid responsive, and if there is a neuropathic component involved.

- You will also need to perform a full assessment of her other symptoms, eg dyspnoea.

History of the presenting problem

It is necessary to know as much as possible about the cause of her pain and how she has been dealing with it prior to seeing you.

- Where is the pain located?

- What is it like? Ask the patient to use descriptive terms, eg 'aching' and 'burning'.

- How severe is it? A score out of 10 can be helpful, particularly because it establishes a scale that enables you to judge the patient's response to a treatment.

- When did it start and is it getting worse?

- Is it constant?

- Does it radiate anywhere?

- What precipitates or relieves it?

- Has she taken any breakthrough medication, and has it dulled or relieved the pain?

- Is the pain worse when she is coughing or inhaling deeply?

If so, musculoskeletal pain or pulmonary embolism are possible.

- Can she sleep at night or does the pain wake her up?

- How has the pain stopped her from continuing her usual routine?

- What does she think the pain is due to? Anxiety of any sort exacerbates pain, and this woman clearly has a great deal to be anxious about.

The presence or absence of other symptoms may help in identifying the cause of her pain. It is also important to determine how she is tolerating current treatment measures. Ask if she has experienced the following.

- Dyspnoea: if present, enquire if it has changed, whether anything exacerbates or relieves it, and if it is associated with the pain she is experiencing.

- Swelling of one or both legs: unilateral swelling would clearly suggest deep vein thrombosis in this context.

- Haemoptysis: could indicate pulmonary embolism, but might also be due to lung involvement with tumour.

- Any fevers, night sweats or purulent sputum that might indicate she has an infection.

- Opioid-related side effects, eg nausea, drowsiness or constipation.

Other relevant history

It is also important to check if there are any past medical or social factors that might be affecting the pain the patient feels now.

- Does she have a history of bony metastases?

- Are there any other factors indicating that she might be at risk from a pulmonary embolus? For example, has she had thromboembolic disease before, or has her mobility and/or performance status deteriorated significantly?

- How is the pain impacting on her activities of daily living? Do her routines involve her doing things that make the pain worse?

Examination

General features

Does the woman look terminally ill? Aside from vital signs, it will clearly be important to note if she is cachectic or frail, if she is currently in pain, and if she is short of breath while at rest.

Respiratory system

Key features to look for include the following.

- Cyanosis.

- Pleural effusion: how large is it?

- Is there any focal tenderness on palpation of her chest wall?

- Check her calves for unilateral swelling or tenderness.

Investigation

- Blood tests: FBC to look for anaemia and/or evidence of infection; creatinine, urea and electrolytes to document renal function; bone profile to look for hypercalcaemia or increased alkaline phosphatase (bone metastases or liver disease); liver profile. Note that measurement of D-dimers is not recommended because it would *not* be helpful in this case: D-dimers are non-specifically elevated in patients with cancer and cannot confirm or exclude a pulmonary embolism in this context.

- ECG: look for evidence of right heart strain that would support a diagnosis of pulmonary embolism, but remember that the ECG is usually normal in this condition.

- CXR will reveal if the effusion has increased and show if there is evidence of rib metastasis and/or pathological fracture.

- Other imaging: spiral CT will be required if you are suspicious of a pulmonary embolism; ventilation–perfusion lung scanning will not be interpretable in this woman. A bone scan may be appropriate if bony metastases are suspected.

Management

The patient's pain could be the result of several factors, so the measures prescribed will depend on the causes determined by your examination. In many cases you will need to use several treatments to bring her symptoms back under control.

Pain

Aim to retitrate the patient with immediate-release opioids, which should help with both dyspnoea and pain control.

If pain is probably caused by progression of pleural disease, consider:

- trial of steroids (dexamethasone 8 mg od);

- addition of an NSAID (eg diclofenac sodium 50 mg tds);

- addition of a specific neuropathic agent (eg amitriptyline hydrochloride 25 mg nightly);

- palliative radiotherapy.

If bony metastases or a rib fracture are causing the pain, consider:

- addition of regular paracetamol;

- addition of an NSAID (eg diclofenac sodium 50 mg tds);

- radiotherapy;

- intercostal nerve block.

Dyspnoea

If the patient is cyanosed or has low oxygen saturation, give her oxygen.

- Dyspnoea may be noticeably relieved by treatment of a reversible cause, eg an infection or pulmonary embolism, but drainage of the effusion is unlikely to be useful in this case given her history of previous effusion and attempted pleurodesis.

- Symptomatic relief can be achieved with a prn opioid, eg regular breakthrough dose of immediate-release morphine, or a benzodiazepine (eg sublingual lorazepam 0.5 mg).

> **For intractable breathlessness in palliative care, use an opioid or benzodiazepine as needed for symptomatic relief.**

Other specific treatments

If the woman is not terminally ill, then the following may be appropriate.

- If there is evidence of infection: antibiotics, regular paracetamol if pyrexial.

- If there is evidence to suggest pulmonary embolism: start a regular course of low-molecular-weight (LMW) heparin, which is the preferred long-term option for anticoagulation in palliative care patients. Also consider an NSAID (eg diclofenac sodium 50 mg tds).

In the context of her disease it will be necessary to establish and explain clear limits to such treatments. For instance, to give oxygen and oral or intravenous antibiotics for chest infection/pneumonia on the general ward would be sensible, but transfer to the intensive care unit for ventilation and inotropic support would not.

> **Continued LMW heparin is the preferred long-term option for anticoagulation in palliative care patients.**

Further comments

What connotation has the patient placed on the increase in pain? Pain is a frightening symptom and a patient will often associate increased pain with disease progression. Patients often need reassurance that their pain can be controlled and may need the correct use of pain medication carefully explained to them, ie regular use of background medication supported by breakthrough medication if required. It is often impossible to achieve good pain control without addressing the patient's psychological, social and spiritual dimensions as well as physical condition.

How often should the patient be reviewed and has adequate breakthrough medication been prescribed to last the patient until this review? Clear instructions need to be given to the patient and nursing staff regarding breakthrough medication. Four hours is the duration of action of immediate-release morphine, *not* the maximum frequency with which it can be given. Doses may need to be repeated up to every hour. It is important that the patient has access to adequate quantities of medication, particularly during the titration phase. If she is gaining no benefit from breakthrough doses or needs multiple doses in a short period of time, then the strength of the doses should be reviewed and her symptoms reassessed.

1.3.2 Breathlessness

Scenario

Mr Will Bradbrook is a 70-year-old ex-smoker with non-small-cell lung cancer that was treated with a right upper lobectomy 18 months previously, followed by palliative chemotherapy 6 months ago for local recurrence with lung metastases. He is sent to the Medical Admissions Unit by his GP with worsening breathlessness.

Introduction

Your main concern is to identify reversible causes of increased breathlessness, but palliation is required if there is no reversible cause. Think about the case in terms of these broad questions, considering the causes listed in Table 2.

- What are the common malignant causes of breathlessness?

- What are the common non-malignant causes of breathlessness that may also occur in cancer patients?

- What are potentially reversible causes of breathlessness?

- What are the main contributory factors to the patient's experience of breathlessness?

Breathlessness in palliative care is frequently associated with anxiety, panic and fear of impending death and will not improve unless these are addressed: asking the patient about their specific fears may itself be therapeutic.

History of the presenting problem

As shown in Table 2, there are many causes of breathlessness to consider in this patient, hence a detailed history is required.

Breathlessness

- When did it start? Is it changing? Breathlessness that comes on

suddenly (in an instant) is more likely due to pneumothorax, bronchial obstruction or (in some cases) pulmonary embolism.

- Is it continuous or intermittent? If the latter, then anxiety could be the problem: this is one of the common causes of fluctuating breathlessness.

- What are the precipitating or relieving factors?

Assess the severity of breathlessness by its impact on the patient. Does it limit his mobility (how far can he walk), his speech or his sleeping?

Associated symptoms

- Pain: pleuritic pain may be due to a pulmonary embolism or pneumonia; metastatic invasion of pleura and/or pleural effusion are more likely to cause a dull, heavy pain.

- Cough, although this may be associated with multiple causes.

- Haemoptysis: if this is massive it suggests erosion of bronchi by secondaries, although the possibility of a pulmonary embolism should also be considered.

- Swelling of leg(s): unilateral swelling suggests deep venous thrombosis; bilateral swelling is often found with cardiac failure, caval obstruction, ascites or hypoproteinaemia.

- Pyrexia would suggest an infection.

- Wheezing may be due to bronchial obstruction, asthma or cardiac failure.

Other relevant history

It is important to ask the patient about his general health and social circumstances.

TABLE 2 CAUSES OF BREATHLESSNESS IN A PATIENT WITH A HISTORY OF LUNG CANCER

Type of cause	Condition	Reversibility
Malignant	Anaemia	Yes
	Bronchial obstruction	Possible in some cases (temporary)
	Pleural effusion	Yes (temporary)
	Pneumothorax	Yes (temporary)
	Lymphangitis	No
	SVC obstruction	Unlikely
	Pericardial effusion	Yes (temporary)
Non-malignant	Anaemia	Yes
	Anxiety	Yes
	Chest infection	Yes (often)
	COPD	Yes (partial)
	Congestive cardiac failure	Yes (partial)
	Pneumothorax	Yes
	Pulmonary embolism	Yes

COPD, chronic obstructive pulmonary disease; SVC, superior vena cava.

- How does he feel when he is at rest?

- Does he have any other problems?

- Is he eating well, and is he losing weight? Anorexia and weight loss suggest advancing malignancy.

- Does he have any bone pain? Consider bony secondaries.

- How does he usually spend his day?

- Does he have relatives and friends?

- What changes have there been in his activities of daily living between now and 1 month ago?

The answers to all these questions are relevant when it comes to deciding how best to manage his breathlessness.

Examination

General features
General impressions are important and will help to determine how his breathlessness is treated. Is he frail and cachectic? How distressing is his dyspnoea? Is he cyanosed?

Check for the following features, which may suggest disseminated or locally invasive malignancy:

- anaemia;

- lymphadenopathy;

- signs of SVC obstruction (eg swelling of the face, neck and arms; plethoric cyanotic facies; non-pulsatile engorgement of veins; collateral vessels over the surface of the shoulders, scapulae and upper chest; and brush venules over the chest wall);

- hepatomegaly.

Respiratory system
Look for the following:

- stridor or wheeze;

- lung collapse and/or consolidation;

- pleural effusion;

- pleural rub.

Cardiovascular system
Look for signs of heart failure and of pericardial effusion, also for unilateral leg swelling.

Investigation
Attention should focus on investigations that may reveal a treatable problem.

- FBC: is he anaemic?

- CXR: is there a pleural effusion? Has there been progression of pulmonary metastases?

- Other investigations could include a CT scan (looking at pulmonary arteries or at tumour/lymph nodes/lung parenchyma) or bronchoscopy as guided by clinical suspicion and findings of preliminary investigations.

Management
This will depend on the type of disease, stage of illness, previous treatment and the performance status of the patient, but possible palliative treatments for his malignancy include radiotherapy, chemotherapy and laser treatment.

Other interventions that might improve breathlessness depend on the cause.

- Anaemia: blood transfusion.

- Pulmonary emboli: anticoagulation, which in most palliative care patients should be with long-term low-molecular-weight heparin rather than warfarin.

- Pleural effusion: drain and consider pleurodesis.

- Infection: antibiotics.

- COPD: optimise medical therapy.

- Obstruction of airway or SVC: course of steroids (eg dexamethasone 8–16 mg daily) and consider stenting.

- Lymphangitis carcinomatosis: course of steroids (eg dexamethasone 8–16 mg daily).

Do not leave the man struggling and breathless without relief; give symptomatic treatment if needed.

- Opioids: low-dose morphine sulphate immediate release (eg Oramorph 2.5 mg prn).

- Benzodiazepines (eg sublingual lorazepam 0.5 mg prn).

Further comments
Communication and explanation is key: discuss the situation with the patient and his family, explaining the current findings and differential diagnosis, and how this impacts on the future treatment plans and prognosis.

Managing anxiety
Help the patient to cope with the acute situation, but also consider the ongoing long-term management of his respiratory symptoms. Relaxation and breathing techniques may counteract intermittent mild dyspnoeic or panic attacks experienced while at rest. Pharmacological therapy could be suggested, eg benzodiazepines (sublingual lorazepam 0.5 mg prn), or an antidepressant licensed for the management of anxiety. If anxiety is a significant and persisting problem, obtain psychiatric advice.

Maximising function
Multidisciplinary input, eg from an occupational therapist, may help with ongoing management to maximise independence and achieve patient-focused goals.

1.3.3 Nausea and vomiting

Scenario

Mrs Sharon Headley is a 52-year-old woman who was diagnosed with ovarian cancer 18 months ago and then treated with a hysterectomy and bilateral salpingo-oophorectomy. She was well and with no evidence of recurrence at her last check-up 3 months ago, but presented to the Emergency Department earlier this week with abdominal pain and distension and was admitted for further investigation. She has a large pelvic mass palpable on abdominal examination. She is now an inpatient on the oncology ward. Her pain is currently well controlled with regular oral morphine, but she has developed nausea and vomiting that is not responding to prn antiemetics. She has also been constipated for the last few days.

Introduction

Nausea and vomiting are common symptoms of many advancing diseases and are frequent in patients with cancer (Table 3). Your aim must be to determine the most likely cause, because only by doing so can the most appropriate management be determined.

Medications should be given by mouth for nausea prophylaxis, but if symptoms are established that have rendered oral absorption ineffective, then drugs must be given parenterally. Any antiemetic should be administered regularly for a period of at least 24 hours to assess the patient's response before changing regimen.

Nausea is a predictable side effect of some treatments, eg chemotherapy and opioid analgesics. Prophylactic antiemetics should be prescribed when starting such treatments, because it is better to prevent the problem than to treat it when vomiting has caused dehydration and metabolic disturbance.

History of the presenting problem

A detailed history of the nausea and vomiting is necessary to establish its aetiology.

- Is the patient actually vomiting or just nauseous? Make her differentiate between nausea and vomiting, and describe the severity of each symptom.

- When and how did the nausea/vomiting start? An insidious onset may mean a metabolic cause, eg renal failure or hypercalcaemia, whereas a rapid onset, particularly if associated with colicky abdominal pain, suggests intestinal obstruction.

- What are the periodicity, volume and content of the vomit? Small volume and infrequent vomiting suggests a metabolic cause. Large-volume vomits of undigested food immediately after oral intake are typical of proximal obstruction; single and infrequent large-volume vomits typify distal bowel obstruction. Vomiting that is worse on waking suggests raised intracranial pressure.

- Relieving factors: if her state of nausea is relieved by vomiting, the problem may be delayed gastric emptying.

- Precipitating factors: if vomiting starts suddenly on waking or when moving from lying down to sitting or standing up, this might be due to raised intracranial pressure caused by cerebral metastases.

- Bowel habit: constipation is a common and easily reversible cause of nausea and vomiting. Was she put on a laxative when she started opioid treatment? When did she last open her bowels? Was it easy to do so?

- Relationship to medications: take note of any recent

TABLE 3 CAUSES OF NAUSEA AND VOMITING IN PATIENTS WITH CANCER

Disease related	Gastrointestinal tumour Bowel obstruction Hepatomegaly Ascites Brain metastases and raised intracranial pressure Metabolic abnormalities: renal failure, hypercalcaemia, liver failure Pain Anxiety (including anticipatory nausea and vomiting)
Treatment related	Chemotherapy Radiotherapy Drugs: opioids, NSAIDs, antibiotics, steroids
Debility related	Constipation Cough
Concurrent problems	Gastroenteritis Infection Gastritis/peptic ulceration

disease-modifying therapies (eg chemotherapy or radiotherapy) or newly introduced drugs. Morphine can cause nausea and many other medications (eg antibiotics, digoxin, selective serotonin reuptake inhibitors) can do so. Check all drugs in the *British National Formulary*.

- What treatments have already been tried for the nausea? Establish doses, routes and combinations.

Other relevant history

A range of issues need to be explored.

- The patient's performance status will influence the choice of management plan: pay particular attention to debility, oral intake and mobility.

- What is the extent of her disease and what treatment has she already had to treat it? The previous surgery may have predisposed her to adhesions and obstruction. Chemo-naive patients with ovarian cancer may gain good symptomatic benefit from palliative treatment.

- Central nervous system: headache, altered vision or any focal weakness would suggest cerebral metastases in this context.

- Respiratory: coughing may precipitate retching or vomiting, rather than these being due to a primary gastrointestinal cause.

- Mood: anxiety may cause or exacerbate nausea and vomiting, eg anticipatory vomiting before chemotherapy.

Examination

General features

General impressions are important and will help you to determine how to appropriately manage the patient's sickness. Aside from vital signs, is she frail and cachexic? Check her hydration status by looking carefully at the mouth and mucous membranes. Jaundice may indicate metastatic disease.

Gastrointestinal system

Look in particular for

- distension due to a tumour or ascites;

- visible peristalsis;

- localised abdominal masses (present in this woman) or organomegaly;

- bowel sounds, which may be high-pitched or absent in the case of obstruction;

- local or general abdominal tenderness.

A rectal examination must be carried out to assess for constipation.

Central nervous system

Nausea and vomiting may be due to pathology in the central nervous system. The key features that would indicate this are:

- papilloedema, which would be evidence of raised intracranial pressure;

- focal neurological deficit, which would suggest cerebral secondaries.

Investigation

Blood tests

Look for both possible causes and consequences of vomiting, and also for evidence of metastases.

- Raised urea and creatinine may result from dehydration, or be due to renal failure of other cause (perhaps obstruction in this case).

- Hypokalaemia may be caused by vomiting and contribute to ileus.

- Hypercalcaemia of malignancy can cause constipation, nausea and vomiting.

- A raised white cell count may indicate infection.

- Abnormal liver tests may indicate hepatic secondaries.

- Serum albumin can be used to assess nutritional status.

Imaging

This is guided by history and differential diagnosis (Table 3). A plain abdominal film with or without an abdominal CT scan should be requested if bowel obstruction is suspected, and a CT brain scan if cerebral metastases are likely. An ultrasound scan would be the appropriate test to look for hydronephrosis if there was renal failure.

Management

If she is able to eat and drink, then advise her to do simple and obvious things such as eat bland food in small portions and encourage hydration with frequent sips (as much as she can tolerate).

If she is actively vomiting, then a combination of drugs is likely to be needed to achieve control: these will need to be given parenterally, with the preferred route for all regular and prn medication being subcutaneous injection.

> Give prophylactic antiemetics orally. In the treatment of nausea and vomiting give antiemetics parenterally.

Use supportive measures to increase the patient's comfort, notably mouth care and intravenous rehydration, as both will have suffered if she has been nauseous and vomiting for any length of time.

Deal with any reversible factors.

- Rationalise medication: stop any drugs precipitating the nausea/vomiting if possible, or switch to less emetogenic alternatives.

- Treat constipation: if the patient is not obstructed, then a regular stimulant laxative is best, eg two tablets of senna once to twice daily if able to tolerate any oral intake. If this does not solve the problem, consider rectal intervention starting with suppositories. Avoid stimulant laxatives and other prokinetic drugs (eg metoclopramide hydrochloride) if there is established obstruction.

- Correct metabolic abnormalities if possible, eg give bisphosphonates for hypercalcaemia.

- Drain the abdomen of ascites through paracentesis.

> ⚠ Avoid stimulant laxatives and other prokinetic drugs, eg metoclopramide, if there is established obstruction.

Choose an antiemetic drug carefully, using timing and method of administration to ensure the best chance of controlling the patient's symptoms:

- use a first-line agent appropriate for the specific cause (Table 4);

- give regularly when symptoms are established (as in this case);

- give parenterally as oral absorption is inadequate once vomiting is established;

- maximise the dose of the first-line drug before adding or switching to a different agent.

Adjust analgesics appropriately: convert to parenteral administration as vomiting will impair oral absorption. If renal function is impaired, caution is needed with opioids that are renally excreted because there is the risk of accumulation and toxicity. Non-renally excreted drugs such as fentanyl or alfentanil may need to be used, but this should only be done under specialist guidance.

Further comments

To ensure optimal symptom control with minimal side effects, it is crucial to adopt a structured approach when choosing an antiemetic drug.

	TABLE 4 COMMONLY USED ANTIEMETICS		
Class	Indication	Example	Starting dose
Antihistamines	Raised intracranial pressure and bowel obstruction	Cyclizine	50 mg po/sc tds
Antidopaminergic agents	For drug-induced and metabolic causes, eg opioid related or hypercalcaemia	Haloperidol Metoclopramide hydrochloride Domperidone Levomepromazine (methotrimeprazine)	1.5 mg po/sc od 10 mg po/sc tds 10 mg po tds–qds 6.25 mg po/sc od
5HT antagonists	For chemotherapy and radiotherapy-induced nausea and vomiting	Granisetron	1–2 mg po/iv od
Prokinetic	For delayed gastric emptying	Metoclopramide hydrochloride Domperidone	10 mg po/sc tds 10 mg po tds–qds
Anticholinergic agents	For vestibular dysfunction	Cyclizine Hyoscine hydrobromide	50 mg po/sc tds 1 mg patch top/72 hours
Benzodiazepines	For anticipatory nausea and vomiting	Lorazepam	0.5–1 mg sl/po od–bd
Broad-spectrum agents (anticholinergic, antidopaminergic and 5HT antagonists)	Unknown aetiology or multiple causes	Levomepromazine (methotrimeprazine)	6.25 mg po/sc od
Mechanism of action uncertain	Resistant nausea and vomiting	Dexamethasone	4 mg po/sc od

5HT, 5-hydroxytryptamine.

- Identify the most likely cause of nausea and vomiting.

- Identify the area of the vomiting pathway by which this cause acts (Table 5).

- Identify which neurotransmitter receptors are involved in this area of the vomiting pathway.

- Choose the most specific antagonist to the receptor identified.

- Choose the most appropriate route of antiemetic administration (oral for prophylaxis, parenteral in established vomiting).

- Give the antiemetic regularly and titrate to maximum dose.

- If symptoms persist, reassess for an additional cause of nausea and vomiting and treat this by following the steps above.

If there is no obvious cause or multiple causes are present, consider a combination of first-line agents or the use of a broad-spectrum agent. However, take care to:

- avoid combining drugs from the same class, eg metoclopramide and domperidone, as this has no therapeutic benefit and increases side effects;

- avoid combining drugs that have antagonistic action, eg prokinetics (metoclopramide and domperidone) and anticholinergics (cyclizine), as these will have opposing actions on the gastrointestinal tract.

Reasons for treatment failure

- Poor drug absorption: nausea alone may affect gastrointestinal absorption of drugs.

- Inadequate dose: if the probable cause of nausea and vomiting is unchanged, then the dose needs to be maximised before a second agent is added or the drug used is switched, eg metoclopramide may be increased up to 60 mg per 24 hours total dose.

- Multiple causes of nausea and vomiting: use either a combination of agents or a broad-spectrum drug, eg levomepromazine.

Anxiety

Nausea and vomiting are frequent symptoms in patients with cancer. Sickness is often related to treatment such as chemotherapy or radiotherapy, and anxiety experienced for any reason at a later stage may also result in anticipatory nausea and vomiting. Discussion and explanation will help to relieve anxiety, and non-pharmacological interventions may also be helpful, eg C bands (acupressure) or acupuncture and relaxation techniques.

1.3.4 Bowel obstruction

Scenario
Mrs Claire Wilson is 76-year-old woman who was diagnosed with Dukes B/C carcinoma of the colon 2 years ago and treated with a hemicolectomy and chemotherapy. She developed liver metastases 9 months ago and had second-line chemotherapy, but her disease has progressed. She has had constipation for some weeks and was under review in the palliative medicine clinic. When she attended the clinic for her follow-up today she reported worsening abdominal pain, colic and vomiting. She has been admitted for further investigation.

Introduction

The main priority is to determine whether the patient has developed subacute or complete bowel obstruction. The common causes of bowel obstruction in patients with cancer, both reversible and irreversible, are listed in Table 6. It is essential to identify any reversible causes and take the appropriate immediate management to correct these and control her symptoms, as well as planning longer-term management.

TABLE 5 NEURAL MECHANISMS CONTROLLING VOMITING

Area of vomiting pathway	Receptors	Causes of nausea and vomiting
Gut wall	$5HT_3$, ACh (muscarinic), dopamine D_2	Bowel obstruction, gastric irritants, chemotherapy, abdominal radiotherapy
Chemoreceptor trigger zone	$5HT_3$, dopamine D_2, α_2-adrenergic	For drug-induced and metabolic causes, eg opioid related or hypercalcaemia
Vestibular	ACh (muscarinic), histamine H_1	Motion sickness
Cerebral cortex	GABA, 5HT	Fear and raised intracranial pressure
Vomiting centre	ACh (muscarinic), histamine H_1, $5HT_2$, μ opioid	Other areas of pathway feed into vomiting centre

ACh, acetylcholine; GABA, γ-aminobutyric acid; 5HT, 5-hydroxytryptamine.

TABLE 6 CAUSES OF BOWEL OBSTRUCTION IN PATIENTS WITH CANCER	
Intraluminal	Polypoid tumour Constipation
Luminal	Neurogenic dysfunction
Extraluminal	Adhesions Intra-abdominal disease, including peritoneal seedlings, pelvic mass and ascites

History of the presenting problem

Establish the severity of the problem.

- What was her normal bowel frequency? The average is three to five bowel movements per week, but there is large variation between individuals.

- When did she last open her bowels?

- What were the characteristics of the last stool she passed (eg loose or formed; small, hard pellets or thin)?

- Does she feel the need to defecate but is unable to? If she does, then she may have hard stool or rectal obstruction. Has she got tenesmoid type pain?

You should also check for other symptoms that may indicate the presence of obstruction.

- Is she vomiting? If so, what are the periodicity, volume and content? See Section 1.3.3 for further discussion

- Does she have pain, and is this colic or not? The patient may have background pain due to her tumour or an intra-abdominal disease.

- Does she have abdominal distension? This is less prevalent in proximal obstruction or in omental disease where the bowel becomes 'stuck down'.

Other relevant history

Ensure you check if there are any potential coexisting factors that might affect management.

- What is the extent of the patient's disease and what treatment has she already had for it? Previous radiotherapy or surgery may have left her predisposed to adhesions and will affect decisions regarding future surgical interventions.

- What is the patient's general condition and performance status? Her nutritional status will affect possible treatment options. Is she well enough for surgery or is she coming to the end of her life?

- Are there existing comorbid conditions? If so, this will affect any treatment decisions that are made.

Examination

General features

General impressions are important and will help you to determine appropriate management. Aside from vital signs, is she frail and cachexic? Check her hydration status by looking carefully at the mouth and mucous membranes. Jaundice may indicate progression of metastatic disease.

Gastrointestinal system

To differentiate between simple constipation and bowel obstruction there are a number of key features to look for.

- Distension.

- Visible peristalsis.

- Local or generalised abdominal tenderness.

- Localised masses.

- Bowel sounds: may be high-pitched or absent altogether.

- Rectal examination: is stool present, how much and is it hard or soft? Can you feel an obstructing mass?

Investigation

Blood tests

- Raised urea and creatinine may result from dehydration, or be due to renal failure of other cause (perhaps urinary tract obstruction in this case).

- Hypokalaemia may be caused by vomiting and contribute to ileus.

- Hypercalcaemia of malignancy can cause constipation, nausea and vomiting.

- A raised white cell count may indicate infection.

- Abnormal liver tests may indicate progression of hepatic secondaries.

- Serum albumin can be used to assess nutritional status.

Imaging

An abdominal X-ray would show dilated bowel and air–fluid levels due to obstruction, and faecal loading if present. Consider a CT scan depending on the treatments being considered: if the patient is to be palliated medically, a scan may not be necessary. Endoscopy or colonoscopy could be considered if other investigations indicate a lesion amenable to stenting.

Management

Bringing the patient's symptoms under control is of primary importance and drugs are the most immediate symptom control measure available. Bear in mind the following when deciding on treatment for immediate results.

- Pain control: for background pain give opioids, eg diamorphine hydrochloride, subcutaneously immediately and consider continuous subcutaneous infusion (dose depends on previous opioid usage). For colic give antispasmodic, eg hyoscine butylbromide (Buscopan), 20 mg sc immediately and consider 60–120 mg continuous subcutaneous infusion over 24 hours.

- Antiemetics: give an antihistamine as first-line therapy, eg cyclizine 50 mg sc immediately and consider 100–150 mg continuous subcutaneous infusion over 24 hours. Avoid using prokinetics in cases of mechanical obstruction.

- Laxatives: give regular softener, eg magnesium hydroxide with liquid paraffin (Milpar) 10 mL bd, if the patient is able to tolerate any oral intake and not in renal failure. Avoid stimulants in cases of mechanical bowel obstruction. If laxatives are ineffective, consider rectal intervention starting with suppositories.

Beyond the drugs used to bring symptoms under control immediately, there are other medical interventions that can be considered for longer-term management.

- Pharmacological options: steroids, eg dexamethasone 12–16 mg sc or iv over 24 hours for a fixed trial of 5–7 days to assess response, and antisecretory agents, eg hyoscine butylbromide (Buscopan). Antisecretory drugs may be helpful if the patient is suffering from large-volume vomiting, but the dose needs to be titrated and usage may worsen symptoms of thirst.

- Interventional methods: nasogastric tube, although it is best to try other medical managements prior to this as the tubes are often uncomfortable; a stent, depending on the location of the obstruction; and venting gastrostomy if symptom control is not achieved with pharmacological management.

It is important to remember that palliative surgical options may be available for bowel obstruction: these should be considered early if at all. For a single level of obstruction, bypass surgery may be possible; if there are multiple levels, stoma formation could be considered. It is important to fully discuss the goals of surgery, and its relative risks and benefits, with the patient before advising surgery (see Section 1.2.4).

Further comments

How do you differentiate between subacute and complete bowel obstruction?

This depends on good history-taking and examination. In subacute obstruction symptoms may be intermittent rather than continuous, and bowel sounds may be hyperactive rather than high-pitched or absent as in complete obstruction. If the patient is in subacute obstruction, then optimal medical management with laxatives and hydration may resolve the problem.

What are the factors that will influence treatment decisions?

It is essential to consider the goals and wishes of the particular patient. Surgery may not prolong survival any longer than medical management and may also involve a long recovery period.

Hydration and nutrition

Consider the treatment goals (ie palliation) and context of the patient receiving care when deciding on appropriate hydration and nutrition. Aggressive hydration may actually worsen symptoms, eg increase vomiting and not help with dry mouth, which is best treated by good regular mouth care. Parenteral nutrition can maintain the patient's current nutritional status, but may not significantly improve it. If a patient undergoes surgery, then this should be considered in the perioperative period, but it is rarely a part of longer-term management.

2.1 Pain

Aetiology

Pain is an unpleasant sensory and emotional experience associated with actual or potential tissue damage, or described in terms of such damage. *(International Association for Study of Pain 1986)*

Pain is a complex physiological and emotional experience. In addition to physical pain, psychosocial, emotional and spiritual pain should be identified and addressed, and the wider impact of any type of pain on the life of a patient considered. Perception of pain may be affected by the patient's mental state; those who are depressed experience more pain and chronic pain often leads to depression. RG Twycross classifies physical pain as 'nociceptive or neuropathic with subdivisions of both into either physiological (functional) and pathological and then further into somatic vs visceral'. Useful terminology for describing pain is shown in Table 7.

Pain in cancer patients may be due to:

- cancer, either primary or secondary;
- debility, eg bed sores and stiffness from inactivity;
- treatments, eg vincristine neuropathy and thoracotomy scar pain;
- concurrent disorders, eg arthritis and osteoporosis.

A simplified schema of the neuroanatomy and neurophysiology of pain, and the sites of action of some analgesics, is shown in Fig. 2. There are nerve endings (nociceptors) in all tissues, which when stimulated by noxious stimuli (mechanical, chemical or thermal) will give rise to pain.

Different types of nerve fibres exist: A, B and C with α, β, δ and γ subcategories. Aα, Aγ and B are motor fibres; Aβ, Aδ and C are sensory fibres. Different nociceptors give rise to different pain, for instance Aδ nociceptors give rise to the first sharp pain of injury, whereas C nociceptors produce a slow throbbing pain. The different types of pain are outlined in Table 8.

Epidemiology

Approximately 75% of patients with cancer experience pain at some time during their final year of life. Many patients have more than one type of pain and/or more than one site of pain. These may be of differing aetiologies and might exhibit differential response to different analgesics.

TABLE 7 TERMINOLOGY OF PAIN

Terminology	Description
Nociception	The activity produced in the nervous system by potential or actual tissue-damaging stimuli: pain is the perception of nociception
Allodynia	Pain due to a stimulus that does not normally provoke pain
Hyperalgesia	Increased response to a stimulus that is normally painful
Hyperpathia	Increased reaction to a stimulus that is normally painful which is accompanied by an increased threshold for that pain

TABLE 8 TYPES OF PAIN

Type	Description
Somatic	Arises from damage to skin and deep tissues. It is usually localised and often of an aching quality
Visceral	Arises from abdominal or thoracic viscera. Such pain is often described as deep or pressure pain, and is poorly localised
Neuropathic	Due to nerve damage either in the peripheral or central nervous system. This may be described as 'burning' or 'stabbing' in quality. Often occurs in an area of abnormal or decreased sensation. Neuropathic pain may respond to opioids, but in many cases co-analgesic drugs are required

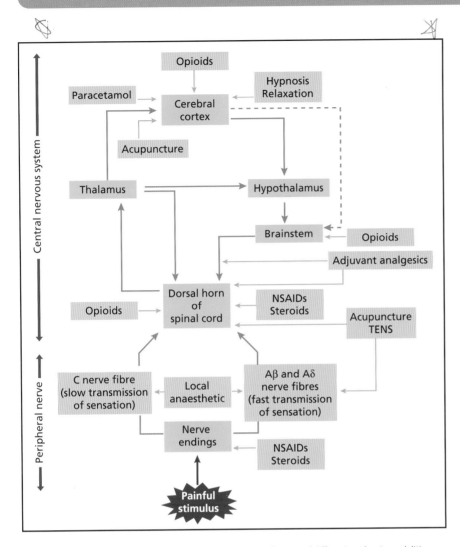

▲ **Fig. 2** A schema of the neuroanatomy of pain and the sites of action of different analgesic modalities. TENS, transcutaneous electrical nerve stimulation.

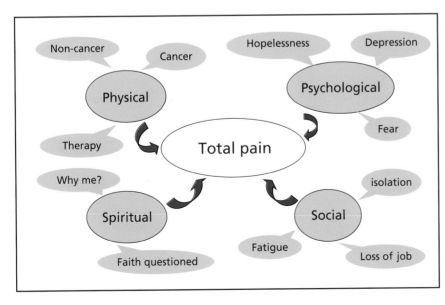

▲ **Fig. 3** Factors contributing to the 'total pain' model.

Clinical presentation

Patients will present in many different ways. The concept of total pain acknowledges the distress a patient with a serious illness experiences and the contribution of psychological, social, spiritual and financial problems to their predicament (Fig. 3). Similarly, dying patients face multiple losses and anxieties, but although pain is just one facet of their disease it is often a constant reminder of their situation. Therefore, some patients will use pain as a benchmark to indicate how their disease is progressing.

Assessment of pain

A clear history and assessment of pain is the basis of treatment. Successful treatment therefore relies on knowledge of the aetiology of a patient's pain and recognition that several types and sites of pain may coexist. Ongoing assessment and evaluation is essential to achieve good pain control.

Obtaining a pain history should include the following questions.

- When did it start?

- Where is it and does it radiate anywhere?

- What is the character of the pain?

- Is it constant or does it fluctuate?

- Does anything alleviate or exacerbate it?

- Which analgesics have been tried and what effect did they have?

- Are there any associated factors?

- What effect does it have on your life?

- Do you have any particular fears or anxieties?

Physical signs

Assess the state of the patient's disease and note palpable evidence

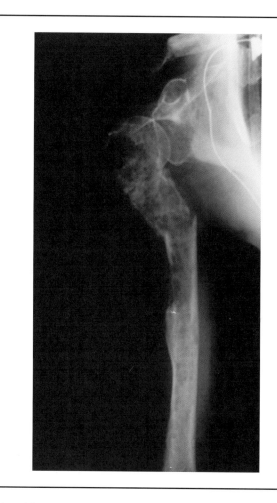

▲ **Fig. 4** A pathological fracture of the upper shaft of the humerus due to multiple lytic deposits.

of its spread. Palpate areas of pain to elicit tenderness, eg from bone secondaries (Fig. 4). Examine the nervous system looking for signs of reduced power and abnormal sensation. Assess the patient's reflexes.

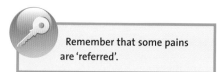

Remember that some pains are 'referred'.

Treatment

Rules for analgesic prescribing are shown in Fig. 1, and can be summarised as follows.

- Continuous pain requires regular doses of analgesics to be effectively suppressed.

- Start simply and follow the analgesic ladder.

- Be patient and give each drug a therapeutic trial at the appropriate dose.

- Anticipate and treat side effects, eg constipation.

- Give drugs orally unless the patient's condition precludes use of this route, eg patient is vomiting or suffering from dysphagia.

- Move up the ladder if the current step is ineffective, but remember that it may be appropriate to add a co-analgesic before moving on to the next step.

Whatever treatment you decide on, take the time to explain carefully to the patient your rationale for choosing it.

Morphine

Morphine is an extremely useful drug and is the opioid of choice for treating moderate to severe cancer pain. The dose should be titrated for each individual patient. There is no upper limit on the dose prescribed.

Titration of morphine The initial dose depends on previous analgesia, age and coexisting medical problems. Renal failure can lead to the accumulation of opioids and their metabolites, which results in toxicity. In such cases immediate-release rather than modified- or slow-release preparations should be prescribed and closely monitored.

Most patients should be started on 5–10 mg orally ever 4 hours, with the same amount prescribed as a breakthrough (or 'rescue') dose whenever needed. Once drug requirements are constant, the patient can be converted to modified-release morphine (eg MST Continus and MXL). However, it is imperative that immediate-release morphine remains as the prescription for breakthrough doses, and that the breakthrough dose is increased in step with the modified-release preparation (ie breakthrough dose should be given at one-sixth of the total 24-hour dose of regular morphine).

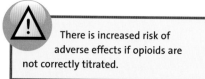

There is increased risk of adverse effects if opioids are not correctly titrated.

Alternative opioids

It should be noted that conversion ratios between different opioids are only a guide, and that marked interindividual variation can thus be seen. Therefore, where possible, titration with immediate-release preparations is recommended, and dose reduction should be considered when switching from one opioid to another.

Oxycodone hydrochloride This is often used as a second-line opioid and is available in immediate-release and modified-release preparations. Patients should be titrated on immediate-release preparations, as they would be with morphine: 5 mg of oxycodone is approximately equivalent to 10 mg of morphine.

Fentanyl A synthetic opioid available as a transdermal patch that is changed every 3 days. It is not suitable for patients with unstable pain requiring dose titration. It has variable pharmacokinetics: dose conversions are estimates only and occasionally patients may need to change patches every 2 days. Useful for patients with difficult constipation or for those unable to take oral medication due to conditions such as head and neck cancer or bowel obstruction. A patch supplying fentanyl 25 mg/hour provides equivalent analgesia to 60–90 mg morphine taken orally over 24 hours.

Methadone hydrochloride Useful for patients with neuropathic pain. It is lipid soluble and accumulates in fat stores resulting in unpredictable pharmacokinetics, so therefore should only be used under specialist guidance. The potency of methadone compared with morphine increases with multiple doses, and is approximately 5–10 times as potent as morphine ingested orally.

Parenteral opioids
Diamorphine hydrochloride The opioid of choice for parenteral use due to its increased solubility. However, if this is unavailable, alternatives are morphine or

oxycodone. The preferred route of administration is subcutaneous unless there are specific contraindications, eg low platelets. Diamorphine should be used when a patient is unable to absorb oral medication. It is approximately three times more potent than oral morphine.

Morphine Parenteral morphine is two times more potent than oral morphine.

Oxycodone Parenteral oxycodone is four times more potent than oral morphine.

Side effects of opioids
The common side effects of opioids are shown in Table 9.

> ⚠ Opioids may accumulate in renal or hepatic failure, resulting in toxicity: caution is needed and specialist advice should be sought.

Fears about morphine and other opioids
Fears over the use of opioids are common in both patients and

doctors. The concerns of both parties can limit appropriate prescription of this safe and useful drug, and may lead to non-compliance unless they are discussed with the patient.

There are a number of common concerns raised by patients when it is suggested that they start treatment with an opioid. These include the misperception that starting morphine is indicative of a short prognosis and heralds the onset of the terminal stage of their illness; fear of addiction to the drug, which does not occur when used correctly for pain control; concern that if morphine is started too early there will be no options left for pain control later in the disease course; and anxiety over possible side effects, such as sedation, that would leave them unable to function normally.

Healthcare professionals may also have unfounded concerns about the side effects of opioids. Sedation is usually transient and other psychogenic side effects, such as confusion, are rare and can be

TABLE 9 COMMON SIDE EFFECTS OF OPIOIDS	
Constipation	Occurs in almost all patients unless there is coexisting malabsorption. All patients should be treated prophylactically with a stimulant laxative plus softener
Nausea	Affects one-third of patients, but in the majority of these is self-limiting to within 1 week. Consider a 1-week course of prophylactic antiemetics if nausea is a problem
Drowsiness	Generally remits after a few days
Dry mouth	A common side effect
Hallucinations	An uncommon side effect. It is often manifested visually, occurring in the peripheral field of vision
Nightmares	Vivid and unpleasant if they occur, but thankfully uncommon
Myoclonic jerks	These may be related to accumulation of morphine metabolites
Respiratory depression	Should not be a problem in patients who are in pain and titrated correctly. However, it can occur if pain is abolished, eg after a nerve block or radiotherapy, or if due to the accumulation secondary to renal failure. Consider using immediate-release preparations in these patients

managed by switching to an alternative opioid. As pain is a respiratory stimulant, as long as opioids are correctly titrated respiratory depression should not occur. If opioids are used appropriately, then none of these fears are justified, and the benefits of their prescription will far outweigh the risks.

> Use open communication to address any concerns about opioid-related side effects and myths to ensure appropriate use of the drugs and compliance with treatment.

Co-analgesics for neuropathic pain

Neuropathic pain may be partially or fully controlled with opioids. However, some patients will need the addition of co-analgesics. These drugs are usually given for alternative indications (eg depression and epilepsy) and it is therefore important to explain to the patient why the drug is being given.

Tricyclic antidepressants These act by blocking the uptake of noradrenaline (norepinephrine) and serotonin. To achieve an analgesic effect, a lower dose is used than for depression and the drugs exert their effect in approximately 4–5 days. Start at a low dose, eg amitriptyline 25 mg nightly, and gradually increase it. Most patients experience transient drowsiness, but some patients have intolerable anticholinergic side effects.

Anticonvulsants Gabapentin, sodium valproate and clonazepam are all used to treat neuropathic pain, but the mechanism of their analgesic effect is not fully understood. They should be started at low doses and gradually increased in order to minimise side effects. The analgesic effect of gabapentin

and clonazepam occurs immediately, whereas sodium valproate takes up to 1 week to have an effect.

Corticosteroids These can be useful in reducing inflammation around tumours, thereby relieving pressure on structures that have been compressed, eg nerve roots and cerebral metastases. They may also have an effect on the prostaglandin pathway. Their usefulness is limited by their side effects, but in the short term they can be a very effective co-analgesic.

Other analgesics

Non-steroidal anti-inflammatory drugs The NSAIDs have analgesic and anti-inflammatory effects because they reduce prostaglandin synthesis. They are used frequently, particularly for bone pain. There are many different groups of NSAIDs and patients who fail to respond to a drug in one group may respond to others from a different group.

Other agents Analgesics used by specialist teams include the following.

- Membrane-stabilising drugs that are used for neuropathic pain, eg lidocaine patches.

- Ketamine: an anaesthetic agent useful for treating neuropathic pain; its intravenous preparation is also made into an oral solution.

- Bisphosphonates: used for the treatment of bone pain.

- Antispasmodics, eg benzodiazepines and baclofen.

> ⚠ There is an increased risk of gastrointestinal bleeding in patients with cancer, so always consider using gastroprotection when prescribing steroids or an NSAID.

Other modalities of pain control

- Epidural and intrathecal opioids: for patients with severe side effects from opioids or pain that requires escalation in the doses of drugs.

- Nerve blocks: for localised pain or pain from one nerve root. Initially injected with local anaesthetic and steroids if successful longer-term relief can be gained from neuroablation.

- Palliative radiotherapy.

- Chemotherapy.

- TENS: electrical stimulation of Aβ fibres which, according to the gate theory of pain, reduces the input from C fibres to the spinal cord.

- Complementary therapies, eg acupuncture.

- Surgery, eg to stabilise a fracture of the spine or a long bone, or prophylactically to prevent an impending fracture.

FURTHER READING

Hanks GW, Conno F, Cherny N, *et al.* Morphine and alternative opioids in cancer pain: the EAPC recommendations. *Br. J. Cancer* 2001; 84: 587–93.

Lussier D, Huskey AG and Portenoy RK. Adjuvant analgesics in cancer pain management. *Oncologist* 2004; 9: 571–91.

Sindrup SH and Jensen TS. Efficacy of pharmacological treatments of neuropathic pain: an update and effect related to mechanism of drug action. *Pain* 1999; 83: 389–400.

Twycross R and Wilcock A. Pain relief. In *Symptom Management in Advanced Cancer*, 3rd edn. Oxford: Radcliffe Medical Press, 2001: 17–68

2.2 Breathlessness

Aetiology

Breathlessness in patients with cancer may be due to either the malignancy itself or comorbid conditions. It may occur as a direct result of a primary tumour or lung secondaries (Fig. 5) or be caused by malignancy-related conditions such as lymphangitis carcinomatosis, pericardial and pleural (Fig. 6) effusions, and superior vena cava (SVC) obstruction. Intra-abdominal disease may also be a contributory factor if ascites and hepatomegaly result in diaphragmatic splinting.

The non-malignant conditions that result in breathlessness may be acute or chronic. Acute infective events occur frequently in those who are ill and immunocompromised, and there is a higher incidence of thromboembolic events in patients with cancer. There could also be coexisting problems such as chronic lung disease or heart failure.

Epidemiology

Breathlessness is a common symptom in cancer, with a prevalence of up to 64% in heterogeneous cancers and 85% in lung cancer. The symptoms increase in frequency and intensity towards the end of life, partly due to deterioration in general performance status, with up to 64% of all patients reporting breathlessness in the last 6 weeks of life.

Clinical presentation

Breathlessness is a complex multidimensional problem that is very distressing to patients. Initially it may be episodic and related solely to exertion, but it can progress to limit the normal activities of daily living. Breathlessness may be accompanied by coughing and haemoptysis.

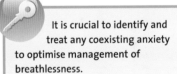

It is crucial to identify and treat any coexisting anxiety to optimise management of breathlessness.

Breathlessness is frequently associated with anxiety, panic and fear of impending death. It is essential to address this panic and asking about specific fears may be therapeutic in itself, eg the sensitive use of questions such as 'I appreciate that you must have many fears and worries, but is there anything in particular that is troubling you?'.

Physical signs

Make sure your examination checks for all the possible signs of breathlessness to enable you to pinpoint the cause. Look for:

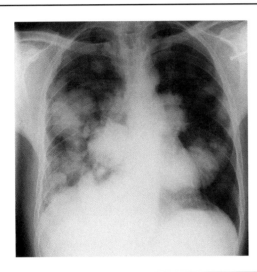

▲ Fig. 5 CXR of a patient with diffuse pleuritic chest pain and breathlessness due to an adenoid cystic carcinoma.

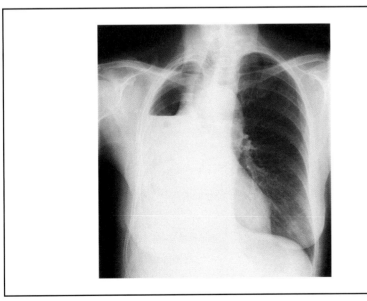

▲ Fig. 6 Carcinoma of the bronchus with pleural effusion and traumatic pneumothorax.

- anaemia;

- bronchospasm;

- signs of collapse and consolidation;

- pleural effusions;

- signs of right- or left-sided heart failure;

- pericardial effusions and pleural rubs;

- SVC obstruction;

- ascites.

Investigations

These should be purposeful and directed at reversible causes of breathlessness, or done to monitor or change specific tumour treatments.

Treatment

The treatment of breathlessness can be difficult. Success depends on determining the aetiology and treating any reversible causes, and then taking care to ameliorate physical symptoms and psychological distress as much as possible. Treatment modalities are shown in Table 10.

> There is often concern about using opioids and benzodiazepines in patients with respiratory disease, but using appropriate drugs in small doses is safe and can have a significant impact on symptom control and quality of life.

Stridor

Stridor is caused by tracheal compression and requires emergency management: give the patient high-concentration oxygen and dexamethasone 16 mg iv. Refer them as an emergency to oncologists for radiotherapy if appropriate, or to head and neck surgeons for tracheostomy if required. Supportive treatments should include nebulised salbutamol and sedation if appropriate. The patient can also be given heliox as a useful alternative to oxygen.

FURTHER READING

Chan K, Sham MMK, Tse DMW and Thorsen A. Palliative medicine in malignant respiratory diseases. In Doyle D, Hanks GWC, Cherny NI and Calman K, eds. *Oxford Textbook of*

Palliative Medicine, 3rd edn. Oxford: Oxford University Press, 2005: 587–618.

Booth S. The management of dyspnoea in advanced cancer. *Hosp. Med.* 1998; 59, 348–9.

2.3 Nausea and vomiting

Aetiology

The emetic pathway is complex, involving many neuronal pathways. A diagram of the pathways controlling vomiting is shown in Fig. 7 and the common causes of such symptoms in cancer patients are listed in Table 3.

Epidemiology

At least three-quarters of patients with cancer will experience nausea and vomiting at some time in their last year of life, as well as 27% of those dying from other causes.

> To optimally control nausea and vomiting it is essential to choose an appropriate antiemetic based on the aetiology. A careful history and examination will guide the choice of drug.

Treatment

It is important to use a logical approach in choosing an antiemetic (commonly used antiemetics are listed in Table 4).

- Identify the most likely cause of nausea and vomiting.

- Identify the area of vomiting pathway by which this cause acts.

- Identify which neurotransmitter receptors are involved in this area of the vomiting pathway.

TABLE 10 TREATMENT OF BREATHLESSNESS	
Treat reversible causes	Tumour modification, eg radiotherapy and chemotherapy/laser treatment Transfusion Anticoagulation Drainage of effusions or ascites Endobronchial or SVC stents
Drug treatments	Bronchodilators Opioids Corticosteroids Benzodiazepines Antibiotics Diuretics Oxygen
Other modalities	Fans to increase airflow in the patient's environment Acupuncture Relaxation therapy Breathlessness clinics

SVC, superior vena cava.

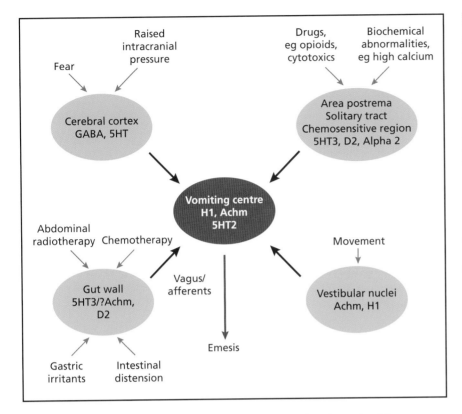

▲ **Fig. 7** Neural mechanisms controlling vomiting. Achm, muscarinic cholinergic receptor; alpha 2, α₂-adrenergic receptor; D2, dopamine receptor type 2; GABA, γ-aminobutyric acid; 5HT, 5-hydroxytryptamine; H1, histamine receptor type 1.

Lichter I. Which antiemetic? *J. Palliative Care* 1993; 9: 42–50.

Mannix K. Palliation of nausea and vomiting. In Doyle D, Hanks GWC, Cherny NI and Calman K, eds. *Oxford Textbook of Palliative Medicine*, 3rd edn. Oxford: Oxford University Press, 2005: 459–68.

- Choose the most specific antagonist to the receptor identified.

- Choose the most appropriate route of antiemetic administration (oral for prophylaxis, parenteral if the patient has established vomiting to ensure absorption).

- Give the antiemetic regularly and titrate to maximum dose.

- Medications should be given regularly for a period of at least 24 hours to assess how the patient responds before any change is made to the regimen.

- If symptoms persist after this time, reassess for an additional cause of nausea and vomiting and treat this by repeating the steps above.

- If there is no obvious cause or multiple causes are present, consider using a combination of first-line agents or a broad-spectrum agent. However, avoid combining drugs from the same class, eg metoclopramide and domperidone, as this has no therapeutic benefit and increases side effects, and avoid combining drugs that have antagonistic action, eg prokinetics (metoclopramide and domperidone) and anticholinergics (cyclizine), as these will have opposing actions on the gastrointestinal tract.

> When choosing drug combinations, avoid using drugs from the same class or those with opposing actions.

FURTHER READING

Ison PJ and Petroutka SJ. Neurotransmitter receptor binding studies predict antiemetic efficacy and side effects. *Cancer Treat. Rep.* 1986; 70: 637–41.

2.4 Constipation

Aetiology

A wide variety of factors can result in constipation. Some common causes in patients with cancer are listed in Table 1.

Epidemiology

Constipation is defined as the passage of small, hard stools less frequently than the patient's usual bowel movements, and with difficulty. It is important to take a good and detailed history of the bowel pattern as patients are often reticent to admit to problems of constipation. However, it is very common in the hospital population, affecting up to 63% of elderly patients and many with cancer.

> It is important to take a good and detailed history of the bowel pattern as patients are often reticent to admit to problems of constipation.

Clinical presentation

Patients may present with abdominal pain, colic, nausea and vomiting, or urinary retention. They may also present with agitation or confusion, particularly in the elderly, or with spurious diarrhoea due to 'overflow'.

Physical signs

Faeces may be palpable either rectally or abdominally. Sometimes this is not obvious and an abdominal radiograph is needed to demonstrate faecal loading.

Treatment

Prevention is better than cure, so it is vital that constipation is treated prophylactically in patients starting opioids. Laxatives should be taken regularly by these patients and not prescribed as prn medication.

When patients do suffer from constipation, reversible causes should be treated and unnecessary medication stopped. Drug treatment may be necessary. Laxatives fall into a number of groups and these may need to be used in combination (combined preparations are available). The laxatives most commonly used are described below.

Stimulants

These should be used for all patients starting opioids, unless there is malabsorption, eg ileostomy or pancreatic insufficiency. It is usual to give a faecal softener as well. Commonly used stimulants are:

- bisacodyl (5–20 mg od–bd);

- senna (start with one to two tablets or 10–20 mL od–bd);

- sodium picosulphate (5–20 mL od–bd).

Softeners

- Docusate sodium (100–200 mg od–bd).

- Liquid paraffin: not recommended for use on its own owing to side effects.

Osmotic

The volume of fluid that needs to be taken with these preparations can limit their use.

- Lactulose (start with 10–20 mL od–bd): this can cause bowel distension with increased abdominal cramps.

- Movicol (polyethylene glycol, start with one sachet od–bd).

Combined preparations

- Softener plus stimulant: co-danthrusate (two tablets od–bd), although this can cause skin burns if taken by someone who is incontinent.

- Softener plus osmotic: magnesium hydroxide and liquid paraffin (10–20 mL od–bd).

Rectal preparations

Suppositories (which may need to be used in combination) include the following:

- glycerol 4 g, one to two suppositories od (softener and mild stimulant);

- bisacodyl 10 mg, one to two suppositories od (stimulant).

Enemas include the following:

- sodium citrate (stimulant);

- phosphate (stimulant);

- arachis oil (softener, use overnight prior to using a stimulant).

Note that bulk laxatives do not have a place in the treatment of seriously ill patients as they require a high liquid intake and can be unpalatable.

> Prevention is better than cure, so it is vital that constipation is treated prophylactically in patients starting opioids. Laxatives should be taken regularly and not prescribed as prn medication.

FURTHER READING

Sykes NP. A clinical comparison of laxatives in a hospice. *Palliative Med.* 1991; 5: 307–14.

- - - - - - - - - - - - - - - - - -

Sykes NP. Constipation and diarrrhoea. In Doyle D, Hanks GWC, Cherney NI and Calman K, eds. *Oxford Textbook of Palliative Medicine*, 3rd edn. Oxford: Oxford University Press, 2005: 483–96.

2.5 Bowel obstruction

Aetiology

Bowel obstruction can occur at any site from the gastric outlet onwards, and can be partial or complete. Obstruction can be due to an intraluminal cause (eg colonic tumour) that usually results in a single level of obstruction, or because of external compression (eg ovarian masses or widespread intraperitoneal disease) that may result in multiple levels of obstruction (Fig. 8). Bowel obstruction in patients with cancer may also be due to non-malignant causes, including postoperative adhesions and radiotherapy-induced fibrosis.

Epidemiology

Bowel obstruction is a well-recognised complication in patients with abdominal and pelvic malignancy. It occurs most frequently in cases of advanced disease, with an incidence of up to 24% in patients with colorectal carcinoma and 42% in those with carcinoma of the ovary.

Clinical presentation

Patients will often present with a combination of pain, colic, nausea and vomiting, and constipation.

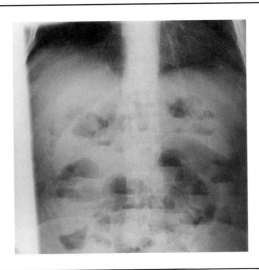

▲**Fig. 8** Malignant bowel obstruction.

Treatment

> 🔑 Do not neglect surgical options for palliation if the patient's wishes and general condition make it appropriate.

Interventional techniques

Endoscopic stent insertion may be an option for single levels of obstruction in the proximal small bowel and distal large bowel. For high levels of obstruction a venting gastrostomy may help palliate symptoms.

Surgery

If the patient is fit, surgery may be appropriate. For single levels of obstruction, bypass surgery may be possible; if there are multiple levels of obstruction, stoma formation, either a colostomy or ileostomy, can be performed. If there is a delay before surgery can proceed, then consideration needs to be given to parenteral nutrition.

Corticosteroids

The role of steroids is unclear. Theoretically, they can reduce oedema around tumour deposits and thereby increase lumen size. A trial of dexamethasone 12–16 mg (sc or iv) can be given for 7 days and then stopped if there is no improvement.

Antisecretory agents

An obstructed bowel will distend further as intraluminal secretions accumulate. A somatostatin analogue such as octreotide (starting at 0.3–0.6 mg csci over 24 hours) inhibits the release of hormones such as gastrin, secretin, vasoactive intestinal polypeptide (VIP) and pepsin, among others. Anticholinergic agents such as hyoscine hydrobromide (60–120 mg csci over 24 hours) may also reduce secretion further. The inhibition of gastrointestinal secretions can break the cycle of distension and increased intraluminal secretions, thereby reducing vomiting and abdominal pain.

Antiemetics

Antiemetics may have varying efficacy but control of nausea and reduction of vomiting can be an achievable goal: first-line agents include cyclizine (100–150 mg per 24 hours). Prokinetic antiemetics should not be used in mechanical obstruction as they can cause bowel perforation.

Analgesics

Subcutaneous diamorphine hydrochloride may control pain fully, although the dose will depend on previous opioid requirements. If colic is present, use subcutaneous hyoscine butylbromide (60–120 mg per 24 hours).

Laxatives

Rectal intervention and faecal softeners should be used if constipation is a problem. Stimulant laxatives should not be used in mechanical obstruction as they can cause bowel perforation.

Nasogastric tubes

These may be occasionally required to relieve symptoms, but are unpleasant and other symptomatic measures should be tried first.

FURTHER READING

Feuer D, Broadley KE, Shepherd JH and Barton DP. Intestinal obstruction from advanced gastrointestinal or gynecological cancer. *Gynecol. Oncol.* 2000; 78: 394–5.

- - - - - - - - - - - - - - - -

Ripamonti C and Mercadante S. Pathophysiology and management of malignant obstruction. In Doyle D, Hanks GWC, Cherny NI and Calman K, eds. *Oxford Textbook of Palliative Medicine*, 3rd edn. Oxford: Oxford University Press, 2005: 496–507.

2.6 Anxiety and depression

Anxiety

Anxiety and difficulty in adjusting to circumstances are common problems for those who have a serious illness. Many patients will cope remarkably robustly with their problems and others will respond to reassurance, but some become increasingly incapacitated by anxiety. This can take many forms, which often focus on symptoms, possible mode of death, the family that will be left behind and issues that are not resolved ('unfinished business').

In many cases anxiety is understandable, and in some may be crippling in its intensity. Patients may declare their anxieties immediately, but many will not do so because they think that they 'should not bother the doctor with them'. If you suspect a patient is suffering from anxiety or his or her reactions do not ring true, then ask 'I know that you must have many fears and worries, but is there anything in particular that is preying on your mind?'

Is treatment needed? Distinguishing anxiety that requires intervention from an expected level of distress or a patient's natural tendencies can be difficult. The patient will often provide insightful comments on his or her temperament, replying 'I've always been an anxious person' or 'this is not like me'.

Treatment

In many cases anxiety responds well to simple non-pharmacological measures, and patients can usually be maintained successfully at home under the care of the primary care team. Psychologists can offer help by suggesting coping strategies and counselling can provide emotional support. Some patients are reassured by meeting others in similar situations to themselves at support groups or in hospitals.

Benzodiazepines are the mainstay of drug treatments for anxiety and can

be given regularly or when needed. Sublingual lorazepam is effective in the event of panic attacks.

Depression

Depression is the most common psychiatric disease in patients with serious illnesses. Its prevalence in the general population is 6–10%, but figures quoted for patients with advanced cancer suggest it is evident in 25–37% of the terminally ill.

Patients at increased risk are those with previous psychiatric problems, poor coping mechanisms and those who feel that communication about their illness, particularly during the 'bad news interview', has not been appropriate for their needs.

Up to 80% of psychological and psychiatric morbidity in cancer patients goes undiagnosed.

> 🔑 **Psychological and psychiatric morbidity often goes undiagnosed in many patients with cancer because of:**
>
> - widespread acceptance of inevitability regarding the patient's situation ('of course they are depressed, they are dying!');
> - nurses and doctors tending to concentrate soley on their patient's physical symptoms.

Clinical presentation

There are no universally accepted criteria for diagnosing depression in the physically ill. In the physically healthy population, depression is diagnosed if patients have a persistent low mood and at least four of the other defined symptoms that are present for most of the days in the 2 weeks preceding their examination.

> 🔑 **Criteria for the diagnosis of depression in the healthy population**
>
> - Diminished interest or pleasure in all or almost all activities.
> - Psychomotor retardation or agitation.
> - Feelings of worthlessness or excessive and inappropriate guilt.
> - Diminished ability to concentrate and think.
> - Recurrent thoughts of death and suicide.
> - Fatigue and loss of energy.
> - Significant weight loss or gain.
> - Insomnia or hypersomnia.

In patients with advanced cancer the experiences of fatigue and loss of energy, significant weight loss or gain, and insomnia or hypersomnia are almost universal. Endicott proposes that somatic symptoms should be substituted with the following states.

- Diminished concentration: cannot be cheered up, does not smile and shows no response to good news or a funny situation.

- Fatigue and loss of energy: brooding, self-pitying and pessimistic.

- Significant weight loss or gain: fearful or depressed appearance in body or face.

- Insomnia or hypersomnia: social withdrawal or decreased talkativeness.

These are useful categories and much of the information needed to make a judgement as to whether the patient is depressed can be obtained by asking simple questions.

- 'How do you spend your day?'

- 'Does any activity give you any pleasure?'

- 'Do you feel depressed?'

The doctor should not be afraid to ask about suicidal thoughts, perhaps

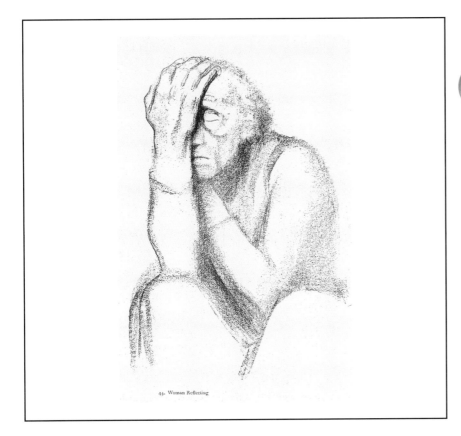

▲ **Fig. 9** *Woman Reflecting* by Kathe Kollwitz.

using the question 'Have things felt so bad that you have had thoughts of harming yourself?' Patients will not be distressed; they will either refute it or show relief that someone has acknowledged the depth of their distress (Fig. 9).

Treatment

Both pharmacological and non-pharmacological therapy should be considered. Pharmacological treatment includes selective serotonin reuptake inhibitors, which are generally well tolerated by patients, and tricyclic antidepressants, which are also used for neuropathic pain and are particularly useful when depression and pain coexist. Newer dual-action antidepressants (eg venlafaxine) may also have some analgesic efficacy. There is no good evidence to support any one drug over another in treating the mental states of cancer patients, but any comorbidities (eg cardiac) and side-

effect profiles (eg sedative effect) may guide the prescriptions for individual patients. Of patients with cancer and depression, 80% respond to antidepressants. It is therefore important to diagnose symptoms and treat them accordingly, even if prognosis for life remaining is only weeks or months.

FURTHER READING

Hotopf M, Chidgey J, Addington-Hall J and Lan Ly K. Depression in advanced disease: a systematic review. Part 1: prevalence and case finding. *Palliative Med.* 2002; 16: 81–97.

- - - - - - - - - - - - - - - - - - -

Lan Ly K, Addington-Hall J, Chidgey J and Hotopf M. Depression in palliative care: a systematic review. Part 2: treatment. *Palliative Med.* 2002; 16: 279–84.

- - - - - - - - - - - - - - - - - - -

Lawrie I, Lloyd-Williams M and Taylor F. How do palliative medicine physicians assess and manage depression. *Palliative Med.* 2004; 18: 234–8.

2.7 Confusion

'What is the answer?' After a short silence, she laughed and added 'Then what is the question?' (Last words of Gertrude Stein, 1946)

Introduction

Acute confusional states are common in patients with advanced malignancy, and increase in prevalence as patients near death. It is important to recognise confusion and to treat its reversible causes. Confusion is distressing for both the patient, who may have lucid periods, and the relatives, who are often fearful and distressed.

Investigation

Any investigation of patients with advanced disease should be purposeful and kept to a minimum. The common treatable causes of confusion need to be excluded rapidly (Table 11). The most likely of these is hypercalcaemia: 10–20% of patients with solid tumours will suffer from this at some point in their illness. Make sure that you exclude any other biochemical abnormalities and hypoxia as possible causes of the confusion.

Confusion without focal neurological signs is an uncommon presentation of cerebral metastases, but does sometimes occur. Investigate with MRI or CT scan if the patient is fit enough to receive high-dose corticosteroids and undergo palliative radiotherapy.

A recent drug history, particularly of any opioids, is important, but do not assume that confusion is opioid-induced.

Include the relatives (and patient if possible) when debating appropriate investigations. A calm and measured approach can do much to allay anxieties.

TABLE 11 COMMON CAUSES OF CONFUSION IN PATIENTS WITH CANCER

Infection	Urinary tract
	Chest
	Fungal
Metabolic	Hypercalcaemia
	Hyponatraemia
	Liver failure
	Uraemia
	Hypoxia from any cause
Drug induced	Opioids (overdose or withdrawal)
	Sedatives, eg benzodiazepines
	Corticosteroids
	Alcohol withdrawal
Neurological	Dementia
	Brain metastases (rarely)
	Postictal
Psychiatric	Paranoid delusional state
Other	Urinary retention
	Constipation

Treatment

Treat all reversible causes as rapidly as possible. You may feel that the patient is dying and that treatment, such as further antibiotics, would be an unnecessary intrusion. It is important to make the diagnosis if terminal agitation is suspected and to palliate appropriately with both adequate analgesia and sedation. Discuss this and the goal of any treatment with the relatives, but do not imply that they are making the decision; they will rarely disagree with a clear and reasoned plan of care.

Drug treatment for confusion is sometimes necessary and the following are suggested.

- Benzodiazepines: sublingual lorazepam 0.5–1 mg or midazolam 2.5–5 mg sc.

- Haloperidol 2–5 mg po/sc tid.

- Levomepromazine 6.25–12.5 mg po/sc (may be sedating).

> Drugs may need to be stopped or opioids changed, eg morphine changed to oxycodone hydrochloride or fentanyl, but do not presume that morphine is always the cause of confusion. It is unlikely to be so if the patient has been taking it without problems previously and renal function is stable.

FURTHER READING

For specific details on confusion in elderly people, see *Medicine for the Elderly*, Sections 1.1.2, 1.2.1, 1.2.2 and 1.4.1.

- - - - - - - - - - - - - - - - - -

Breitbart W, Chochinov H and Passik S, Cognitive disorders in the terminally ill. In Doyle D, Hanks GWC, Cherny NI and Calman K, eds. *Oxford Textbook of Palliative Medicine*, 3rd edn. Oxford: Oxford University Press, 2005: 758–64.

- - - - - - - - - - - - - - - - - -

De Stoutz N. *Topics in Palliative Care.* New York: Oxford University Press, 1997.

2.8 End-of-life care: the dying patient

> I'm not afraid to die, I just don't want to be there when it happens. (Woody Allen, *Getting Even*)

Continuing careful management once it is clear the patient is dying is important for both the patient and the family. The aim of such treatment is comfort for the patient and reduction of the relatives' distress. There is only one chance to get this right.

Planning end-of-life care

> Clear explanations to the patient and relatives are essential.

Often at the end of life there is an identifiable terminal phase. It is important to recognise this so that the focus of care can be changed, with a redefinition of goals, appraisal of symptoms and provision of the opportunity to identify and address the needs of the patient and the family.

Changing the focus of care

Once it has been recognised that the patient is entering the terminal stage of illness, the focus of care changes to ensuring optimal symptom control and comfort for the patient, and ongoing support for the family. At this point a number of treatment decisions need to be made and to guide this process it is helpful to consider the following.

- Would any intervention help alleviate the patient's symptoms?

- Would any treatments cause harm?

- The continuation of activities that had previously been a routine part of the patient's treatment, eg observations, may now be intrusive and not contribute to active care. If so, they should be stopped.

An approach based on these considerations usually results in a treatment plan that is acceptable to the patient and the family.

Withholding and withdrawing treatment

At the end of life all inappropriate interventions should be discontinued. This applies to observations (blood pressure and temperature) and investigations (blood tests and imaging) as well as medical treatments. The place of medical interventions such as antibiotics, artificial hydration and nutrition should be assessed on an individual basis. For example, it may be appropriate to discontinue intravenous fluids in a patient who is not thirsty and remains comfortable with good mouth care, but you may decide to prescribe antibiotics to a dying patient who is distressed by copious amounts of unpleasant bronchial secretions.

Prescribing

Regular medication should be prescribed for existing symptoms and additional medication prescribed on an 'as needed' basis for potential and/or anticipated symptoms. Different routes of administration may be needed if the patient has difficulty in swallowing. The preferred parenteral route in palliative care patients is subcutaneous, either a continuous infusion via a syringe driver or bolus doses. The effect of bolus doses can be used to determine the likely dose of any prescription that would be needed over 24 hours. When you begin prescribing for the end of life, rationalise existing medication. Previously 'essential' medications, such as antihypertensives, may

TABLE 12 CAUSES OF TERMINAL AGITATION	
Nature of problem	**Problem**
Physical	Pain
	Uncomfortable mouth
	Full bladder
	Full rectum
	'General stiffness'
	Inability to move
	Inability to communicate
Emotional	Fear of dying
	Distress on leaving family
	Unfinished business
Any cause of confusion	See Table 11

now be stopped and the goal of prescriptions shifted to patient comfort and symptom control.

Communication

It is important to ensure good communication with the patient and family throughout in order to assess their insight into the situation, identify and address any concerns they might have and enable explanation of management plans. Clear explanations are needed, particularly about treatment issues such as hydration when the family will almost certainly need to be reassured that the patient is not dying because of dehydration but because of the disease. If possible, have conversations early when the patient is well enough to be involved and before the difficult issues arise.

Symptom control

Common symptoms at the end of life include pain, breathlessness, nausea and vomiting, terminal agitation and respiratory secretions. Appropriate assessment and management of these is key in ensuring a comfortable final stage of life. It is essential to regularly reassess the symptoms, as they will change.

Terminal agitation

Due to a combination of physical and psychosocial factors (Table 12),

some patients may become agitated or restless as death approaches. Because of these potential problems the following points are important.

- Have the patient continue with analgesia and other drugs for symptom control.

- If the patient has a full bladder, manage this with catheterisation.

- Suppositories or an enema may be necessary to relieve constipation.

- More than ever, the patient will need a calm environment and good nursing care.

- Unnecessary treatments should be stopped.

If these measures do not control agitation, specific drug treatments may be needed (Table 13).

Respiratory secretions

Respiratory secretions may accumulate in patients who are too weak to cough, resulting in a 'rattling' noise. This can be a cause of distress to both the patient and the relatives. If this does occur, consider non-pharmacological measures first, such as positioning the patient on their side. If drug treatment is required it can include the following.

- Hyoscine hydrobromide 0.4 mg sc prn or 1.2–2.4 mg continuous

TABLE 13 DRUG TREATMENT OF TERMINAL RESTLESSNESS AND AGITATION

Drug	Preferred route of administration	Dose
Midazolam (anxiety and distress)	Subcutaneous	10–60 mg continuous infusion over 24 hours
Levomepromazine (anxiety, distress, more sedating and antiemetic)	Subcutaneous	12.5–250 mg continuous infusion over 24 hours
Haloperidol (also antiemetic)	Subcutaneous	1.5–10 mg continuous infusion over 24 hours
Lorazepam (anxiety and breathlessness)	Sublingual	0.5–3.0 mg od

FURTHER READING

Back IN. Terminal restlessness in patients with advanced disease. *Palliative Med.* 1992; 6: 292–8.

Bennett M, Lucas V, Brennan M, *et al.* Using anti-muscarinic drugs in the management of death rattle: evidence-based guidelines for palliative care. *Palliative Med.* 2002; 16: 369–74.

Higgs R. The diagnosis of dying. *J. R. Coll. Physicians Lond.* 1999; 2: 110–12.

NHS End of Life Care initiative. Available at http://www.endoflifecare.nhs.uk/.

subcutaneous infusion over 24 hours. Such a dose may be sedative and in rare cases can result in agitation.

- Glycopyrronium bromide 0.4 mg sc prn or 1.2–2.4 mg continuous subcutaneous infusion over 24 hours. This has a slower onset of action than hyoscine hydrobromide, but has a longer duration of action and is less sedating.

Holistic care

It is essential that all the needs of the patient and the family are met, not just the physical ones. Identify and address any outstanding psychosocial issues and ask whether there are particular religious or spiritual requirements for the patient when coming to the end of life.

Place of care

Many patients wish to die at home, but despite this only around 25% do so. Whilst patients do spend the majority of their last year of life at home, they tend to die in institutions such as hospitals, nursing homes and hospices. There are several reasons for this.

- Patients may change their minds about the care they need as death approaches.

- Many come to feel that their illness is too great a burden for their relatives.

- There is a lack of nursing care available for patients at home.

- The patient's symptoms have worsened.

- Requests for hospital admissions are sometimes made from deputising services or other GPs who are unfamiliar with the patient and his or her wishes.

A number of new initiatives have been introduced to try to optimise the provision and planning of care for patients with life-limiting illnesses at key stages of their disease journey: the Gold Standards Framework focuses on care in the community in the last year of life, the Liverpool Care Pathway gives guidance on care in the last few days of life and the Preferred Place of Care project attempts to identify a patient's wishes on their place of death and facilitate this. With advance planning it is often possible to support patients at home for their end-of-life care and prevent unnecessary or unwanted hospital admissions.

2.9 Specialist palliative care services

Specialist palliative care is available in all settings: hospital, hospice and community. Both the NHS and voluntary sector provide palliative care services, with the precise configuration varying by region. This care is holistic and covers four domains: physical, psychological, social and spiritual. It is provided by a multiprofessional team, the core members of which are specialist doctors and nurses, with extended input coming from other groups including social workers, physiotherapists, occupational therapists, spiritual advisors and psychologists.

Inpatient units

Specialist palliative care inpatient units are found in a number of locations. They may be attached to acute NHS hospitals or be stand-alone units on separate sites, which are often funded by the voluntary sector. Patients are admitted for symptom control, rehabilitation and end-of-life care; some units also offer respite care for the benefit of

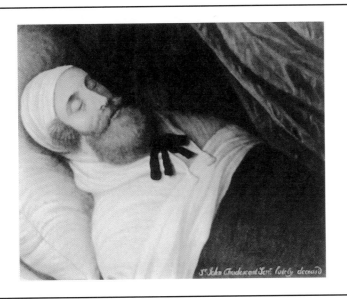

▲ **Fig. 10** St John Transcendent, lately deceased.

'hands-on' nursing care, either as part of a Hospice at Home scheme or via Marie Curie nurses, that can provide some night-time care in the home.

Hospital palliative care teams

These have palliative medicine consultants and specialist nurses as their core members. They are usually advisory services, working with the different hospital teams to assist in the management of patients with palliative care needs.

FURTHER READING

Doyle D. The provision of palliative care. In Doyle D, Hanks GWC and MacDonald N, eds. *Oxford Textbook of Palliative Medicine*, 2nd edn. Oxford: Oxford Medical Publications, 1997: 41–55.

NHS End of Life Care initiative. Available at http://www.endoflifecare.nhs.uk/.

patients and carers. The emphasis of the treatment these units provide is on improving quality of life and dealing with symptoms effectively. The units may also offer other services, such as day therapy and outpatient services, which can provide medical and nursing input, lymphoedema management, complementary therapies and psychological and bereavement support.

Community nurses

Clinical nurse specialists in palliative care (sometimes called Macmillan nurses) work locally in an advisory capacity, providing advice and support to the primary care team on managing the palliative care needs of community patients. A wider multiprofessional team, based at a local hospice or hospital, usually supports the community nurses. Some areas are also able to offer

Final note

If possible, death should be peaceful (Fig. 10).

3.1 Self-assessment questions

Question 1

Clinical scenario

A woman with advanced carcinoma of the breast is admitted with new symptoms of drowsiness and confusion. She had been discharged from hospital 3 weeks previously following a pathological fracture of her humerus. Pain control during her previous admission had been difficult but is now well controlled on MST Continus 200 mg bd, which she has been taking for 4 weeks.

Question

What is the most likely cause of her symptoms?

Answers

A The large dose of morphine prescribed

B Hypercalcaemia

C Morphine accumulation due to renal failure

D An opioid overdose

E Cerebral metastases

Question 2

Clinical scenario

A 78-year-old woman with carcinoma of the ovary presents with colicky abdominal pain and nausea and vomiting. Her abdomen is distended with reduced bowel sounds.

Question

Which of the following is the most appropriate antiemetic?

Answers

A Cyclizine 50 mg sc

B Domperidone 20 mg po

C Metoclopramide 10 mg sc

D Granisetron 1 mg iv

E Cyclizine 50 mg po

Question 3

Clinical scenario

A 60-year-old man with metastatic renal cell carcinoma presents with increased lower back pain and shooting pain radiating down his left leg. He is taking MST Continus 30 mg bd and the pain has not responded to two breakthrough doses of Oramorph 10 mg.

Question

Which of the following is the most appropriate change to his analgesia?

Answers

A Increase MST Continus to 50 mg bd

B Add paracetamol 1 g qds

C Add diclofenac 75 mg bd

D Switch to fentanyl patch 25 µg/hour

E Add gabapentin 100 mg tds

Question 4

Clinical scenario

A 75-year-old man with metastatic prostate cancer is in the terminal phase of his illness and has been unresponsive but settled for 48 hours. His pain has been controlled for the past 24 hours with morphine 15 mg sc via a syringe driver. The nurses have reported that he has become increasingly agitated overnight with no response to a stat dose of morphine 2.5 mg sc.

Question

What initial change to his management is appropriate?

Answers

A Increase morphine in syringe driver to 20 mg

B Increase frequency of prn doses of morphine

C Trial of a prn dose of midazolam 2.5 mg sc

D Addition of midazolam 10 mg to syringe driver

E Trial of prn lorazepam 0.5 mg sl

Question 5

Clinical scenario

A 73-year-old man with carcinoma of the bronchus is admitted with worsening dyspnoea and severe pleuritic chest pain. He last left his house 4 weeks ago and spends much of the day in bed. You suspect a pulmonary embolism; the CXR is unhelpful.

Question

What would you consider the most appropriate treatment option?

Answers

A None, pending the result of a ventilation–perfusion scan

B Give analgesia, but no investigation or treatment

C Start an NSAID and commence warfarin

D Low-molecular-weight (LMW) heparin until ventilation–perfusion scan confirms or refutes diagnosis

E Give analgesia and start LMW heparin

Question 6

Clinical scenario

A 35-year-old woman with non-Hodgkin's lymphoma was commenced by her GP on MST Continus 30 mg bd for pain last week. Her pain is now controlled but her bowels have not been opened for 3 days.

Question

What is the most appropriate management?

Answers

A Phosphate enema

B Glycerin suppositories

C Stat dose of senna

D Fybogel

E Regular senna

Question 7

Clinical scenario

A 52-year-old man with prostate cancer has been commenced on modified-release oxycodone 60 mg bd for his bony pain with good effect. He has not been given any breakthrough medication.

Question

What should you prescribe?

Answers

A Oxycodone modified release 20 mg

B Codeine 30 mg prn

C Oxycodone immediate release 20 mg

D Paracetamol 1 g

E Morphine immediate release 40 mg

Question 8

Clinical scenario

A 35-year-old woman having palliative chemotherapy for breast cancer still has persistent nausea 5 days after her chemotherapy despite domperidone and dexamethasone prophylaxis.

Question

What is the most appropriate drug to bring her nausea under control?

Answers

A Granisetron 1 mg po

B Metoclopramide 10 mg po

C Haloperidol 1.5 mg po

D Cyclizine 50 mg po

E Prochlorperazine 25 mg po

Question 9

Clinical scenario

A 57-year-old woman with multiple myeloma is taking immediate-release morphine 15 mg 4-hourly that is controlling her pain but she finds the frequent dosing regimen burdensome.

Question

What alteration would you make to her drug regimen?

Answers

A Change to morphine immediate release 20 mg qds

B Change to morphine modified release 45 mg bd

C Change to fentanyl patch 75 µg/hour

D Change to morphine modified release 30 mg bd

E Change to morphine immediate release 15 mg qds

Question 10

Clinical scenario

A 55-year-old man with multiple myeloma is experiencing increased bony pain in his lumbar spine. His current FBC shows haemoglobin 9.6 g/dL (normal range 11–16), white cell count 14×10^9/L (normal range 4–11) and platelets 76×10^9/L (normal range 150–400). He is currently taking two co-codamol tablets qds. You are asked to advise regarding his pain medications.

Question

What would you prescribe?

Answers

A Diclofenac SR 75 mg bd

B Paracetamol 1 g qds

C Morphine modified release 30 mg bd

D Zoledronic acid 4 mg iv.

E Morphine immediate release 10 mg 4-hourly

Question 11

Clinical scenario

A 25-year-old woman with acute myeloid leukaemia has been experiencing episodes of difficulty breathing in the evenings that predominantly occur when her husband leaves for his night shift. Investigations have shown no physiological cause for her breathlessness. Her GP has referred her for psychological support and her first appointment is in 2 weeks' time.

Question

What would be the most appropriate intervention while she awaits counselling?

Answers

A Morphine immediate release 15 mg prn

B Lorazepam 0.5 mg sl prn

C Temazepam 10 mg nightly

D Home oxygen

E Amitriptyline 25 mg nightly

Question 12

Clinical scenario

The nursing staff report that a 45-year-old woman with metastatic breast cancer is low in mood and has been non-compliant with her analgesic medication.

Question

Select which two of the following are criteria for the diagnosis of depression in this patient?

Answers

A Fatigue

B Weight loss of 13 kg in the previous month

C Tearful response when questioned about her prognosis

D Expressing thoughts about ending her life

E Poor mobility

F Loss of appetite

G Past history of depression as a teenager

H Weight gain of 6.5 kg in the past month

I No interest in seeing her new grand-daughter

J Refusal of further chemotherapy

Question 13

Clinical scenario

A 68-year-old man with carcinoma of the bronchus and chronic obstructive pulmonary disease (COPD) presents with worsening breathlessness and pleuritic chest pain. He is afebrile. On a previous admission he had been noted to have a small pleural effusion and mild right heart failure.

Question

What are the two most likely diagnoses in this patient?

Answers

A Progression of his carcinoma of the bronchus

B Chest infection

C COPD exacerbation

D Pulmonary emboli

E Worsening right heart failure

F Anxiety

G Superior vena cava obstruction

H Acute coronary syndrome

I Increasing pleural effusion

J Radiotherapy-induced fibrosis

Question 14

Clinical scenario

It is Friday afternoon and you are reviewing the patients before the weekend. You see an 82-year-old woman who has adenocarcinoma of an unknown primary and who has been slowly deteriorating over the past week to the point of being bedbound and struggling with oral intake. Her pain is well controlled with regular oral morphine but the nurses report that she has become more chesty today and they feel that she is getting worse.

Question

What are the two most important measures you would take in case of further deterioration over the weekend?

Answers

A Start intravenous fluids

B CXR

C Prescribe prn subcutaneous morphine

D Refer her to a dietitian

E Broad-spectrum intravenous antibiotics to cover chest sepsis

F Convert oral morphine to fentanyl patch

G Prescribe prn subcutaneous glycopyrronium

H Insert nasogastric tube for feeding and medications

I Increase frequency of nursing observations to monitor for deterioration

J Refer for chest physiotherapy

Question 15

Clinical scenario

You are asked to review a 40-year-old woman with metastatic ovarian carcinoma. A CT scan shows multiple levels of obstruction and dilated loops of small bowel. She is only managing sips of water orally and has intermittent vomiting. She is complaining of constipation and generalised aching abdominal pain. She has been taking co-codamol only.

Question

What are the two most important immediate-management steps?

Answers

A Insert nasogastric tube

B Urgent surgical opinion

C Metoclopramide 30 mg continuous subcutaneous infusion over 24 hours

D Senna two tablets bd

E Buscopan 60 mg continuous subcutaneous infusion over 24 hours

F Immediate-release morphine 10 mg po 4-hourly

G Paracetamol 1 g iv qds

H Diamorphine 10 mg continuous subcutaneous infusion over 24 hours

I Co-danthramer liquid 10 mL po bd

J Cyclizine 150 mg continuous subcutaneous infusion over 24 hours

Question 16

Clinical scenario

A 66-year-old man with oesophageal carcinoma and bony metastases is now unable to swallow his oral medication. He is on the ward awaiting insertion of a percutaneous enterogastrostomy (PEG) tube for feeding. His pain was previously well controlled on MST Continus 45 mg bd.

Question

Which two of the following would be appropriate regular and breakthrough analgesics in this case?

Answers

A Fentanyl patch 25 µg/hour and diamorphine 5 mg sc prn

B Diamorphine 30 mg csci over 24 hours and morphine immediate release 15 mg po prn

C Diamorphine 90 mg csci over 24 hours and diamorphine 15 mg sc prn

D Fentanyl 25 µg/hour and morphine immediate release 15 mg po prn

E Diamorphine 30 mg csci over
24 hours and diamorphine
5 mg sc prn

F Oxycodone 60 mg csci over
24 hours and oxycodone
10 mg sc prn

G Fentanyl patch 50 µg/hour and
diamorphine 5 mg sc prn

H Morphine 45 mg iv background
over 24 hours via a patient-
controlled analgesia pump
with 2–5 mg bolus

I Diamorphine 30 mg csci over
24 hours and diamorphine
10 mg sc prn

J Morphine 90 mg csci over
24 hours and morphine 15 mg
sc prn

3.2 Answers to self-assessment questions

Answer to Question 1

B

Hypercalcaemia is a common
problem in patients with breast
cancer and bony metastases;
drowsiness and confusion are
common presenting symptoms.
The large dose of morphine
prescribed is an unlikely cause
because the patient has been on
a stable dose and sedation occurs
at the start of opioid therapy or
when a dose is changed. Morphine
accumulation due to renal failure
is an unlikely cause as there are no
other symptoms of opioid toxicity
reported, eg myoclonus, which
would occur with renal failure
and opioid metabolite accumulation.
An opioid overdose is also an
unlikely cause as the patient is
on a stable dose and has no other
symptoms or signs of opioid toxicity.
There is no other history given to
indicate that cerebral metastases
are the cause.

Answer to Question 2

A

Cyclizine is first-line choice for
nausea and vomiting in bowel
obstruction. Prokinetics such as
domperidone and metoclopramide
are contraindicated in bowel
obstruction due to the risk of
perforation. Granisetron should
be used for chemo-induced nausea
and vomiting, and can worsen
constipation. With regard to
cyclizine, if vomiting is established
then a parenteral route should be
used as oral absorption will be
compromised.

Answer to Question 3

E

The history is typical of
neuropathic pain and gabapentin
is an appropriate co-analgesic to be
commenced. If pain is not opioid
sensitive, then increasing the dose or
changing the intake route is unlikely
to improve symptom control.
Paracetamol and diclofenac are of
limited benefit for neuropathic pain.

Answer to Question 4

C

Benzodiazepines are the first-line
management for terminal agitation
and a trial of parenteral therapy is
indicated to assess response before
commencing regular therapy. A
parenteral route is more appropriate
at this stage of the patient's illness. If
agitation is not due to pain, opioids
are unhelpful and may worsen
agitation.

Answer to Question 5

E

It is essential to commence
symptomatic management as well
as appropriate disease-modifying
therapy. It is important to treat
the pain as well as the underlying
cause. Diagnosis will help to guide
appropriate long-term therapy: this
is important even in patients who
are being managed palliatively.
Ventilation–perfusion scan is unlikely
to be helpful given the underlying
pulmonary disease. Warfarin and
NSAIDs should not be used together
as there is a significant risk of
bleeding; LMW heparin is the drug
of choice for anticoagulation in
palliative patients.

Answer to Question 6

E

A regular laxative should be
commenced on initiation of regular
opioid therapy. Oral therapy is first
choice in this situation. Laxatives
should always be given regularly, and
a prn dose will not control symptoms.
Bulk-forming laxatives are unpleasant
to take and of limited use.

Answer to Question 7

C

Breakthrough analgesia should be
one-sixth of the total 24-hour dose
and should be an immediate-release
formulation such as oxycodone
20 mg. Modified-release preparations
are for regular use only, not prn
administration. If a patient is on
a regular strong opioid, then
breakthrough medication should
also be a strong opioid. Where
possible, the same opioid should
be used for both regular and
breakthrough doses.

Answer to Question 8

A

$5HT_3$ antagonists are first-line
therapy in treating chemotherapy-
related nausea and vomiting.
Metoclopramide, haloperidol
and cyclizine may be helpful as
adjuncts but not as first-line

treatment. Prochlorperazine is of limited use in palliative care.

Answer to Question 9

B

The modified-release dose should be the total 24-hour dose divided by 2, ie $15 \times 6 = 90$ mg/24 hours, so $90/2 = 45$ mg bd. There is no benefit in increasing the dose at a decreased frequency, as it will provide inadequate pain relief: a regular immediate-release preparation should be given 4-hourly. As symptoms are well controlled with oral morphine, there is no indication that the drug should be changed and the dose of fentanyl sugested is significantly higher than the current morphine dose.

Answer to Question 10

E

Titration with an immediate-release strong opioid is the management of choice. Diclofenac is contraindicated with anaemia and low platelet count. Paracetamol is inappropriate as co-codamol already contains a therapeutic dose of paracetamol. Zoledronic acid is a long-term intervention and will not improve immediate symptoms.

Answer to Question 11

B

Short-acting benzodiazepines are indicated for the management of acute anxiety. Opioids are used in low doses for the management of breathlessness. Temazepam is good for night sedation but less useful in acute anxiety. This pattern of symptoms is unlikely to be due to hypoxia and should not be treated with oxygen. Amitriptyline is not first-line treatment for anxiety.

Answer to Question 12

D and I

Suicidal thoughts should always be taken seriously and explored to gauge actual suicidal risk. Her reaction to her grand-daughter shows an uncharacteristic lack of interest in a positive family event. These two factors should raise a high index of suspicion of depression. Fatigue, weight loss, poor mobility, loss of appetite and weight gain are all non-specific symptoms that may be related to the underlying malignancy. A tearful response is a normal response to a life-limiting illness. Teenage depression is not predictive of adult psychiatric pathology. Refusal of further chemotherapy may be a rational decision in the context of her illness.

Answer to Question 13

A and D

Coexisting breathlessness with a pleuritic-type pain are characteristic of local disease progression involving the pleura or pulmonary emboli. Absence of pyrexia or other symptoms of infection make chest infection less likely. COPD exacerbation, worsening right heart failure, superior vena cava obstruction, increasing pleural effusion and radiotherapy-induced fibrosis would not explain concurrent pleuritic chest pain. Anxiety may present with chest pain but this is unlikely to be pleuritic in character. In acute coronary syndrome, pain is not typically pleuritic and other symptoms are likely to be present.

Answer to Question 14

C and G

The patient is clearly in the terminal phase of her illness and the focus should be on symptomatic palliation with the provision of adequate analgesia and other symptom control measures to combat probable symptoms. Starting intravenous fluids will not benefit symptoms or increase prognosis. CXR will not change management plan and is a burdensome investigation. Decreased oral intake is a normal phenomenon at the end of life. Broad-spectrum intravenous antibiotics, nasogastric tube and chest physiotherapy would be burdensome and unlikely to improve symptom control at this stage of the illness. The preferred route of administration of analgesics in the terminal phase is by subcutaneous infusion. Routine observations should be discontinued but regular clinical review with the focus on symptom control is required.

Answer to Question 15

H and J

Symptoms are established, so analgesics and antiemetics should be given regularly. The preferred route is by continuous subcutaneous infusion. Optimal medical management to control symptoms is indicated before invasive interventions such as a nasogastric tube are required. Surgery is less likely to be helpful when multiple levels of disease are present. Prokinetics are contraindicated in mechanical bowel obstruction due to the risk of perforation. Stimulant laxatives are also contraindicated in mechanical bowel obstruction due to the risk of perforation. Buscopan is helpful for colicky rather than background abdominal pain. She has established vomiting so medication should be given parenterally. Patients who are already established on opioids (co-codamol) should continue with opioids via an appropriate route (sc).

Answer to Question 16

A and E

The preferred route for medication should be parenteral; subcutaneous or transdermal (in stable pain only). The intravenous route is rarely indicated in palliative care patients. The oral route should be avoided here as the patient has dysphagia. A fentanyl patch 25 µg/hour is equivalent to oral morphine (60–90 mg/24 hours) so it is the correct starting dose. Appropriate breakthrough diamorphine should be prescribed: the correct dose conversion from oral morphine to diamorphine is one-third of the total oral dose in 24 hours (45 × 2 = 90 mg/24 hours, 90/3 = 30 mg). The correct breakthrough dose is one-sixth of the total 24-hour dose (30/6 = 5 mg prn).

The correct dose conversion from oral morphine to parenteral oxycodone is one-quarter of the total oral dose in 24 hours (45 × 2 = 90 mg/24 hours, 90/4 = 20–25 mg).

The correct dose conversion from oral morphine to parenteral morphine is half of the total oral dose in 24 hours (45 × 2 = 90 mg/24 hours, 90/2 = 45 mg).

MEDICINE FOR THE ELDERLY

Authors:

R Morgan, CG Nicholl and KJ Wilson

Editor:

CG Nicholl

Editor-in-Chief:

JD Firth

1.1 History-taking

1.1.1 Frequent falls

Letter of referral to elderly care outpatient clinic

Dear Doctor,

Re: Mrs Angela Benning, aged 83 years

Thank you for seeing this retired headmistress who lives alone and is normally fully independent. However, over the past 2 months she has fallen over several times. She makes light of the problem, but when she fell last week she severely bruised her left hip and has not been able to leave her flat since. She has a long history of hypertension and takes bendroflumethiazide 2.5 mg once daily; she also has osteoarthritis of her hips and knees for which she takes paracetamol regularly. She is registered as partially sighted secondary to age-related macular degeneration. She has no other significant past medical history and takes no other medication.

Her daughter (who is a health visitor) spends every other weekend locally, but she lives 80 miles away. She has become increasingly concerned about these falls and is keen for them to be sorted out.

Yours sincerely,

Introduction

Falls in older people are usually multifactorial. As described in Section 2.1, the effect of her various diseases and drugs (Table 1) will interact with the background of ageing changes, loss of fitness and social factors. The effects of normal ageing (eg increased postural sway) make falls more common with advancing years and potentially more serious (eg osteoporosis). Toddlers fall, but they are designed to! Sorting out falls requires a multidisciplinary, multi-agency approach and good communication with the patient and her family.

- Why is she falling?
- What other factors may be contributing?
- Have there been any serious consequences?
- Is she on bone protection?

History of the presenting problem

There may be clues in the patient's history to explain why she falls. In routine clinical practice it would be essential to obtain a corroborative story from the patient's daughter (although she may not know exact details or the cause), carers or GP. This will not be available in the context of PACES, but specifically ask the following questions.

- How many falls have there been, and over what period? If the falls are new, then there may be an acute precipitating event, such as MI, hypotension secondary to a gastrointestinal bleed or a change in function because of a urinary tract infection.

- Do the falls occur outside (this means a better prognosis as she is still able to get out) or in the home?

TABLE 1 RISK FACTORS FOR FALLING	
Risk factor	**Notes**
Osteoarthritis	Most common contributing factor to falls
Polypharmacy	Remember to ask about over-the-counter medication and alcohol intake
Visual impairment	Presbyopia, glaucoma, age-related macular degeneration (ARMD), cataracts
Cognitive impairment/dementia	Directly, due to lack of awareness regarding limitations and dangers, ataxia, apraxia, visuospatial problems, wandering and agnosia; indirectly, secondary to psychotropic medications
Postural hypotension	Commonest causes are medications, cardiovascular disease, diabetes and Parkinson's-plus syndromes
Acute event leading to hypotension	Myocardial infarction (MI), pulmonary embolism or gastrointestinal bleed
Gait abnormality	Parkinson's disease, previous stroke, cerebellar disease and fixed joints due to osteoarthritis

- What was she doing before the falls? For example, standing up (consider postural hypotension), turning or reaching up for something (consider vertebrobasilar insufficiency).

- Do the falls occur at a similar time?

- Was there a prodrome of nausea, sweating and feeling hot? (Indicates vasovagal event/syncope.)

- Did she feel dizzy? (Indicates cardiac/drug problem.)

- Does the patient have any palpitations? Remember, however, that intermittent atrial flutter/fibrillation is common and not necessarily the cause of her falls (Fig. 1).

- Is there true vertigo, ie the illusion of rotatory movement? (Indicates ear/brainstem lesions.)

- Has she ever blacked out and if so for how long? (A transient loss of consciousness suggests a vasovagal event/syncope.)

- Was she able to get up herself or did she have to wait for help?

- Was she confused when she came round? (This would make syncope less likely.)

- Were there features of an epileptic fit, such as incontinence or tongue biting?

- What injuries have been sustained? Take particular note of fractures, but do not forget subdural haematoma and anaemia secondary to a large haematoma.

- Was she pushed? (Indicates elder abuse.)

> **To obtain full information about the fall, remember SPLATT:**
>
> *Symptoms at the time*
> *Previous falls*
> *Location*
> *Activity at the time*
> *Time*
> *Trauma sustained*

Other relevant history

- Symptoms to suggest underlying neurological or cardiac pathology, eg symptoms of Parkinson's disease. This is associated with high risk of falls secondary to poor postural control, loss of autonomic reflexes and shuffling gait.

- Degree of visual impairment: has with vision deteriorated recently?

- Loss of height, history of maternal hip fracture and early menopause: should she be on treatment for osteoporosis?

Past medical history
Ask about the following.

- Strokes, evident if CT brain scan shows multiple infarcts (Fig. 2).

- Epilepsy.

- History of cognitive impairment: she may tell you she has been worried about her memory lately.

- Ischaemic heart disease.

- Arthritis: knees, hips and the lower back are the most important areas in this context, but arms are helpful for getting up out of a chair.

- Previous fractures: think about osteoporosis.

Social history
Detailed information is essential.

- Does she live in a house with stairs, a bungalow (which may still have steps between rooms), sheltered accommodation, a ground- or a first-floor flat, or a residential home?

- Are there rails, bath aids, etc?

- Is there good lighting – especially important in stairways?

- Can she get out of her house? Even in the UK, sunshine is the major source of vitamin D.

- How much alcohol does she normally drink? Has her supply been cut since she has been housebound?

- Elderly people with no psychiatric illness sometimes live surrounded by all manner of junk in the 'senile squalor' (Diogenes) syndrome, which makes it hard not to trip.

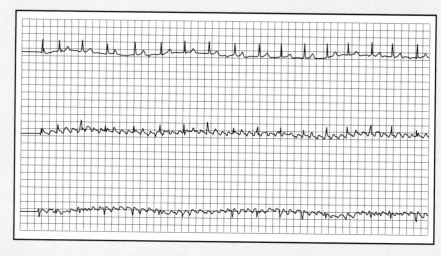

▲**Fig. 1** ECG showing atrial flutter/fibrillation.

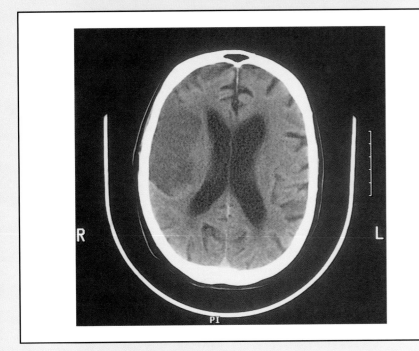

▲ **Fig. 2** CT scan of the brain showing multiple infarcts.

Drug history

Older people are more susceptible to drug side effects, and are also more likely to suffer serious consequences because of them. Many of the elderly are on many different medications, and this raises the additional possibility of drug interactions. Remember to ask about over-the-counter medications, eg decongestants and antihistamines are sedative.

Plan for investigation and management

In routine clinical practice you would perform a full physical examination. In PACES it would be sensible to explain to the patient that you would do this, before proposing investigations and management to help prevent further falls and reduce the consequences if they do occur.

Investigations should be guided by the history, but consider the following.

Blood tests to exclude 'silent' illnesses

- FBC: anaemia, macrocytosis of vitamin B_{12} deficiency or high alcohol intake, and neutrophilia.

- C-reactive protein: acute-phase response to infection.

- Creatinine, urea and electrolytes, glucose: renal function, dehydration and hypoglycaemia/ hyperglycaemia.

- Troponin: if it is an acute presentation, this may reveal silent MI.

- Creatine kinase (CK): if it is an acute presentation, rhabdomyolysis is a risk after a long lie.

- Liver profile: in an acute presentation a rise in alanine transaminase, which occurs later than a rise in troponin or CK after MI, may be found incidentally; an elevated value may also raise suspicion of alcoholism.

- Bone profile: raised alkaline phosphatase in vitamin D deficiency.

- Thyroid function.

Exclude infection (if an acute presentation)

- Midstream urine.

- CXR: look for rib fractures, pneumonia and kyphosis suggesting osteoporosis.

Cardiac tests

- ECG: rhythm, ischaemia and conduction defect. Check for long QT interval.

- 24-hour Holter monitoring: check for arrhythmias and long pauses. Ask the patient to keep a diary of symptoms (if there are any) when on the monitor to aid interpretation. Although the detection rate is low, this is a relatively cheap and non-invasive test.

Neurological tests

- CT brain scan: look in particular for evidence of vascular disease, space-occupying lesion and normal pressure hydrocephalus.

- Electroencephalography: if there is clinical suspicion of epilepsy.

Other tests

If the history is suggestive of carotid sinus sensitivity or neurocardiogenic syncope, perform the following.

- Check the patient's BP lying down, immediately on standing, and then repeat over 3 minutes: you will get more reproducible results if you do it yourself!

- Carotid sinus massage: first check that there is no history of recent MI or previous ventricular tachycardia. There is also debate on what to do if there is a carotid bruit: it is accepted that a bruit does not correlate well with carotid stenosis, but if you are concerned then arrange carotid Doppler first (the risk of neurological sequelae is quoted to be 0.14%).

- Tilt-table testing: this measures the BP with every beat of the heart, both when the patient is lying flat and when tilted at 70°. You need to explain to the patient that she will be strapped to the bed and have ECG leads in place, together with a BP cuff and a finger sensor. You should warn the patient that the test will continue until she blacks out or it is clear that there is no neurocardiogenic cause.

Management

Multiple interventions work best, which would generally include:

- review of all medications, stopping any hypotensive agents that are unnecessary and switching other drugs to those less likely to lower BP if possible;

- physiotherapy review;

- occupational therapy review.

Once you have considered all the causes for her falls (Table 1), identify those that are amenable to treatment. Treat specific diseases, for example is the problem worse now because she also has cataracts? If this is the case, should she be referred for surgery now? In contrast, if her visual problem is irreversible (eg worsening of ARMD), should she now be registered blind? If visual impairment is a significant issue, she should also be referred to a visual aids centre.

In the broader context, think about the following.

- Manage other problems that increase the risk of falls.

- Improve general health and fitness (there is some evidence that Tai Chi improves balance).

- Treat osteoporosis in case she falls again.

- Provide education and support (for both the patient and her daughter): aim to reduce the likelihood of another fall and minimise the consequences if it does happen. A phone and duvet on the floor can be life-saving. Try to educate the daughter to support her mother's right to take a risk and remain in her own home.

- Provide contact numbers for patient-based societies, eg Parkinson's Disease Society and the Stroke Association.

The multidisciplinary team has a key role in assessment and management (see Section 1.4.2). The benefits of reducing the risks of further falls include the prevention of injuries (including fractures) and therefore hospital admission, and also promotion of the independence of elderly people in the community.

Usually the patient will be fit enough to go home and you can arrange follow-up, preferably in a falls prevention clinic with physiotherapy for balance training. However, you should admit patients who have blacked out with features of a pure cardiac cause, of syncope causing severe injury or of frequent recurrent syncope.

Further discussion

There are many consequences of falls, both acute and chronic:

- hypostatic pneumonia, pressure sores and hypothermia (if she spends time immobile on the ground);

- burns (if she falls near a fire or radiator);

- fear of falling syndrome;

- depression;

- loss of independence and, in more extreme cases, institutionalisation.

The best management of this patient would involve a complete screen to identify her risk factors for falling. All possible risk factors would be addressed; this might include stopping her diuretic, changing her glasses (remembering that bifocal lenses are associated with tripping over pavements), treating cataracts, stopping inappropriate medications and preventing or treating osteoporosis.

1.1.2 Recent onset of confusion

> ### Letter of referral to rapid access medicine for the elderly clinic
>
> Dear Doctor,
>
> **Re: Mrs Debra Bell, aged 89 years**
>
> Thank you for seeing this 89 year old. She recently moved into a warden-supervised flat in this area. Her neighbour became concerned because she was found wandering in the street. She is new to our practice but according to her records her past history includes myocardial infarction (MI), diabetes and arthritis. She had a right total hip replacement 3 months ago. Her medication includes aspirin, lisinopril, digoxin, gliclazide and co-codamol.
>
> On examination, she does seem rather vague and muddled but does not look unwell. Her pulse

is irregular and 78/minute, her
BP is 135/94 mmHg and she has
some crackles at her left base.
I am concerned that she is
developing a chest infection.
I have started her on amoxicillin
500 mg tds, but would appreciate
your urgent assessment of
whether she can remain in
her flat.

Yours sincerely,

Introduction

A diagnosis is essential for
appropriate management. You need
to decide whether this patient is
confused, if this is likely to be acute
or chronic, what the likely cause is
and how ill she is. Whether she can
return home today will depend on
the available support as well as
her clinical state. Well-presented
clothing, clean styled hair and
well-manicured nails speak volumes:
either this is an acute problem or
she has an assiduous carer (who
would usually have brought her
to the clinic).

There are numerous causes of
confusion in older people (Table 2);
in this case the GP suspects a
chest infection, but there are many
possibilities. In the PACES setting
the patient/surrogate will have been
selected or briefed to be able to give
you some information, but this may
not be the case when you are on
take.

History of the presenting problem

Try to get a history from the patient.
Make sure she can hear you. Ask her
about what has happened. Does she
remember meeting her neighbour in
the street and can she explain what
she was doing there? Does she have
any symptoms of a chest infection or
heart failure?

**When taking a history from a
confused patient:**

- keep the questions short;
- sound encouraging and try not to
  rush the patient;
- ask questions in a logical order and
  signpost when you are moving on to
  another area;
- check that you have got the story
  straight.

Other relevant history

The recent move to a warden-
supervised flat suggests significant
pre-existing physical or mental
impairment. Why did she move?
Most acute confusion occurs on a
background of dementia, and you
are looking for evidence of global
cognitive decline. Note her
orientation and short-term memory,
and observe her use of language and
speed of comprehension as you take
the history. However, you will need
information from other sources
before you can make a diagnosis of
dementia. Do not carry out a formal
mental test here (this is part of the
examination), but ask about mood;
the move may have led to isolation
and low spirits. Depression can be
confused with dementia, but they
also frequently coexist.

Assuming there has been a recent
change in the patient's symptoms or
function, the time course will give
you clues to the aetiology: infection
usually takes its toll in a couple of
days, stroke and MI even more
rapidly.

Past history

- Ischaemic heart disease: this
  makes her more likely to have
  cardiac failure, uncontrolled AF or
  MI. Has she been short of breath,
  noticed her pulse racing or had
  any chest pain?

- Diabetes: this increases the
  patient's risk of developing a
  non-ketotic hyperosmolar state,
  having an MI or a stroke, or of
  developing infection such as
  cellulitis. Impaired vision due to
  retinopathy would make her more
  prone to delirium, and impaired
  renal function due to nephropathy
  would increase the risk of toxicity
  from renally excreted drugs.

- Total hip replacement: was
  this because of a fracture
  (suggesting falls and osteoporosis)
  or arthritis? Has she fallen again
  since the operation, hit her
  head and sustained a subdural
  haematoma? If her mobility has
  been poor since her hip surgery,
  then she will be at high risk of
  pulmonary embolism, with her
  confusion perhaps due to hypoxia.
  Are there any features to support
  this diagnosis, eg calf pain,
  pleuritic chest pain, haemoptysis
  or breathlessness?

Drug history

Can she list her drugs for you? The
medications listed in the GP's letter
include aspirin, lisinopril, digoxin
and gliclazide. Consider the
following.

- Ask directly about over-the-
  counter medications, eg ibuprofen
  for joint pain. An NSAID plus
  aspirin may lead to chronic blood
  loss, and severe anaemia may
  present with confusion, although
  more often with lethargy or
  breathlessness.

- Lisinopril: may be responsible for
  electrolyte imbalance or uraemia.

- Digoxin: toxicity usually presents
  with nausea, but this may also
  cause confusion.

- Gliclazide: may have resulted in
  hypoglycaemia, and profound
  nocturnal hypoglycaemia may

TABLE 2 CAUSES OF AN ACUTE CONFUSIONAL STATE

Condition/mechanism		Example	Watch for
Intracranial pathology			
Vascular	Stroke		Frontal stroke with little paresis
Raised pressure	Space-occupying lesion	Primary or secondary malignancy, subdural haematoma or abscess	Cerebral atrophy may minimise mass effect
Parkinson's disease			Subtle signs: the disease, its complications and its treatment all predispose to confusion
Epileptic fit	Post-seizure or status		May present with focal signs
Infection	Meningitis Encephalitis		Neck stiffness may be absent Cranial herpes zoster with few skin lesions
Head injury	Concussion		Elder abuse is more common in confused individuals
Systemic pathology			
Infections	Chest, urine and cellulitis		Pyrexia absent or masked by mouth breathing. Tachypnoea/tachycardia as the only signs of pneumonia. Infectious endocarditis is not common but easily missed
Metabolic	Fluid, electrolyte or acid–base disturbance	Hyponatraemia Hypernatraemia	Drugs, eg thiazides, SSRIs and SIADH Thirst may be blunted in elderly people
	Hypercalcaemia	Hyperparathyroidism Metastatic malignancy Myeloma Excessive antacids	Check for mass in the breast or thyroid, lymphadenopathy and 'invisible' surgical scars (neat healing in elderly people)
	Organ failure		Liver failure is usually obvious, uraemia less so
Endocrine	Diabetes	Hypoglycaemia Hyperglycaemia	Prolonged with glibenclamide Elderly people may present with HONC
	Thyroid	Hypothyroidism Hyperthyroidism	'Myxoedema madness' Confusion often exacerbated by AF
	Addison's disease		
Shock/hypoxia	Pump failure	MI	Chest pain may be absent. The mechanism may be hypotension, LVF or both
		Tachydysrhythmias or bradydysrhythmias	Always exclude hyperthyroidism in fast AF
	Respiratory failure	COPD and end-stage fibrosis	In severe COPD, give nebulisers with air
	Loss of blood volume	Gastrointestinal bleed or a bleed into a hip fracture	Usually apparent, but melaena may be delayed in severe constipation Warfarin, NSAIDs and aspirin are common drugs
	Loss of vascular tone		Overwhelming sepsis (eg intra-abdominal emergency): perforation, obstruction (check for femoral hernia) and mesenteric ischaemia (acidosis and high K^+)
	Severe anaemia		Usually chronic
	Carbon monoxide poisoning		Husband and wife may present together
Nutritional deficiencies		Wernicke's encephalopathy (thiamine deficiency)	Other deficiencies, eg nicotinic acid and vitamin B_{12}, tend to present as chronic confusion
Hypothermia			Check rectal temperature with low-reading thermometer
Unreported discomfort	Hip or pelvic fracture		Missed in agitated confused patients with other pathology, eg stroke
	Faecal impaction/ urinary retention		Rectal examination is essential
Drugs and withdrawal			Prescribed and over-the-counter drugs. Remember steroid psychosis Accidental or intentional overdose
Alcohol and withdrawal			A few days' illness may have prevented the usual intake of alcohol

AF, atrial fibrillation; COPD, chronic obstructive pulmonary disease; HONC, hyperosmolar non-ketotic coma; LVF, left ventricular failure; MI, myocardial infarction; SIADH, syndrome of inappropriate antidiuretic hormone secretion; SSRI, selective serotonin reuptake inhibitor.

result in extended periods of confusion in older people. This is one reason that longer-acting sulphonylureas such as glibenclamide are not recommended in this age group.

- Co-codamol: this contains either 8 or 30 mg codeine with 500 mg paracetamol per tablet. Therapeutic doses of codeine are a potent cause of confusion and constipation in older people, but if the patient is muddled and in pain from her hip then she may have taken an accidental overdose.

If you are unsure whether a drug can cause confusion, always check in the *British National Formulary* (BNF). In PACES it would be fair to tell the examiner that you would do this, but if pushed on the matter try to remember if the drug gets into the brain, or whether its action or side effects could upset homeostasis. You may recall that digoxin toxicity can be associated with altered colour perception: this could be due to an effect on the retinal cones, but it suggests that digoxin crosses the blood–brain barrier; there is a long list of central effects in the BNF. All drugs designed to have an effect on the brain, such as antidepressants, sedatives, antipsychotics, analgesics, drugs for Parkinson's and Alzheimer's disease, and antiepileptics, have confusion as a common side effect.

> 🔑 **Drugs are one of the commonest causes of confusion in the elderly.**

Social history

- Ask about her job before she retired: this may not be helpful, but if she had a responsible job it provides a benchmark to gauge cognitive change.

- Get details about her accommodation: occasionally warden-supervised flats are on the first floor with no lift.

- Assess her functional abilities: check mobility (including with a stick or frame).

- Is she independent or does she have carers and, if so, how many times a day do they visit?

- Is she known to a community psychiatric nurse? If so, make contact later to obtain details of previous psychiatric assessments.

Smoking and drinking

Ask elderly ex-smokers when they gave up: if the patient gave up 20 years ago she may still have notched up considerable pack-years. Elderly alcoholics rarely binge or appear drunk, but they may develop withdrawal symptoms if they stop drinking because of an intercurrent illness or hospital admission. Alcohol and drug withdrawal (or indeed overdose) are often overlooked in old age.

Plan for investigation and management

Explain to the patient that you would perform a full physical examination before organising blood tests, a CXR and a heart tracing. During PACES you should explain in subsequent discussion with the examiner that your examination would include a simple test of cognition, (eg Abbreviated Mental Test or Mini-Mental State Examination), that you would need to get more information before deciding if she can go home (so would ask her permission to ring her warden or any other contacts she has mentioned), and also that if any of the investigations are done in different departments she will need to be taken there by a healthcare

assistant (you should suggest a cup of tea while she is waiting).

Investigations

These will depend on the clinical features, but as non-specific presentation is common the tests marked in italics are advisable in almost all patients.

- *FBC*: anaemia and low mean corpuscular volume (MCV) suggest iron deficiency; high MCV suggests vitamin B_{12} or folate deficiency, hypothyroidism, alcoholism or myelodysplasia (predisposes to infection); neutrophilia suggests infection.

- *Urea, electrolytes and creatinine.*

- *Liver and bone profiles*: γ-glutamyl transpeptidase may need to be measured if alcoholism is suspected, or urgent calcium if for example there is a history of breast cancer.

- Amylase.

- *Cardiac enzymes.*

- D-dimer, but only if there is a history, vital signs or examination findings that could be related to deep vein thrombosis or pulmonary embolism.

- *Glucose.*

- *Thyroid function*: thyroid-stimulating hormone is the best screening test.

- *C-reactive protein.*

- Blood cultures.

- Syphilis serology: rare in the UK (the cases that have caused the recent increase are not in older people); can be confused with yaws in the West Indian population; consent for HIV serology if indicated.

- *Dipstick urine*: a midstream urine or clean catch specimen may be difficult to obtain.

- *ECG.*

- *CXR.*

- *Oxygen saturation*: check arterial blood gases in cases of pneumonia, deranged acid–base balance or hyperglycaemia.

- Carboxyhaemoglobin.

- Blood and urine for drug screen.

- CT brain scan.

- Lumbar puncture.

Management

This will depend on the patient's clinical state (ascertained from history, examination and rapid basic investigations) and what you can find out about her support in the community. If there is no serious acute pathology (eg your findings support the GP's diagnosis), then a return home is the best option, after speaking to the warden and GP (see Section 1.4.1 for further discussion).

1.1.3 Urinary incontinence and immobility

Letter of referral to elderly care outpatient clinic

Dear Doctor,

Re: Mrs Jane Paris, aged 79 years

Please would you review this elderly housewife who is not well known to me. She came to see me last week because she is finding it increasingly difficult to cope at home. She admits that she has been incontinent of urine for the past 18 months, but has been buying pads for herself at her local pharmacist and trying to ignore it. The situation has only come to a head because she has now become immobile, and

is therefore unable to get out of the house. She has a history of hypertension and takes co-amilofruse 5/40 once daily.

Many thanks for your help in the management of her incontinence.

Yours sincerely,

Introduction

Consider the problems of incontinence and immobility separately at first, although one diagnosis could explain both, eg incontinence is an early finding in normal-pressure hydrocephalus and Parkinson's disease (PD) is a common cause of urge incontinence.

> Chronic disease may be undetected in elderly people because both they and their carers accept problems such as poor mobility, deteriorating memory and incontinence as a normal part of ageing. It is only when the family can no longer cope that medical advice is sought.

History of the presenting problem: immobility

Common causes of immobility are shown in Table 3. The major system limiting mobility will usually be clear.

Neurological

- Onset of symptoms: sudden with a cerebrovascular accident, gradual with PD, progressive with motor neuron disease and stepwise with multi-infarct dementia.

- Specific symptoms: difficulty turning over in bed, freezing or dribbling suggest PD.

Remember that neurological problems affecting motor function may be painful if there is altered tone or muscle wasting that leave joints unsupported.

Musculoskeletal

- Joint pains associated with joint swelling and early-morning stiffness: consider rheumatoid arthritis.

- Pain, deformity and crepitus in knees and hips suggests osteoarthritis.

TABLE 3 COMMON CAUSES OF IMMOBILITY

Cause	Common examples	Less common examples
Neurological	Stroke PD Peripheral neuropathy Cord lesion	Normal-pressure hydrocephalus Cerebellar disease Motor neuron disease
Musculoskeletal	All types of arthritis Painful feet Myopathy	Myositis
Psychiatric	Depression Dementia	
Cardiorespiratory	Cardiac failure Angina Chronic lung disease Peripheral vascular disease	
Morbid obesity		

PD, Parkinson's disease.

- Difficulty rising from a chair may indicate proximal myopathy (eg thyrotoxicosis and vitamin D deficiency) or muscle discomfort (eg polymyalgia or polymyositis).

- Bone pain: this may overlap with neurological symptoms, eg vertebral secondaries can present with gradual or sudden cord compression.

Psychiatric

- Loss of appetite, insomnia, poor concentration and anhedonia: suspect depression if these signs are present.

- Poor memory and disorientation: this probably indicates acute or chronic confusion.

Whatever the main cause, a number of factors may contribute and a vicious cycle may have developed so that loss of fitness becomes a major component. Recurrent falls of any cause lead to reduced mobility due to fear of further falls.

Other relevant history: immobility

Is there anything to suggest major organ pathology, a rheumatic disorder or an underlying malignancy?

Past history

Very severe osteoarthritis may be the sequel of childhood conditions (eg congenital dislocation of the hip and osteomyelitis), and a short leg invariably leads to scoliosis. Has the patient had multiple hip or knee replacements, or an inflammatory arthritis?

Drugs

Statins are now the commonest cause of muscle pain. Also, is she experiencing postural hypotension due to her co-amilofruse?

History of the presenting problem: incontinence

There are several types of incontinence, which are managed differently, so a correct diagnosis is essential.

> Distinguish between urge, stress and overflow incontinence, or a mixed picture: the managements are different.

The history usually helps determine the probable cause, so ask the patient to keep a continence diary recording times and volumes of voiding, and any accidents. Ask specifically about the following.

- Does she have a frequent, sudden and overwhelming desire to pass urine, often not reaching the toilet in time? Does she have to pass urine frequently during the night?

Either circumstance would indicate urge incontinence.

- Does she pass small amounts of urine on coughing, laughing or exercising? If so, this suggests stress incontinence.

- Is she constipated? This can cause urinary retention and overflow incontinence.

- Does she have dysuria and frequency? If so, indicates urinary tract infection.

Ask men about poor stream, dribbling and nocturia suggestive of prostatism.

Other relevant history: incontinence

Past history

Ask about the number and size of any babies the patient had and about trauma to the perineum. Also enquire about any pelvic surgery, particularly hysterectomy and oophorectomy. Symptoms such as vaginal dryness and dyspareunia correlate better with atrophic vaginitis than mucosal appearance.

Drug history

Remember that alcohol, caffeine and aspartame all irritate the bladder (Table 4). Check her list of drugs, looking especially for diuretics, anticholinergic drugs and

	Bladder irritation	Sedative effect	Urinary retention	Diuretic effect	Relaxation of prostatic smooth muscle
Alcohol	✓	✓	—	✓	—
Caffeine	✓	—	—	✓	—
Antipsychotic medication (eg chlorpromazine)	—	✓	✓	—	—
Antidepressants (eg lofepramine)	—	✓	✓	—	—
Benzodiazepines (eg diazepam)	—	✓	—	—	—
Alpha-blockers (eg doxazosin)	—	—	—	—	✓
Diuretics (eg furosemide)	—	—	—	✓	—

TABLE 4 DRUGS THAT INCREASE THE RISK OF INCONTINENCE

Station 2: History Taking

sedatives. Does she need to keep taking her co-amilofruse?

Plan for investigation and management

Explain sensitively that you are going to try to find the cause of her difficulty keeping dry because it may be possible to cure the problem, and it can certainly be made less troublesome. She will understand that whatever the cause of the continence problem, her decreased mobility makes it harder to get to the toilet in time: describe a multidisciplinary plan to improve her mobility. Bladder tests will need full explanation and input from a specialist continence nurse would be helpful from diagnosis to management.

> The secret of success is early liaison with the hospital or community continence adviser.

Investigations

These will be dictated by clinical findings, but a range of screening and specific blood tests looking for underlying causes of incontinence and impaired mobility will be appropriate. She will also need appropriate imaging, eg radiographs of affected joints and a CT brain scan.

Specific investigations for her incontinence include the following.

- Urine dipstick: if there are nitrites or leucocytes, send a midstream urine sample. Haematuria needs renal tract ultrasonography and urological assessment.

- Ultrasonography: to assess chronic retention and residual volume.

- Urodynamic studies: these are indicated if there is no improvement in her symptoms

after simple interventions (see Section 2.4).

Management

A generic plan to improve mobility will include the following.

- Treat underlying medical conditions where possible.

- Regular analgesia if pain is a limiting factor.

- Information: education, advice and support to patient and carer (remember patient-based societies).

- Physiotherapist: gait practice, exercise and balance work, also assessment for aids.

- Occupational therapist: providing assessment of the patient and her home.

- Social worker: to assess for benefits (see Section 2.12) and tailor a package of care around the patient's needs.

A generic plan to improve continence will include the following.

- Stopping drugs: any drugs that may contribute to the problem (see Table 4) should be discontinued unless there are pressing reasons why this cannot be done.

- Regular toileting and bladder retraining.

- Improving mobility will help in the management of incontinence of any cause.

- Urge incontinence: the patient will usually benefit from anticholinergic therapy, eg oxybutynin or tolterodine. Start with the lowest dose to reduce the risk of side effects such as confusion.

- Stress incontinence: encourage pelvic floor exercises, but if these

produce no improvement and she is fit for surgery then refer her to a urogynaecologist for bladder neck surgery.

- If all of the above fail, consider pad and pants or an indwelling catheter.

1.1.4 Collapse

Letter of referral to medicine for the elderly outpatient clinic

Dear Doctor,

Re: Mrs Christine Mitchell, aged 79 years

Thank you for seeing this retired accountant who has had several funny turns. She thinks she had one last August, when she remembers finding herself on the sitting room floor, but she did not seek medical help. She had no more trouble until this month, since when she has had two further episodes, both in her own home. On the second occasion her son was with her; he heard a crash and went in to the kitchen to find her on the floor. She had hit her head on the radiator and cut her forehead, but otherwise seemed fine.

Her past history includes hypertension, hiatus hernia, diverticular disease, a left knee replacement in 1999 and a left mastectomy in 1995. Her medication is bendroflumethiazide 2.5 mg, amlodipine 10 mg and furosemide 40 mg *mane*, on which her BP control has been excellent: BP 132/83 mmHg and heart rate 82 bpm regular. On examination she looks well: there is a systolic murmur, but her chest is clear and there is no ankle oedema.

She is remarkably well for her age but admits that she feels anxious about going out in case she collapses in public. I would appreciate your opinion about the likely diagnosis.

Yours sincerely,

Introduction

> A patient who claims 'I must have fallen' may have blacked out briefly.

Collapse with loss of consciousness ranges in severity from sudden death to repeated brief episodes, so it is not surprising that it can be caused by a wide range of conditions. Terminology in this area is confusing and used inconsistently.

- 'Blackout' implies temporary loss of consciousness but says nothing more.

- 'Syncope' is defined as a transient loss of consciousness with the loss of postural tone due to an abrupt reduction of cerebral perfusion. The commonest cause is neurocardiogenic syncope or the common faint (also called vasovagal or vasodepressor syncope), but 'faint' is sometimes used less precisely. Multiple episodes of syncope or near-syncope (a feeling of being about to lose consciousness) are often called 'funny turns' until a definitive diagnostic label can be given. There is considerable overlap between 'syncope' and

'falls' because there is often retrograde amnesia for the loss of consciousness.

- 'Drop attack' describes a dramatic condition in which a patient (usually an elderly woman) drops to the ground without alteration of alertness but finds it impossible to get up straight away: the mechanism is said to be vertebrobasilar insufficiency resulting in brainstem ischaemia (eg compression of the vertebral arteries by cervical osteophytes when the patient looks up).

- 'Adams–Stokes attack' (also called Stokes–Adams or Morgagni–Adams–Stokes disease) is a term reserved for transient collapse with loss of consciousness due to heart block and bradycardia.

In order to remain conscious and upright, an individual needs a functional pump, unimpeded arteries, adequate blood pressure, oxygenated blood containing glucose, cerebral function and normal postural tone. Consideration of these parameters enables the causes of collapse to be listed in a logical fashion (Table 5). The pathogenesis of a collapse may involve several components. Remember that there can be quite marked limb jerking in any form of syncope due to cerebral hypoxia and that, particularly in older people with poor circle of Willis function, hypoxia may lead to an epileptic fit.

History of the presenting problem
Clarify the number of episodes and what the patient was doing at the time of each. Key issues include the following.

- Is there a common pattern? Recurrent episodes with rapid recovery make it most unlikely that a major problem is causing sudden severe hypotension (eg

myocardial infarction, pulmonary embolism or gastrointestinal bleed). If she is always using the vacuum cleaner (or performing some other vigorous activity) when she has an episode, then this is 'effort syncope', and aortic stenosis is relatively common at this age. If an attack is brought on by watching TV, then consider epilepsy. If she can have an attack when lying down and having a nap, then this is not syncope. If she is typically standing up after a meal, postural hypotension is likely; a variety of factors may predispose to this, including drugs for hypertension, diuretics, intercurrent illness (infection), salt and water depletion (diarrhoea and vomiting), neuropathies, recent prolonged bed-rest and Addison's disease.

- Does she get any warning of her attacks and does she have 'near misses' when she manages to sit and avert an attack? These often occur in patients with neurocardiogenic syncope or postural hypotension, but not always.

- Are there any associated symptoms? Ask if she notices a fast or slow heart beat, breathlessness or an aura ('Is anything unusual . . . any odd feelings, funny smells or sounds, or do you see anything funny?').

- How long do her episodes last? When she comes to, has anything happened? Urinary incontinence may occur in syncope as well as epilepsy, but a bitten tongue is very suggestive of a fit.

- Is she back to normal immediately after an episode, apart from being bruised and shaken? It is very rare for transient ischaemia to cause loss of consciousness without leaving significant focal

TABLE 5 CAUSES OF COLLAPSE WITH LOSS OF CONSCIOUSNESS

Overall requirement	Components of normal function	Possible cause of problem
Functional pump	Cardiac muscle function	Ischaemia
	Heart able to contract and relax	Tamponade
	Heart rate	Tachycardia[1]/bradycardia[1] (Adams–Stokes attack)/mixed[1]
	Flow through right heart	Pulmonary stenosis
	Circulation through lungs	Pulmonary hypertension, pulmonary emboli
	Flow through left heart	Mitral stenosis, aortic stenosis, hypertrophic obstructive cardiomyopathy, atrial myxoma
	Flow into great vessels	Aortic dissection, subclavian steal
Adequate venous return to heart		Cough and micturition syncope[1]
Peripheral resistance maintaining BP	Intact autonomic nervous system	Neurocardiogenic syncope[1], many drugs[1], orthostatic hypotension[1], carotid sinus hypersensitivity[1], primary and secondary autonomic failure[1], multisystem atrophy, septic shock
Adequate gas exchange	Breathing and gas exchange	Carbon monoxide poisoning, choking, lung pathology
Adequate oxygen-carrying capacity of blood	Circulating volume and haemoglobin	Major gastrointestinal bleed, severe anaemia
Adequate blood sugar		Hypoglycaemia (usually due to medication for diabetes)
Intact circulation to the brain	Carotids, vertebrals and circle of Willis	Vertebrobasilar insufficiency[1], carotid stenosis[1], stroke
Normal brain function	Normal function of reticular activating system	Epilepsy[1] and drug/alcohol overdose or withdrawal
Normal postural tone	Reciprocal activation of extensors and flexors	Neurocardiogenic syncope[1]

1. Commoner causes of recurrent syncope. The other conditions listed can cause collapse with loss of consciousness, but are unlikely to do so recurrently or are rare.

neurological signs (and a transient ischaemic attack cannot be diagnosed in the absence of clear focal neurological symptoms or signs). Muscle pain and extensive bruising would suggest a tonic–clonic fit, and confusion is usual postictally.

> A diagnosis of transient ischaemic attack should never be made in the absence of a clear history or findings of focal neurological signs.

In routine clinical practice (although clearly not possible in PACES) you would certainly try to confirm the history with the patient's son, particularly asking about his mother's colour during the attack, its duration and the speed of her recovery.

Other relevant history

Check that there was no intercurrent illness at the times of these attacks, and also ask about any other major change in the patient's health. Her breast cancer was over 10 years ago, but unfortunately late recurrences occur with this disease so probe for any symptoms of a brain secondary. Does she have a progressive neurological problem? Does she have any other cardiac symptoms suggestive of aortic stenosis or an arrhythmia?

Review her drugs: have there been any recent changes to what she is taking? Is she drinking excessive alcohol?

Plan for investigation and management

In routine clinical practice you would examine the patient looking for cardiovascular or neurological signs; check for postural hypotension after she has been standing for 3 minutes.

Depending on your findings, you would arrange a basic blood screen (FBC, electrolytes and creatinine, liver and bone profile, glucose, cholesterol and thyroid-stimulating hormone), CXR and 12-lead ECG.

Further investigations may be appropriate if there are clear leads in the history or on examination, in which case consider a 24-hour tape (limited evidence of usefulness) or a cardiac event monitor, echocardiography, carotid sinus massage, tilt test (but carotid sinus hypersensitivity is common in older persons, even those with no history of syncope, dizziness or falls), brain CT scan or electroencephalography.

Assuming you find nothing untoward and confirm (or suspect) postural hypotension, plan to reduce her amlodipine to 5 mg and stop the furosemide. Add a 3-month course of calcium and vitamin D as she has not been leaving her house (although the evidence for this is debated) and arrange to see her in a month to check that her symptoms have resolved.

Further discussion

Driving
Always check whether any patient experiencing blackouts is driving; if you are in doubt as to the regulations (there is a range of time bans depending on the probable cause of the blackouts) always say that you will discuss with your consultant and check details on the Driver and Vehicle Licensing Agency (DVLA) website (http://www.dvla.gov.uk/). People are supposed to inform the DVLA and their insurance company of any significant change in health, so it is safe to recommend that she informs both.

What is the mechanism of neurocardiogenic syncope?
The pathophysiology commonly involves venous pooling and reduced venous return to the heart on standing. Reduced cardiac output and blood pressure stimulate arterial baroreceptors, resulting in increased sympathetic activity and catecholamine levels. The vigorous contraction of relatively empty ventricles results in the activation of left ventricular wall mechanoreceptors that normally respond to stretch. Afferent nerve fibres to the medulla activate the reflex withdrawal of peripheral sympathetic tone and increase vagal parasympathetic activity. The resultant vasodilatation and bradycardia cause reduced cerebral perfusion to the reticular activating system with loss of consciousness.

1.1.5 Vague aches and pains

Letter of referral to the elderly care outpatient clinic

Dear Doctor,

Re: Mr Patrick Bannister, aged 80 years

Thank you for seeing this retired town councillor. He complains of a 1-month history of sudden-onset, but vague, aches and pains, weight loss and generally feeling under the weather. He takes glipizide for type 2 diabetes, atorvastatin for hypercholesterolaemia and ibuprofen for back pain secondary to 'wear and tear'. He says that he feels generally weak, but I could not elicit any definite signs. However, some of his blood tests are abnormal: haemoglobin is 10.8 g/dL (mean corpuscular volume 85 fL, normal range 80–100 fL); urea and electrolytes are normal; and erythrocyte sedimentation rate (ESR) is raised at 95 mm/hour.

I would be grateful for your help with the diagnosis and management of this man who is normally reasonably fit.

Yours sincerely,

Introduction
The differential diagnosis here is wide, and there may be more than one problem (Table 6).

History of the presenting problem

> ⚠️
> - The risk of blindness makes GCA a diagnosis that must not be missed.
> - Of patients with PMR, 15–20% develop GCA.

Ask the patient about the following.

- Onset of the symptoms: classically PMR is acute, but occasionally it has an insidious onset. If the patient is very clear about a sudden onset, then this strongly suggests PMR.

- Distribution of the aches and stiffness: PMR usually affects the neck and shoulder girdle first, then the pelvic girdle; the patient may describe difficulty combing his hair.

- Change in vision and reduced acuity: diplopia and visual hallucinations are less common features of GCA.

- Pain in the jaw when chewing or tenderness of the scalp when combing the hair would support the diagnosis of GCA.

- Influenza-like symptoms: indicate that there may be a prodromal illness in PMR or GCA.

TABLE 6 DIFFERENTIAL DIAGNOSIS OF ACHES AND PAINS WITH RAISED ESR IN AN ELDERLY PATIENT

Type of condition	Common	Less common
Rheumatological	Polymyalgia rheumatica (PMR) Giant cell arteritis (GCA)	Late-onset rheumatoid arthritis Systemic lupus erythematosus Polymyositis (myopathies are neuromuscular disorders in which the primary symptom is muscle weakness due to muscle fibre dysfunction; myositis is an inflammatory myopathy)
Malignant	Myeloma Carcinoma of the prostate or colon, and other malignancies Lymphoma or low-grade leukaemia	Lambert–Eaton myasthenic syndrome (LEMS)
Infective		Chronic infection, eg tuberculosis and endocarditis
Other	Osteoarthritis, especially cervical spondylosis or frozen shoulder with a non-rheumatological cause of raised ESR Depression with non-rheumatological cause of raised ESR Poorly controlled diabetes with chronic infection (even subacute bacterial endocarditis) and neuropathy	

- Early-morning stiffness: if this is persistent beyond 30 minutes, consider rheumatoid arthritis.

- Change in bowel habit and/or blood in the stool: these are clear pointers to bowel malignancy.

- Symptoms of depression.

- Muscle pain and general weakness, with initial improvement on exercise suggests LEMS (which is very rare).

- When was the atorvastatin prescribed? Myositis is an uncommon but significant side effect of statins.

Other relevant history

This will cover a wide area, looking for evidence of chronic inflammatory disease or infection, underlying malignancy or multisystem disorder.

Drug history

Many drugs have been associated with myopathy or myositis: statins are the most common cause, but others include fibrates, chloroquine, steroids and alcohol. Drugs may also cause lupus; this usually occurs after at least 3 months on treatment and the top three culprits are procainamide, hydralazine and quinidine.

Plan for investigation and management

Investigations

In routine clinical practice you would examine the patient fully, but the diagnosis of PMR is a clinical one: in this case the symptoms are very suggestive and his GP has already confirmed that his ESR is raised. However, there are some other illnesses you would wish to exclude with further tests, and it would be sensible to check (or recheck) the following.

- C-reactive protein (CRP) and repeat ESR.

- FBC and film.

- Liver and bone biochemistry: hepatic alkaline phosphatase is often raised in GCA.

- Muscle creatine kinase.

- Rheumatoid factor.

- Glycosylated haemoglobin: to check diabetic control.

- CXR: for primary lung cancer or secondaries, and also tuberculosis.

- Prostate-specific antigen and radiograph of lumbar spine.

- Myeloma screen: immunoglobulins and protein electrophoresis, urinary Bence Jones proteins and skeletal survey.

Depending on the clinical picture and the results of the tests indicated above, then the following may also be required.

- Blood cultures and echocardiography: if you are concerned about infection or there is a murmur.

- Radiographs of joints: as indicated by examination.

- Abdominal CT scan or barium enema/colonoscopy: if there is a high index of suspicion of gastroenterological malignancy.

- Temporal artery biopsy: there is debate as to whether this is indicated in PMR. A positive result confirms the diagnosis, but a negative result does not exclude it and in most cases the experienced clinician will reserve temporal artery biopsy for cases that are not clinically clear-cut.

- Electromyography or nerve conduction studies: if myositis or neuropathy is suspected.

- Voltage-gated calcium channel antibodies: if the extremely rare condition of LEMS is suspected.

Management

Once blood tests and basic imaging have been organised you would need to decide whether you are going to start steroids straight away, or a week later when you have most results. Do not delay steroid treatment if GCA is a possibility: if a temporal artery biopsy is going to be positive, it still will be after a 'few' days on treatment (there is controversy in the literature about how long a 'few' days can be). PMR responds to a much lower dose of prednisolone than GCA does, usually between 15 and 20 mg daily for 1 month (as opposed to 60–80 mg prednisolone daily for GCA). Ask the patient to report any visual symptoms at once and explain why. The patient may appreciate an information leaflet (from the Arthritis and Rheumatism Council) as it is an 'unusual' illness, and will definitely need a steroid card, consideration of ulcer risk and bone protection.

A trial of steroids in PMR

If the diagnosis of PMR is correct, symptoms of malaise and stiffness will melt away 'like magic' in 2–3 days on prednisolone 20 mg daily. *If this does not occur, reconsider your diagnosis.* Note that a clinical response is more useful diagnostically (and therapeutically!) than a fall in CRP or ESR, because these usually fall on administration of steroids whatever the underlying condition.

If treating this man for PMR, do the following.

- Start prednisolone 20 mg daily.

- Replace ibuprofen with regular paracetamol since the risk of gastrointestinal bleeding with use of an NSAID along with steroids in this age group is high.

- Start gastric protection with a histamine H_2-receptor blocker or proton pump inhibitor: the patient is generally weak, anaemic and has been on ibuprofen, so this is advisable even in the absence of a history of peptic ulcer (often silent).

- Review requirement for atorvastatin: this is not a cause of PMR, but it would seem reasonable to stop any drug that is a possible cause of muscle pain unless there is a pressing need to continue.

Note that there are no good prospective trials that provide clear information about the dose and duration of steroid treatment for PMR. A standard approach would be to reduce the prednisolone dose by 2.5 mg every 2–4 weeks until it is down to 10 mg/day, and then by 1 mg every 4–6 weeks after that, guided mainly by the patient's symptoms. Many patients require treatment for 3–4 years, but one-third to a half may be able to stop after 2 years. Try to stop steroids at this point and then watch for relapse.

Further discussion

Steroids are an important cause of mortality and morbidity in older people. Important points include the following.

- Difficulty in weaning from steroids: because of the clinical nature of the diagnosis of polymyalgia, it is often difficult

to wean patients off steroids, with many saying that they feel worse as the dose is reduced. As a result there is a real risk that over-liberal treatment of an elderly population for 'PMR' may do more harm than good.

- Bone prophylaxis: it is essential to prescribe a bisphosphonate (risedronate or alendronate), calcium and vitamin D (eg Calceos); or just calcium and vitamin D if bisphosphonates are poorly tolerated or if the patient is house-bound.

- Diabetic control: the hyperglycaemic action of prednisolone is likely to impair diabetic control, which should be monitored carefully.

- Steroid side effects: elderly people are more susceptible to all the side effects of steroids (eg psychosis, fluid retention/ cardiac failure, increased susceptibility to infection, weight gain and masking of perforated viscus) and there is a case for using steroid-sparing drugs such as azathioprine.

- Intercurrent acute illness: the steroid dose should be increased during periods of stress, eg severe illness and perioperatively.

1.1.6 Swollen legs and back pain

Letter of referral to elderly care outpatient clinic

Dear Doctor,

Re: Mr Walter Quashie, aged 79 years

Thank you for seeing this man who is a rare attender in the surgery. He tells me that he has had severe low backache, fatigue and leg swelling which has caused decreased mobility for 6 weeks. He has lived alone all his life and previously has only consulted occasionally for respiratory tract infections in the winter months.

I would be grateful for your help with the diagnosis as I am concerned there may be some serious pathology here.

Yours sincerely,

TABLE 7 CAUSES OF PERIPHERAL OEDEMA

Cause	Comment
Gravitational	Result of immobility, a common cause in elderly people
Chronic venous insufficiency	Will exacerbate gravitational effects or any other cause of peripheral oedema
Side effects of drugs causing fluid retention or vasodilatation	Steroids, NSAIDs and fludrocortisone; also calcium channel blockers
Congestive heart failure	
Chronic renal failure (advanced)	The retention of sufficient salt and water to cause oedema is not a feature of mild chronic renal impairment
Hypoalbuminaemia	Undernutrition, chronic liver disease and nephrotic syndrome
Venous obstruction	Thrombosis or external compression by pelvic malignant disease
Lymphatic obstruction	External compression by pelvic malignant disease

Introduction

The symptoms may be linked or due to separate pathologies, hence a full clinical history is essential. First consider the causes of leg swelling (Table 7) and back pain (Table 8).

History of the presenting problem

Peripheral oedema

Consider the causes listed in Table 7 as you take the history, in particular probing for evidence of cardiac failure.

- Dyspnoea: this is less common in elderly people because their exercise tolerance is often limited for other reasons.

- Orthopnoea: however, older people may sleep propped up for reasons other than breathlessness.

- Paroxysmal nocturnal dyspnoea and nocturnal cough: can be confused with asthma, or the major problem may be waking early with depression and then feeling breathless as usual.

- Fatigue and lethargy: common in heart failure but non-specific because they are common in many chronic diseases and in cancer.

TABLE 8 CAUSES OF LOWER BACKACHE IN AN ELDERLY PATIENT

Cause	Comment
Lumbar spondylosis	Osteoarthritis, disc degeneration and osteophytes; very common
Malignant disease	Consider metastatic carcinoma (prostate, bladder or colon) and myeloma; also consider meningioma (although this is rare)
Osteoporosis	Usually considered in women but older men are also at risk, particularly if they have been treated with steroids. Pain from an osteoporotic fracture usually improves in about 3 weeks, but sequential vertebral crush fractures may present as chronic back pain
Herniated disc	Particularly if the patient has a history of sciatica (pain radiating into the leg that worsens with coughing, Valsalva manoeuvre or sneezing); also beware cauda equina syndrome
Cauda equina syndrome	This rare condition is usually caused by a tumour or massive midline disc herniation. Urinary retention with overflow incontinence is usually present, often in association with sensory loss in a saddle distribution, leg weakness and bilateral sciatica
Spinal stenosis	Pseudoclaudication describes persistent back and leg pain that improves with spinal flexion, eg going up stairs
Infection	Consider osteomyelitis (disciitis) and paraspinous abscess eg Pott's tumour if there is fever and general malaise
Inflammatory arthritis	Often associated with HLA-B27, eg inflammatory bowel disease

HLA, human leucocyte antigen.

- Nausea and vomiting: this may raise the suspicion of gastrointestinal pathology, but is relatively common in heart failure as a result of gastric congestion.

- Possible aetiology: remember that there are often multiple predisposing and precipitating factors. Specific questions may give clues, eg sudden onset of breathlessness with the ankle swelling 6 weeks ago may have followed a painless infarct. Or palpitations and a more gradual development of oedema may have followed the onset of atrial fibrillation (AF); in old age the atrial contribution compensates for impaired diastolic filling, so loss of this with AF may precipitate heart failure. As with breathlessness, angina may not be a problem because of impaired mobility.

Common causes of heart failure

- Coronary heart disease: prevalence increasing with better treatment of myocardial infarction (MI).
- Hypertension.
- Cardiomyopathy: dilated (can be idiopathic or due to alcohol).
- Valve disease.
- Drugs: cardiac depressant drug, eg calcium antagonists and beta-blockers.
- Arrhythmias: both tachyarrhythmias and bradyarrhythmias can precipitate heart failure.
- Right heart failure, eg recurrent pulmonary emboli and cor pulmonale.

Less common causes of heart failure

- Cardiomyopathy: hypertrophic and restrictive (amyloidosis and haemochromatosis).
- Myocarditis: usually viral, eg coxsackievirus and influenza.
- Pericardial disease.
- High-output states, eg anaemia, thyrotoxicosis and Paget's disease.

With regard to other possibilities, pursue evidence for the following.

- Drug side effects: have any new medications been started?
- Renal disease: has the urine become frothy, indicating the

development of substantial proteinuria?

- Liver disease: has the patient become jaundiced etc?
- Malignancy causing venous or lymphatic obstruction: features may be general or specific, as described below.

Backache

Consider the causes listed in Table 8 and ask particularly about the following.

- Trauma/falls: the sudden onset of back pain, particularly after trauma or falling, strongly suggests a fracture, most commonly associated with osteoporosis.
- Any general features to suggest an underlying cancer, eg malaise, anorexia or unexplained weight loss.
- Any features of specific cancers: prostatic cancer (urgency, nocturia, poor stream and terminal dribbling); myeloma (symptoms of hypercalcaemia, eg polyuria, polydipsia and constipation); bladder neoplasm (haematuria); colonic malignancy (altered bowel habit, abdominal pain, blood and mucus *per rectum*).

Patients whose low back pain is due to infection or cancer usually have no relief from their back pain when they lie flat.

Other relevant history

Consider risk factors for ischaemic heart disease, particularly smoking, hypertension and diabetes. But remember that other factors which may be very significant in a young patient are less important in

older people, eg family history and hyperlipidaemia. Is there other evidence that would indicate vascular disease such as history of transient ischaemic attacks, stroke or intermittent claudication?

Elderly people still present with the sequelae of rheumatic heart disease, so ask about childhood rheumatic fever. However, most valve disease is now the result of the effects of degenerative and ischaemic heart disease.

Also ask directly about any history of kidney disease: previous blood or urine tests (and any comments that a doctor made about them: the offhand remark 'there's a bit of protein in the urine' made 10 years ago suggests long-standing renal disease), haematuria, urinary stones and previous episodes of swelling.

Social history

This man appears to have had little contact with any social services: this may be because he has been fit and not needed any help, but it may also be that he is very isolated. It is important to establish how he is managing.

- Does he need more support at home, and if he needs admission for investigation and treatment will there be any immediate problems (eg pets) to consider?
- Is he able to perform the activities of daily living (washing, dressing and food preparation)?
- Does he have a family who can help him?
- Will he need social support, eg meals on wheels and home help?
- Is he eligible for extra income, eg attendance allowance? (See Section 2.12.)

Station 2: History Taking

> Is alcohol a problem? This may be at the root of this man's presentation, with cardiac failure explaining oedema and the falls leading to vertebral fractures.

Drug history

What analgesia has the patient been using? This might inform you about the severity of the pain and the relevant complications may contribute to the clinical picture, eg NSAIDs may cause fluid retention, and renal impairment and chronic gastrointestinal blood loss may have led to severe anaemia. Has he been left on steroids after his 'bronchitis'? Remember to think about all routes of administration: beta-blockers in eye drops can exacerbate cardiac failure and asthma. Is he on any drugs that can cause oedema (Table 7)?

Plan for investigation and management

In routine clinical practice you would perform a full physical examination, with abnormal findings directing the focus of investigation.

While you are planning the investigations prescribe regular and top-up analgesics, and plan a strategy, eg returning to the GP if he remains in pain. Draw his attention to any red flag symptoms he may develop, eg the sudden onset of difficulty passing urine or leg weakness, and give specific instructions about who to contact if these occur. If he needs admission to hospital, remember to institute preventative measures immediately, eg subcutaneous low-molecular-weight heparin, pressure-relieving mattress and nutritional supplements.

Investigations

Peripheral oedema Check the following.

- Blood tests: FBC, electrolytes and renal function, liver and bone function, glucose and thyroid function tests. Check troponin if a recent MI is suspected. It is uncertain whether it is worth measuring lipids at the age of 79 years: there is little evidence for the efficacy of treatment, but this is not the same as evidence of no benefit.

- CXR, ECG and, if cardiac failure is suspected, echocardiogram: 24-hour Holter monitoring is useful if intermittent arrhythmias are suspected.

Figures 3 and 4 show typical CXR findings in a case of cardiac failure. The ECG is abnormal in 90% of cases, with common abnormalities including Q waves, T- and ST-segment changes, left ventricular hypertrophy, bundle-branch block and AF. The ST elevation may indicate recent infarction but, if

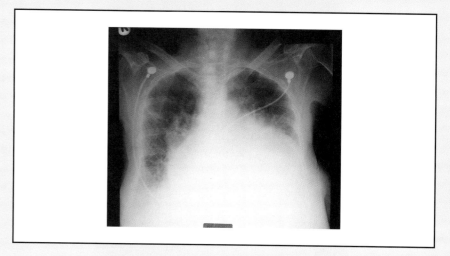

▲**Fig. 3** CXR showing gross cardiomegaly and pulmonary oedema.

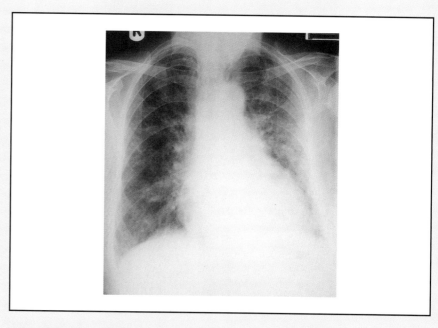

▲**Fig. 4** CXR showing cardiomegaly and early pulmonary oedema with upper lobe diversion and increased lung markings of interalveolar oedema (Kerley B lines).

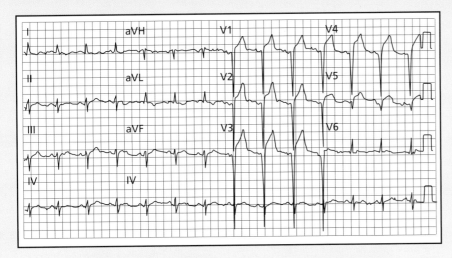

▲**Fig. 5** ECG showing anteroseptal ST elevation (leads V₁–V₅) in a patient with a left ventricular aneurysm.

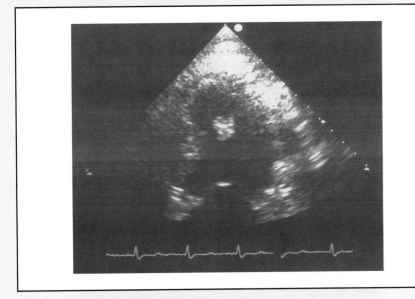

▲**Fig. 6** Two-dimensional echocardiogram showing a left ventricle that is aneurysmal at its apex. The high density around the lesion in the apex is a thrombus in the aneurysm.

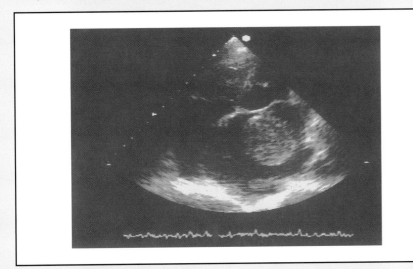

▲**Fig. 7** Two-dimensional echocardiogram: parasternal long-axis view. The round 'tennis ball'-like density in the left atrium is an atrial myxoma.

persistent, is a sign of a left ventricular aneurysm that can also be complicated by heart failure (Figs 5 and 6). The echocardiogram is a useful non-invasive test to detect and assess valvular disease and left ventricular function, and can also detect some rare causes of heart failure, eg atrial myxoma (Fig. 7).

Back pain Most simple low back pain settles within 2–3 weeks; failure to improve after 4–6 weeks, especially in a man of this age, should prompt investigation.

- Plain radiograph of spine: look for vertebral fracture, but note that plain radiographs are not very sensitive for infection or cancer.

- Blood tests: erythrocyte sedimentation rate, C-reactive protein, prostate-specific antigen (PSA) and myeloma screen (see Section 1.1.5).

- Other imaging: CT and MRI are more sensitive than plain radiography for the detection of early spinal infection or cancer, and may also reveal herniated discs and spinal stenosis. Bone scintigraphy may reveal secondary deposits. These imaging tests should be reserved for patients in whom there is a strong clinical suggestion of infection, cancer or neurological deficit.

Management
The requirements are effective analgesia in addition to measures directed towards the specific causes of the oedema and back pain.

> If a patient has severe heart failure and prostate cancer, then he is likely to die of the heart disease and not of the cancer: good symptom control is often neglected in terminal heart and lung disease.

Station 2: History Taking **125**

Heart failure Management is similar to that in younger patients (see *Cardiology*, Section 2.3), but with a different emphasis. Lifestyle changes and drugs for secondary prevention are only worthwhile if the patient has a reasonable prognosis. Encourage patients with cardiac cachexia to eat whatever they fancy and graze! Exercise programmes may be particularly valuable in elderly people in whom lack of fitness may make a major contribution to their symptoms.

Heart failure is so common that you must be familiar with the details and subtleties of pharmacological management in older people.

- Diuretics: thiazide or loop diuretics are usually used as first-line treatment to control symptoms, but have never been shown to reduce mortality. Intravenous treatment may be needed initially if there is gastric congestion. Watch the potassium, especially if the patient is on digoxin. In severe resistant oedema, the combination of metolazone and a loop diuretic may be very effective. However, start with metolazone 2.5 mg every other day because the diuresis may be drastic; then review frequently and reduce the diuretics before the patient reaches his 'dry weight' or you will overshoot. When the patient is stable, metolazone may be useful intermittently, eg twice a week.

- Angiotensin-converting enzyme (ACE) inhibitors: all patients with left ventricular systolic dysfunction should receive these drugs (unless there is a contraindication) because many studies have shown that they reduce morbidity, mortality and hospital admissions.

- Angiotensin receptor blockers: until recently these were used if an ACE inhibitor was not tolerated, eg due to cough. The CHARM study suggested there was benefit when candesartan was added to treatment with an ACE inhibitor.

Use of ACE inhibitors

Proceed with caution when starting these drugs: aortic and renal artery stenoses are more common in old age. If the patient is not dry and has adequate blood pressure, start with the lowest dose of your preferred once-daily ACE inhibitor and watch for hypotension and renal impairment (by checking serum creatinine after 7 days). If the drug is well tolerated, increase the dose to the therapeutic range.

Risks of ACE inhibitors

A dose that is well tolerated when a patient is stable may cause renal failure if a problem such as volume depletion caused by diarrhoea and vomiting or a chest infection supervenes. If a patient becomes acutely unwell, check creatinine and if this has risen significantly stop the ACE inhibitor (and any other drugs that will reduce glomerular filtration rate, eg NSAIDs). Consider restarting the ACE inhibitor if and when the patient recovers.

- Nitrates and hydralazine: if the patient is intolerant of ACE inhibitors, then this combination could be considered because it has been shown to reduce mortality, but is rarely used.

- Digoxin: this is a drug of choice to control the rate in established AF, and it has also been shown to be inotropic in the presence of sinus rhythm. It reduces hospital admissions in those with heart failure, but has not been shown to have an effect on mortality.

Anticoagulation

In AF or paroxysmal AF prescribe warfarin unless there is a reason not to, but use common sense: warfarin is more likely to do harm than good in the patient with failing memory and frequent falls.

- Spironolactone: provided there are no contraindications, the addition of spironolactone to treatment with diuretics, ACE inhibitors and digoxin has been shown to reduce mortality in instances of moderate to severe heart failure. Watch the potassium.

- Beta-blockers: these drugs have been shown to reduce morbidity and mortality. They should be used with care by a specialist and may be contraindicated in many elderly smokers because of chronic obstructive pulmonary disease and peripheral vascular disease.

'But I don't feel better'

Your patient has lost 10 kg in weight, his ankles are slim, his blood pressure is acceptable and his electrolytes and renal function are satisfactory. You are delighted but he insists that he still feels awful. Do not despair but encourage him: patients often take about a week to feel better.

'I'm on too many drugs'

The patient could well be right! The circulation of an 80 year old with heart failure may find it difficult to cope with the combination of a diuretic, ACE inhibitor, spironolactone and beta-blocker: he may have excellent blood pressure and few abnormal physical signs when you examine him, but then collapse on his way to the shops, which is not a therapeutic triumph. Temper justice with mercy.

Prostate cancer This is usually suspected because of an elevated PSA on screening or the findings on digital rectal examination. Transrectal needle biopsy guided by ultrasound is needed to obtain a tissue diagnosis and prognostic score; 90% of prostatic metastases involve the spine, with the lumbar spine affected three times more often than the cervical spine because of the paravertebral venous plexus. Metastases that lead to spinal cord compression are located in the vertebra (85%) or the paravertebral space (15%). Metastases to the lungs and brain are seen in a few cases, and paraneoplastic syndromes may also occur.

Management should involve the urologists and cancer services, and will probably include a gonadorelin analogue along with initial antiandrogen cover to prevent flare, pain control and radiotherapy. If spinal cord compression is suspected, the key is speed: urgent MRI, neurosurgical opinion, possibly dexamethasone and radiotherapy or urgent decompression.

1.1.7 Failure to thrive: gradual decline and weight loss

Letter of referral to elderly care outpatient clinic

Dear Doctor,

Re: Mrs Gloria Brown, aged 78 years

Could you please see this elderly woman who has been generally declining for the past 12 months? She has lost at least 6 kg in weight and according to her family has a poor appetite. She has chronic obstructive pulmonary disease (COPD)

and hypertension, and takes a salbutamol inhaler on a prn basis and bendroflumethiazide. Despite her lung troubles she still smokes, but has reduced the number of cigarettes to five a day. She has a productive cough most days but thinks her breathlessness has gradually worsened over the last 6 months. She has recently noticed intermittent haemoptysis.

I should appreciate your opinion on how far we should investigate here.

Yours sincerely,

Introduction

'Failure to thrive' is a term often used to refer to older patients who are losing weight, have declining functional status and are affected by processes that often culminate in death. Ageing and clinical and psychosocial factors may set up a cycle of weight loss and poor nutrition, with muscle wasting causing reduced functional status and increased susceptibility to acute illness. Weight loss is a significant marker for increased risk of disease, disability and death.

Possible mechanisms of failure to thrive include changes in neurohumoral regulation that occur in normal ageing, an increase in cytokine activity and a reduction in anabolic activity. A decline in growth hormone results in a decline in lean body mass, which may be reduced by up to 40% by 80 years of age, with a decrease in muscle strength and bone mineral density. In men this is exacerbated by a fall in testosterone levels.

While both depression and dementia can lead to failure to thrive, it is important to exclude a range of underlying illnesses.

In an older person who is losing weight consider the following.

- Disease: acute or chronic.
- Depression: may be the sole cause of disability, malnutrition and weight loss, or a contributing factor.
- Dementia: Alzheimer's disease is a cause of weight loss in later life.
- Drugs.
- Dentition, usually lack of.
- Dysgeusia (impaired taste).
- Dysphagia: neurological (eg stroke or motor neuron disease) or obstructive (eg oesophageal cancer).
- Dyspepsia: may lead to avoidance of eating.
- Diarrhoea: malabsorption and neoplasm.
- Dysfunction, eg arthritis and poor mobility, which leaves patients unable to feed themselves.

Causes of drowsiness/ tiredness in the elderly

- Drugs: 'hangover' effect of sedatives, antidepressants and neuroleptics; side effects of other drugs, eg anticonvulsants and codeine.
- Alcohol.
- Psychiatric problems, particularly depression and dementia.
- Infections, eg urinary tract after pneumonia or influenza.
- Chronic disease, especially with an acute-phase response, eg malignancy and rheumatoid disease.
- Metabolic and endocrine problems, eg hypothyroidism, diabetes mellitus and hyponatraemia.
- Intracranial pathology, especially lesions causing a pressure effect, eg frontal tumour, subdural haematoma, tuberculous meningitis in rare instances or a brain abscess.
- Chronic organ failure (eg respiratory failure, renal failure and cardiac failure) may present insidiously.
- Severe anaemia.

Station 2: History Taking **127**

History of the presenting problem

Weight loss can occur for a number of reasons, but weight loss associated with anorexia should always lead to investigation for an underlying neoplasm. Here, haemoptysis should raise the possibility of a bronchial carcinoma or tuberculosis (TB). However, the symptoms could be due to a combination of diseases, eg bronchiectasis and depression. You will clearly want to ask in detail about the following.

- Amount and colour of haemoptysis: a little fresh red blood at the end of a severe coughing bout may not be sinister, merely reflecting broken capillaries; brisk red haemoptysis suggests a cavity; frothy pink sputum suggests cardiac failure; streaking with very copious sputum production could indicate bronchiectasis.

- Breathlessness: is it present all the time, or does it vary with time of day, posture, activity and weather?

- Cough: productive or non-productive?

- Sputum: colour and volume. Has there been any change, and what is normal for her?

- Wheeze: diurnal variation may occur in asthma and heart failure.

- Chest pain: may or may not be pleuritic in nature.

- Hoarse voice: any change in voice that she or her family has noticed? This would clearly increase suspicion of malignancy (but do not forget hypothyroidism).

- Are there any new pains around her wrists or ankles? This would suggest hypertrophic pulmonary osteoarthropathy.

- New lumps or swellings would suggest a malignant process.

- Night sweats are an obvious pointer towards infection, perhaps TB.

Other relevant history

A full functional history is required and should focus on symptoms of the diagnostic possibilities listed in the Key point box above. A lung lesion is likely if the haemoptysis is significant, so check for a past history of TB or any recent contacts with the disease, and also confirm the smoking history.

A full social history is required (see Section 1.1.6).

Plan for investigation and management

Failure to thrive should prompt a focused examination for diseases that may have gone undetected and which are potentially treatable. Many patients with this condition have multifactorial causes, with a sentinel event superimposed on a background of comorbidity and age-associated changes.

Prognosis of failure to thrive

Although identification of a likely cause is helpful, and appropriate intervention may improve outcome for some patients, failure to thrive is unfortunately an inexorable terminal process.

Investigation

The following would be appropriate as an initial screen.

- Electrolytes and creatinine.

- Liver function tests.

- Serum calcium/bone function tests.

- FBC.

- Glucose.

- Thyroid function tests.

- C-reactive protein.

- Sputum for cytology, culture and sensitivity, including for acid alcohol fast bacilli (TB culture).

- 12-lead ECG.

- CXR looking for pulmonary mass, effusion, consolidation, collapse and enlargement of mediastinal lymph nodes.

- Lung function tests to establish severity of COPD: if present, inhaled long-acting β_2 agonist/steroid and antimuscarinics may help.

Further investigations would be as directed by clinical suspicion, eg if there were new-onset joint pain then conduct radiography of the wrists looking for periosteal thickening from hypertrophic pulmonary osteoarthropathy, or CT of the chest if any abnormalities were seen on plain radiography.

Management

This will clearly depend on the cause. If the patient is found to have lung cancer, then refer her to appropriate specialist services, such as the palliative care team, and arrange nutritional support and Attendance Allowance under the special rules. Explain to her that the focus is on symptom control and explain who will visit, eg Macmillan nurse. Ask her if she would like you to discuss the situation with her family. Phone her GP so there is no delay in imparting this news, and ask for urgent assessment by social services.

However, the diagnosis may not be of malignancy, and other acute and chronic problems may benefit from treatment in this case, including the following.

- COPD: optimising treatment may improve functional capacity; consider respiratory referral for an assessment for long-term oxygen therapy or for support from a specialist nurse if appropriate.

- Chest infection: this could have precipitated presentation to the GP but is unlikely to explain decline over many months, unless the patient has TB.

- Lack of well-fitting dentures: blindingly obvious, but often neglected.

- Depression.

Increased support at home is likely to be required whatever the cause of this woman's decline, so organise assessment by an occupational therapist, a care package, nutritional support and benefits assessment, etc.

1.2 Clinical examination

Elderly patients commonly appear in the physical examination stations of PACES and there is an increasing tendency for actual patients admitted a few days before the exam to appear, eg the woman admitted after a fall may, depending on the reason for it, be suitable as a cardiac, neurological or musculoskeletal case. This means that there is greater probability of encountering common pathology than there used to be and examiners are more likely to direct questions towards 'on-take' investigation and management. This can be challenging if the candidate has spent more time on courses than the wards. This section offers tips for the examination of an older patient but it does not aim to be comprehensive: use the individual *Medical Masterclass* modules for more detail.

When dealing with all the examination scenarios below, remember that older patients may have several problems and it may not be possible to make everything 'fit' into one neat diagnosis. You will always need to give the differential diagnosis of your main findings, but you should not neglect to mention other abnormal physical signs in the (almost invariably) futile hope that the examiners will not have noticed them. You should comment on anything else you are sure you found, even if you cannot make it 'fit'. Be prepared to discuss possible mechanisms for why the patient with a given pathology presented with falls/confusion/failure to thrive. The disease or the drugs used to treat it may explain the presentation.

After explaining your physical findings and differential diagnosis, you will be invited to discuss investigations and management. Stick to a generic plan of investigation as when dealing with younger patients, grouping related investigations and starting with the basics (eg blood tests, urine, ECG and imaging) before proceeding to specialist tests. However, when dealing with management of the elderly, remember that this is much more than drugs. For any chronic disease, are there opportunities for educating the patient or relatives, or are there any relevant patient organisations or local support groups? Is benefit to be had from attempts to improve the patient's general health (eg nutrition)? And always comment on the need to improve communication by ensuring, for example, that the patient has the correct glasses and that the hearing aid has a battery. Could the physiotherapist, occupational therapist or speech and language therapist contribute? What would social services have to offer?

Are there any legal considerations? For example, if the patient has had a stroke or a myocardial infarction then you would need to check whether he or she is still driving. Only then start discussing drugs, but if the examiner interrupts, do listen and answer the point, speeding up if you are told to.

1.2.1 Confusion (respiratory)

Instruction

This elderly man presented with confusion. Please examine his chest.

General features

Hypoxia, hypercapnia, chest sepsis or a brain secondary from lung cancer are all possible mechanisms for confusion due to chest pathology. When examining the patient, check the following.

- Is he cyanosed, tachypnoeic at rest or using accessory muscles?

- Does his chest shape, plethoric appearance, hair colour (white tinged with yellow is due to the tar in cigarettes not the nicotine) suggest chronic obstructive pulmonary disease (COPD)?

- Is he markedly kyphotic, suggesting restrictive lung disease?

Patients with chronic chest disease are often emaciated, but gross obesity presents its own chest problems (eg sleep apnoea). Swollen legs, particularly if unilateral, may suggest embolic disease. Mesothelioma is becoming steadily more common as the cohort effect of industrial asbestos exposure takes its toll. Look around: if the patient is in the exam all morning he may have left his inhalers on the bedside locker, and there may be a peak flow meter in case you want to use it (offer to take the hint).

Respiratory examination

Check for clubbing, tar-stained fingers, flap, a raised JVP (a high JVP with no waves, plethora, conjunctival oedema and collateral veins suggest superior vena cava obstruction), cervical lymphadenopathy or skin nodules due to metastases, and then examine the chest (having briefly checked for thoracotomy scars or post-radiotherapy telangiectasia). If you begin to suspect lung cancer, glance back at the pupils – don't miss Horner's syndrome.

Common findings are signs of infection superimposed on chronic lung disease such as COPD, bronchiectasis (coarse crackles, often asymmetrical, with a full sputum pot) or fibrotic lung disease (symmetrical fine end-inspiratory 'Velcro' crackles). If you hear crackles, ask the patient to cough to check that they persist; older people may have crackles of no pathological significance just because they do not breathe deeply.

> 🔑 Look at the sputum pot if there are a lot of crackles in the chest: if there is sputum, then the diagnosis is almost certainly bronchiectasis; if there isn't, then the diagnosis is probably interstitial lung disease.

A large unilateral pleural effusion (look for previous drain site) may be due to mesothelioma.

Look for likely drug side effects: is the patient with COPD shaky and tachycardic due to salbutamol or does the appearance, kyphosis and fragile skin suggest steroid treatment?

Further discussion

Be familiar with the guidelines for the treatment of COPD, drug side effects, exercise programmes and practicalities of long-term oxygen therapy.

1.2.2 Confusion (abdominal)

Instruction

This elderly woman presented with confusion. Please examine her abdomen.

General features

In the Emergency Department patients with an acute abdomen of any cause may present with confusion. Patients with acute abdominal problems are too ill for examination and will not be found in PACES, but chronic liver disease or other chronic abdominal pathology that may be complicated by infection would be possible given the scenario of confusion. So, when in the exam look for the following.

- Anaemia.

- Evidence of chronic liver disease: jaundice, anaemia, liver flap (suggesting hepatic decompensation), clubbing, Dupuytren's contracture, liver palms, xanthelasma and spider naevi.

- Evidence of chronic renal disease: vascular access for dialysis.

Abdominal examination

Note scars, swelling and any abnormal veins (check the direction of blood flow, eg away from the umbilicus in caput medusae).

If you detect ascites check the JVP and for swollen legs, review for peripheral signs of chronic liver disease and palpate for lymphadenopathy in the neck.

This will help you decide between congestive cardiac failure/constrictive pericarditis, chronic liver disease, intra-abdominal neoplasm (check for pelvic mass in women) and nephrotic syndrome.

A large liver and spleen suggests haematological malignancy, where anaemia or infection could explain confusion.

Remember that some patients with polycystic kidneys live until old age with normal renal function, but also that increasing numbers of elderly patients are receiving treatment for end-stage renal failure. Look for signs of dialysis treatment (arteriovenous fistulae in forearms/elbows, indwelling central venous catheters, peritoneal dialysis catheters or scars from any of these), and palpate under any scars in the iliac fossa for a renal transplant. If you find what you think is a large kidney, check the other side again – polycystic kidneys may be asymmetrical but are usually palpable bilaterally (if at all) – and then recheck for a large (polycystic) liver. Confusion in a patient with polycystic kidney disease could be due to infection (all anatomically abnormal kidneys are vulnerable) or be a result of a subarachnoid haemorrhage from an intracranial aneurysm.

> 🔑 **Five differences between a kidney and a spleen**
>
> - You can get above a kidney but not a spleen.
> - The kidney moves down with respiration; the spleen moves towards the right iliac fossa.
> - A kidney is ballotable but a spleen is not.
> - The kidney is resonant to percussion, whereas the spleen is dull.
> - The spleen may have a notch.

Further discussion

Chronic liver disease in the elderly is commonly due to alcohol, and hepatitis C is also increasing in prevalence. In the PACES exam, primary biliary cirrhosis is over-represented (in older women). If you do not drink alcohol, make sure you know a range of popular drinks and what constitutes 1 unit.

Polycystic kidneys make frequent appearances in PACES, so be familiar with the genetics and disease associations.

> Don't miss serious abdominal pathology in the confused elderly patient: remember that findings of peritonitis that are typical in a middle-aged patient may be absent in an old person. Also remember that perforation may present with an unremarkable abdominal examination and only be recognised when the routine CXR shows air under the diaphragm.

1.2.3 Failure to thrive (abdominal)

Instruction

This elderly woman presented with weight loss and increasing frailty. Please examine her abdomen.

General features

Does she look unwell, cachectic, pale or jaundiced? Although the instruction suggests an underlying malignancy, she may have less serious pathology such as malabsorption (eg late-onset coeliac disease).

Abdominal examination

You are looking for signs of malignancy, particularly the following.

- Lymph nodes in the left supraclavicular fossa.

- Scars: these may indicate surgery for a primary, so assess what might have been removed from the position and consider whether it is very old or more recent (although it is not always easy to tell).

- General shape of the abdomen: is it scaphoid, or do the shape, full flanks and purple striae suggest recent abdominal distension?

- Liver enlargement: if present, is it knobbly?

- Splenic enlargement: lymphomas are relatively common in older people and often not treated aggressively because of a relatively indolent course and the poor results of chemotherapy.

- Renal mass.

- Pelvis: palpate carefully for an ovarian mass or distended bladder.

- Ascites.

- Lymph nodes in the groin.

- Rectal examination: tell the examiner that in routine clinical practice you would perform a digital rectal examination, and also test the patient's urine.

Further discussion

You might be asked about whether it is worth investigating the abdomen further as the patient will be too frail for surgery. So remember that making a diagnosis is useful in other ways: you may be able to help the patient and her family to plan ahead, and perhaps avoid inappropriate emergency surgery at a later date. Start off by suggesting simple but informative tests.

1.2.4 Frequent falls (cardiovascular)

Instruction

This man has a history of multiple falls. Please examine his cardiovascular system to determine why.

General features

The most obvious cardiovascular causes for falls would include aortic stenosis and postural hypotension. Look specifically for parkinsonian features in case the patient has multiple system atrophy or Shy–Drager syndrome.

Cardiovascular examination

Atrial fibrillation is very common in the elderly. Check for a slow rising pulse. Ask to measure the blood pressure both when the patient is lying down and standing up, looking for a narrow pulse pressure and/or a postural drop (the examiner may well ask you why you want to do so, but then tell you to proceed with the rest of the cardiovascular examination). Listen for an ejection systolic murmur, best heard in the right second intercostal space and radiating to the carotids, which is characteristic of aortic stenosis.

> How do you distinguish between aortic stenosis and aortic sclerosis?
>
> | | Stenosis | Sclerosis |
> | --- | --- | --- |
> | Pulse character | Slow rising | Normal |
> | Pulse pressure | Narrow | Normal |
> | Radiation of murmur | To the neck | Not to the neck |
> | Carotid thrill | Yes | No |

Further discussion

Signs of valve disease may be attenuated in the older patient. The slow rising pulse and narrow pulse pressure of aortic stenosis may be affected by decreased arterial compliance. The altered shape of the chest wall in kyphosis and chronic lung disease alters the classic radiation of murmurs and the position of the apex beat. Basal crackles in the chest are non-specific.

In a cardiovascular station the falls are probably collapses (remember that a loss of consciousness is often not recalled) and the examiner's question here is likely to be whether or not the patient would benefit from aortic valve replacement. Factors to be considered will be the patient's general fitness and comorbidities: clearly a frail patient with multiple problems will not tolerate general anaesthesia, nor will someone with severe heart failure or ischaemic heart disease. An echocardiogram would be useful for estimating the degree of stenosis and left ventricular function, which would help with decision-making.

1.2.5 Confusion (cardiovascular)

Instruction

This elderly man presented with confusion. Please examine his heart.

General features

Heart failure and – a presentation that is over-represented in PACES – infectious endocarditis as a complication of valvular heart disease, perhaps with a prosthetic valve, would both be possible diagnoses to explain a presentation with confusion. Although it is more common to see congenital heart disease in younger adults, this is still rare in elderly patients apart

from a bicuspid aortic valve, which often becomes stenotic in old age. Degenerative conditions are now more common than rheumatic heart disease, with aortic stenosis at the top of the list. Overt heart failure will probably be apparent from the end of the bed (Fig. 8).

Cardiovascular examination

Check for the stigmata of infectious endocarditis. (Does the patient have a venflon? If not, think again.) If you suspect this diagnosis offer to palpate for a spleen, dipstick the urine and look at the fundi (Roth's spots are retinal haemorrhages with paler middles).

Most midline sternotomy scars are the result of operations done for coronary grafts. If there is a metallic valve, look for bruising (a side effect of warfarin).

Further discussion

- Know the indications and instructions (usually amoxicillin 3 g po 2 hours before dental surgery) for antibiotic prophylaxis.
- Be able to discuss the management of a patient receiving warfarin.

1.2.6 Frequent falls (neurological)

Instruction

This 79-year-old woman has fallen over many times. Please examine her gait.

General features

Rapidly assess her general health: is she cachectic and frail suggesting chronic illness? Look for obvious signs of Parkinson's disease (PD) such as mask-like facies, resting tremor and a flexed posture. Look

for signs of a stroke: drooping of one side of her face or a flexed arm. Look for cerebellar signs: does she miss your hand when you hold it out to shake hands?

Neurological examination

Offer the patient her walking aid. Assess her rising, walking and turning.

Parkinsonian gait

The patient is stooped, is flexed at the knees and hips, has difficulty getting going and tends to speed up during motion. The gait is shuffling and there is reduced arm swing. The patient has difficulty turning around and foot clearance may be poor, leading to increased trips. Look for propulsion and retropulsion.

Steppage gait/foot drop

Watch carefully: the patient with long-standing foot drop will have adapted to it by lifting the leg high. Additional signs will include reduced tone and glove/stocking sensory loss. If there is bilateral foot drop, think of hereditary sensorimotor syndrome type II (Charcot–Marie–Tooth); polio and lateral popliteal nerve palsy are causes of unilateral foot drop.

Spastic hemiplegic gait

Check to see whether the affected arm is held immobile, close to the chest and with the elbow, wrist and interphalangeal joints flexed. The ipsilateral leg will circumduct, ie the toes will be dragged in a sideways circle. The usual cause is stroke.

Scissors gait

This is caused by bilateral spastic paresis of the legs. The gait is stiff and the legs tend to cross over each other because the hips and knees are flexed and adducted with extension of the ankles, leading to 'scissoring'.

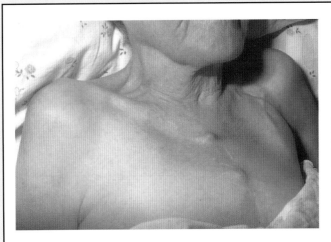

(a)

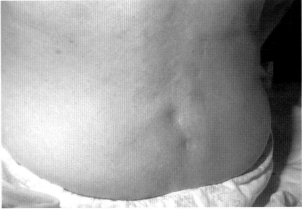

(b)

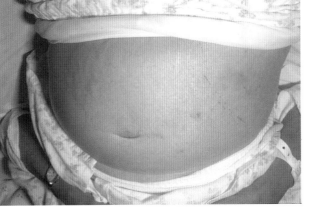

(c)

▲ **Fig. 8** This elderly woman was admitted with an exacerbation of heart failure. She had undergone a mitral valve replacement 20 years previously: her sternotomy scar can be seen, and she also has a permanent pacemaker that can be seen as a bulge in the left upper chest wall (**a**). Her JVP was elevated and she had sacral oedema (**b**), ascites (**c**) and peripheral oedema (**d**). The abdominal distension has resulted in striae; the purple discoloration of her legs is varicose eczema caused by chronic venous insufficiency.

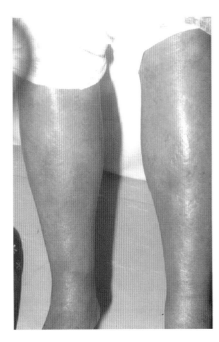

(d)

Check for a sensory level. Consider late-onset multiple sclerosis (MS) and cord compression.

Sensory ataxia

The gait is broad-based and unsteady. Patients look at the ground for feedback as they have lost joint position sense. Consider diabetes and subacute combined degeneration of the cord due to vitamin B_{12} deficiency. Patients with Friedreich's ataxia rarely reach old age.

Cerebellar ataxia

The gait is wide-based and staggering, with particular loss of balance turning around. Check for nystagmus, dysarthria and past-pointing. A cerebellar degeneration or a non-metastatic manifestation of cancer is likely. Spasticity is usually the dominant feature in late-onset MS.

Myopathic gait

Waddling gait due to muscle weakness leads to the pelvic girdle tilting to the non-weight-bearing side. Some hereditary muscular dystrophies present very late. Steroids, osteomalacia and diabetic amyotrophy are possible causes.

Further discussion

Consider the following.

- What can be done to improve the patient's mobility?

- Physiotherapy to try to re-educate the gait where possible.

TABLE 9 WALKING AIDS

Walking aid	Description	Use	Disadvantages
Stick	Wood or aluminium. Correct length essential for functional gait pattern. Can be used singly or in pairs. Individually moulded hand grip may improve function	Widens base of support, supporting up to 25% body weight. Use on the opposite side from the pain in cases of arthritic knee or hip	Has to be propped up or laid flat when not in use, thus becoming a trip hazard
Tripod or quadrupod	Aluminium with three or four feet	Gives more support than a stick and stands up on its own. Used on the side of hemiplegia	
Elbow crutches	Aluminium crutches with forearm support. Used in pairs	Can support 80% of body weight. Useful for non-weight bearing on a lower limb, eg because of amputation or fracture	Risk of tripping as with a stick. Patient needs to have enough cognitive function to use safely
Axillary crutches	Crutches which bear the weight under the arms	More often used for younger patients. Can enable a patient to achieve a speed greater than that of normal walking	Brachial nerve palsy if used too much
Zimmer frame	Aluminium tubing with four rubber feet	Offer maximum support to patient	Patient has to be able to learn new gait pattern: the frame is lifted up and forward, and the patient then steps into the frame. Encourages poor posture
Rollator	As with the Zimmer frame, but there are wheels on the two front legs	Patient can push the frame continuously	Poor posture, slow gait and problems walking outdoors
Gutter frame	Has support for the forearms	Useful for patients with rheumatoid arthritis affecting their wrists and/or wrist injuries	As with the rollator
Delta frame	Usually a three-wheeled foldaway frame, often with a seat/space for shopping	More robust so can be used outside	Heavy

- Use correct walking aids (Table 9).
- Drugs for PD and spasticity.

1.2.7 Confusion (neurological)

Instruction

This elderly man presented with confusion. Please examine his nervous system.

General features

In the Emergency Department there are many neurological causes for a presentation with confusion, ranging from the common (eg post-ictal state, alcohol excess/withdrawal and drugs) to the rare (eg encephalitis). Many of these are most unlikely to appear in PACES, but an obvious hemiparesis, more limited facial droop or parkinsonism may be apparent.

Neurological examination

Consider parkinsonism

Poverty of facial expression, a stooped posture and pill-rolling resting tremor, usually worse on one side, indicate a parkinsonian syndrome. The written instruction may specify which part of the neurological system you are to examine, but checking tone, rapid alternating movements and something functional (eg doing up buttons or offering a pen to assess writing) along with offering to assess gait would be important.

Abnormal eye movements (more than mild reduction in up-gaze) would suggest progressive supranuclear palsy; cerebellar and pyramidal signs would suggest multisystem atrophy; and marked postural hypotension would point to Shy–Drager syndrome.

If you are confident that there is parkinsonism, you may wish to ask your examiner whether you should complete your usual neurological examination by examining sensation, even though you are not expecting to find an obvious sensory problem. However, elderly patients may have multiple pathologies: a patient with parkinsonism may also have diabetic peripheral neuropathy.

Consider hemiparesis

If you suspect hemiparesis, eliciting pronator drift is a good place to start. Ischaemic stroke is the commonest cause, but a subdural haematoma or a space-occupying lesion (especially a meningioma in exam conditions) is possible.

Noting that the patient has presented with confusion, pay attention to language and cognition. Explain that you are going to ask a few questions to check whether he is having any difficulties with speech; check for receptive dysphasia with a one-stage command and then with a two-stage command, and then check for a nominal dysphasia. The 'draw a clock' test has the merit that it will not strain your memory in an exam setting.

Further discussion

Make sure that you can explain the difference between dysphasia, dysarthria and dysphonia, and also that you can talk about the tests you could use to assess cognition.

1.2.8 Impaired mobility (neurological)

Instruction

This 82-year-old man has had difficulty walking for several weeks. Please examine his legs neurologically to determine why.

General features

Does the patient look comfortable or distressed? Is he adopting a particular posture for comfort? Is he cachectic or malnourished? Has he got a neurological condition such as Parkinson's disease (PD)? Think about whether the arms look normal.

Neurological examination

Begin by offering to examine the patient's gait (the examiner may decline, but it is the obvious place to start the assessment if the patient's problem is difficulty walking and you will score points in the examiner's mind for having asked) and then perform a full neurological examination of the legs, looking for clues like muscle wasting, asymmetry or fasciculation as you begin. If there is weakness, expect some incoordination. Look for patterns of neurological findings, but remember that there may be two pathologies in the elderly: common lesions could also include peripheral neuropathy, stroke, PD, spastic paraparesis or myopathy. A slipped disc is less common in old age, but the L5 and S1 roots are involved in 95% of lumbar disc herniations. Motor neuron disease is possible.

> ⚠ If a limb is weak, tests of coordination will be impaired. However, do not overdiagnose incoordination of a weak limb.

Further discussion

Have a ready list of causes of neuropathies, but do not forget common conditions such as diabetes, alcohol, paraneoplastic, vitamin B_{12} deficiency and drugs (isoniazid in slow acetylators, phenytoin and nitrofurantoin).

> 🔑 Make sure that you can explain the different findings in cauda equina syndrome and cord compression.
>
> - Cauda equina syndrome: bowel or bladder dysfunction, numbness in the perineum and medial thighs (saddle distribution), bilateral leg weakness and flexor plantars (lesion is lower motor neuron).
> - Cord compression: weakness and extensor plantars with a sensory level.

As well as the neurological findings be prepared to discuss the consequences for this man in terms of impairment, handicap and disability, and the role members of the multidisciplinary team could play in his management.

1.2.9 Confusion (skin)

Instruction

This elderly woman presented with confusion. Please examine her skin.

General features

Cellulitis, leg ulcers or herpes zoster (particularly involving cranial dermatomes) could all cause confusion. Zoster is not likely to come up in an exam because of the element of judgement as to when the lesions it causes are all crusted and hence non-infectious. In contrast, patients with cellulitis and leg ulcers are always to be found on the ward if an invited patient cannot attend, and they often floor candidates who are smooth in their descriptions of the rare.

Skin examination

Describe what you see in precise terms. If there is an ulcer, is it likely to be due to pressure, venous or arterial disease, or is the site typical of diabetes? Check foot pulses, and offer to check for neuropathy and to test the urine. If there is infection, look between the toe webs for tinea. Cellulitis (like all infections) is more common where there is 'stagnation', ie poor venous or lymphatic return.

Lymphoedema is usually distinguishable from 'pitting' oedema, but chronic pitting oedema pits less well and is thus harder to spot. If the leg is swollen up to the thigh, then feel for a tender thrombosed vein and inguinal lymph nodes, and check for sacral oedema. Cellulitis and deep venous thrombosis may have caused the swelling or be a complication of cardiac failure.

> • Gross leg oedema may be missed if previous recurrent cellulitis has made the ankles so 'woody' that the skin cannot expand. Look further up the leg.
> • If one leg is more swollen than the other, check for deep venous thrombosis or a previous history (scar of hip surgery or a stroke that affected that side) or check for a tremor (eg Parkinson's disease) affecting the 'thin' leg.

Further discussion
Why do older people often complain of itch? This usually occurs because skin becomes drier with age. As well as the discomfort and risk of falls if antihistamines are used, dry skin can develop into asteatotic eczema and this (or athlete's foot) is a common route of infection for cellulitis.

1.2.10 Frequent falls (locomotor)

Instruction
This woman has fallen over several times. Please examine her joints.

General features
Look at her hands for signs of rheumatoid arthritis or osteoarthritis (OA). Does she have marked dorsal kyphosis?

Locomotor examination
You should be looking for evidence of chronic bony swelling suggestive of severe OA of the knee. Feel for crepitus. Don't forget that even if the patient has rheumatoid arthritis, she is still at risk of OA of the knees.

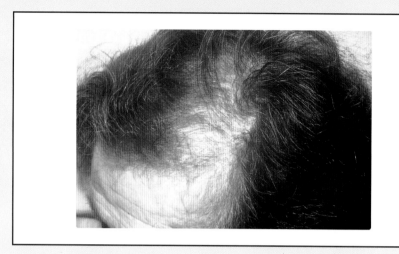

▲**Fig. 9** Diffuse alopecia.

Look to see if there are scars from previous hip replacements. Do not underestimate the importance of good shoulder strength and function in getting out of a chair or off a bed.

Further discussion
Examination here will often be quick, but 5 minutes must be filled in the locomotor station of PACES. Make sure you can discuss the current situation with NSAIDs and 'coxibs' (cyclooxygenase-2 inhibitors) with regard to their side effects and long-term risks.

1.2.11 Confusion (endocrine)

Instruction
This elderly woman presented with confusion. Please examine her neck.

General features
Both hyperthyroidism and hypothyroidism may present with confusion in older people.

Endocrine examination
Examine the neck in the usual way, taking particular care to look for the scar of a thyroidectomy. Check the pulse for atrial fibrillation and assess the outstretched hands for tremor, as

well as for evidence of carpal tunnel surgery. Look at the eyes, the hair for alopecia (Fig. 9), and the skin for pretibial myxoedema, erythema ab igne (Fig. 10) or vitiligo (Fig. 11). Check the patient's reflexes: are they brisk or slow relaxing?

If asked whether the patient is euthyroid, say what you think, although it is reasonable to add the rider that it would be sensible to check the thyroid-stimulating hormone.

> ⚠ Thyroidectomy scars can be very difficult to see, so look carefully.

Further discussion
Remember that in hypothyroidism with coexisting ischaemic heart disease, the initial dose of levothyroxine should be 25 µg for 2–4 weeks, depending on the severity of both the myxoedema and the ischaemia.

1.2.12 Confusion (eye)

Instruction
This elderly woman presented with confusion. Please examine her eyes.

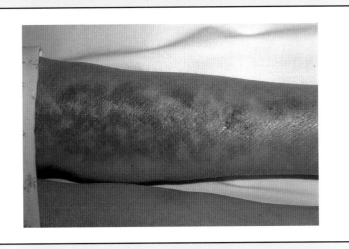

▲**Fig. 10** Erythema ab igne: excoriation can be seen in this lesion, which needs to be monitored because malignancy occasionally occurs.

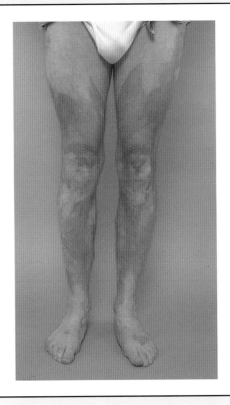

▲**Fig. 11** Vitiligo.

General features

This station is often used to assess skills with the ophthalmoscope, but do not forget to examine visual acuity, pupils and visual fields.

Eye examination

Before you start, check that the patient can count fingers with each eye. If one eye is blind, much time can be wasted doing fields before the truth dawns. A homonymous hemianopia (look at limb posture for likely hemiparesis), optic atrophy (look for craniotomy scar) or papilloedema would be possible physical signs here.

Further discussion

Be prepared to discuss the systemic effects of eye drops. Be aware of the variety of aids for the visually impaired (very bright lights, magnifying sheets and talking watches, etc.).

1.3 Communication skills and ethics

1.3.1 Frequent falls

Scenario

Role: you are a junior doctor working on a general medical ward.

Mrs Elizabeth Dunn is aged 74 years and has been admitted after a fall. Her daughter asks to speak to you. She has heard that the occupational therapist is taking her mother on a home visit tomorrow. Mrs Dunn's daughter, who lives 50 miles away and rarely sees her mother, does not think she should go home, but should be discharged to a residential home.

Mrs Dunn was admitted after a trip at home, following which she sustained bruising to her arms and face. She had no postural drop in blood pressure, a 12-lead ECG showed sinus rhythm and she has not fallen while on the ward. She has been started on prophylaxis against osteoporosis. She has no mental health issues, wants to go home and it is the view of the multidisciplinary team that it is reasonable for her to do so. She gives you permission to talk to her daughter.

Your task: to explain to Mrs Dunn's daughter that Mrs Dunn wants to go home and has the right to make her own decisions.

Key issues to explore

- The patient's autonomy.

- The patient's right to choose where she goes on discharge.

- The patient's capacity to choose where she goes on discharge.

- The patient's safety.

Key points to establish

- That Mrs Dunn is happy for you to discuss her discharge plans with her daughter: introduce the session by explaining that you have specifically sought permission from Mrs Dunn to talk to her daughter. This sometimes comes as a surprise: families may infantilise older members and need reminding gently that they have the same rights to confidentiality as other adults.

- The daughter's understanding of the situation.

- That Mrs Dunn has the capacity to decide to go home: capacity is situation specific, ie she may be able to go home safely but may not have the capacity to change her will.

- That 'safety' cannot mean absence of any risk.

Appropriate responses to likely questions

Daughter: you cannot let my mother go home. She will fall over again and might break her hip next time.

Doctor: we have looked into the reasons why your mother fell and we think that she tripped. We have checked out her heart with an ECG – an electrical recording – and everything seems to be in order. Furthermore, there is nothing to suggest that she had a fit or anything like that. But I am afraid that I cannot give you a guarantee that she won't fall again: there will always be some risk, but admitting her to a residential home would not stop her from falling. The aim of the home visit is to assess her home for hazards and find out what care package, if any, she needs to support her, and to make arrangements to keep her as safe as possible.

Daughter: but I'm terrified that she'll break her hip. That's what happened to her mother.

Doctor: I can understand why you are worried about this. I agree that she is at risk, as is pretty well every old person, of breaking her hip. To cut down the risk we can assess her home to try and deal with things that might trip her up, and we can provide aids like walking sticks and a frame if that would be helpful. Also, we have started her on some tablets to treat thinning of the bones, so that they'll be stronger if she does have a fall.

Daughter: my mother gets confused at times, so how can she make her own decisions about this?

Doctor: she is not confused at the moment. She is able to retain information and is able to weigh up risks about her discharge. Why don't you arrange to go on the home visit with your mother and the occupational therapist? Then you can see what she is able to do safely and say what you are concerned she will have difficulty with. After that you could discuss the amount of care that would make you feel confident with the social worker and your mother.

If Mrs Dunn's daughter is still not happy, offer to arrange a meeting with your consultant.

1.3.2 Confusion

Key issues to explore

- The patient's autonomy: frail older people still have rights despite cognitive impairment.

- The patient's right to choose where she goes on discharge.

- The patient's capacity to choose where she goes on discharge, which in this case is reduced.

- The patient's safety: a patient can fall and break a hip in a hospital or care home as well as at home.

Key points to establish

- Ask the daughter in detail about how her mother was coping prior to admission. She may have non-specific concerns and be anxious (and often guilty) that she can do little of practical help as she lives at a distance. If she has specific worries, then make a list as you need to address each one, eg if she fears her mother might leave the gas hob on, then the gas can be turned off and carers can provide hot meals with a thermos flask for hot drinks between their visits.

- Explain why Mrs James was admitted and that, although there is a degree of dementia, she is less confused now. If her daughter knows nothing about dementia, give a brief explanation and a source for more information (eg Alzheimer's Disease Society).

- Explain that her mother will have a full multidisciplinary assessment and that an appropriate care package will be arranged before she is discharged. Say that as her mother only had care once a day before admission, you anticipate that with more care she should do well at home.

- Explain the drawback of residential care: institutionalisation often leads to

rapid decline in early-to-moderate dementia. Also, it will be difficult to find a home that will accept the cat, a key component of Mrs James' quality of life, and this may affect her longevity.

Appropriate responses to likely questions

Daughter: but surely my mother would be much safer in a home?

Doctor: I can understand why you think that, but because of her dementia she is likely to find it difficult to adjust to a new environment. She may become more muddled and likely to fall. She really misses her cat and is determined to go home, and although we accept that she is not fully able to weigh all the risks involved we have to try to respect your mother's strongly held wishes.

Daughter: how will she manage? The staff nurse says her memory score is only 5/10.

Doctor: the score tells us that her memory and orientation are not perfect, but what really matters is how much she can do towards looking after herself. She is walking steadily with her frame, but did find it difficult to make a hot drink in the kitchen here. That is why the occupational therapist is planning on taking her on a visit home. The therapist will put her through her paces in a familiar environment to assess how much regular care she needs. I know it's a long journey, but do you want to take part in the visit to see how she manages for yourself? Would you like me to ask the occupational therapist to contact you?

Daughter: how will you decide if she can manage?

Doctor: that is the purpose of the home visit. The occupational

therapist will take her home to see how she manages: whether she can get into the house, how she can move around inside it, whether she can get herself into and out of bed, whether she can use the toilet and whether she can use the kettle and the cooker – all the basic things that someone needs to be able to do to look after themselves. If she can't do any of these things, then help would need to be provided to enable her to get home. Without the help, she would not be able to go.

Daughter: I'm sorry, but I disagree. She is my mother and she cannot go home.

Doctor: of course you know her best and I know this is a difficult situation, but we cannot force her to go into a home against her will. Can I fix an appointment for you to see her consultant?

1.3.3 Collapse

Scenario
Role: you are a junior doctor working on a medicine for the elderly ward. Mr Davis was admitted to your ward 10 days ago with a dense right hemiparesis, right homonymous hemianopia and a degree of receptive and expressive dysphasia. He is 94 years old, but prior to this stroke was living independently at home. Initially he was treated with intravenous benzylpenicillin, ciprofloxacin and metronidazole for 7 days for aspiration pneumonia. He is still on intravenous fluids and has remained drowsy since admission, but he had been more alert for the last couple of days.

Today his chest sounds worse, his oxygen saturations have dropped and his score on the Glasgow Coma Scale has fallen again. The view of the medical and nursing team is that he should be kept comfortable. His daughter and grand-daughter are upset about his deterioration and the nurse in charge of the ward asks you to speak to them.

Your task: to meet the family on the ward and discuss their concerns.

Key issues to explore

This is a major stroke in a very old man. Although he was previously fit for his age, his homeostatic reserve will now be limited: whatever you do he is very likely to die, and you want him to have a dignified death that is not prolonged by pointless medical intervention. Key ethical aspects are beneficence, non-maleficence and justice. Ethical aspects that many doctors still avoid are the actual cost of his treatment if it is futile and the opportunity cost, eg if he is put in intensive care, this may deny the bed to another.

Key points to establish

- The names of the daughter and grand-daughter: much confusion and many complaints arise when the notes record 'discussed with daughter', and it is only discovered later that there are three daughters with very different views.

- Establish the background: as always, encourage the daughter and grand-daughter to talk first. This may provide an easier route to delivering your bad news and you will be able to assess the appropriate level of complexity for your replies. For example, ask how Mr Davis was coping before admission: even though he was independent, he might have been struggling with developing dementia, failing vision or a recent bereavement. Ask what his views were ('He was such an independent, outdoor man'). Ask what their experience on the ward has been so far. If they have a major concern, however unlikely, about the care (eg 'He has caught pneumonia from the man next to him'), they will not be interested in what you have to say until this is addressed.

- Mr Davis is dying and no treatment will prevent this.

- Aggressive medical attempts to prolong life would be futile and wrong, and you intend Mr Davis' comfort to be the priority.

Appropriate responses to likely questions

Daughter: dad's not so awake and his chest seems really terrible again.

Doctor: I'm afraid you are right. As you know it was a very big stroke and almost straight away he developed a chest infection. We have treated that and his chest improved, but he is certainly very chesty again today. He may be getting another infection, or because he cannot move his legs he may have developed a clot in the leg veins which has gone to the lungs.

Grand-daughter: well, what are you going to do?

Doctor: that's what I wanted to talk to you about. Even when your granddad was getting over the first infection there wasn't much sign of improvement in his stroke, so there is obviously a lot of damage to his brain. It's disappointing that he has got another problem with his chest so quickly, but I think this is telling us just how seriously ill he is.

Daughter: I suppose you will just give him some antibiotics then?

Doctor: treatment with antibiotics usually works only along with other measures such as physiotherapy to clear the chest. This would not be very effective because your father cannot work with the therapist and having physiotherapy – shaking his chest and sucking out his throat – would almost certainly be uncomfortable or distressing for him, particularly as we cannot explain to him what we are trying to do. It is also getting difficult to find a vein for his drip and that is quite uncomfortable for him as well.

Daughter: what if it's a clot?

Doctor: the only way of being sure of that would be to send your father down to the X-ray department for a special scan, but his is too poorly for that at the moment and there wouldn't be any point. If it was a clot, we would not be able to treat it: the treatment for a clot on the lung is to thin the blood and this would probably cause bleeding into the brain which would make things even worse.

Daughter: so you're telling me you can't do anything and we just have to watch him suffer until he dies?

Doctor: I'm sorry, but I think you are right that he is probably going to die. If that is going to happen, I don't think there is anything we can do to change it and we don't want to make things more uncomfortable for him. But we certainly do not want him to suffer: we will move him into a side room so that you and the rest of the family can come and go as you wish. The nurses know him well now and they will carry on with his mouth care so that he doesn't feel dry and thirsty. They will also turn him regularly on his special mattress. If he seems to be in discomfort or any distress, we can give him a little diamorphine to make sure he is comfortable. Just occasionally patients surprise us and rally, so we won't be doing anything that we can't change. But I think we need to make him comfortable now and see how he goes.

Offer tissues, cups of tea, a visit from the chaplain, a chance to pop back to see the patient later and beds in the hostel if the family are not local. If things are not going well, do what you should in real life: offer a senior opinion and propose arrangements to ensure this happens.

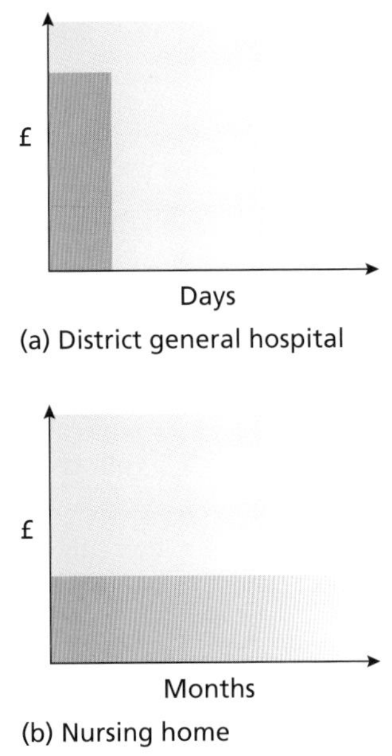

1.4 Acute scenarios

This section offers tips for when the patient being examined is older, but does not aim to be comprehensive: use the individual *Medical Masterclass* modules to obtain more detailed information.

1.4.1 Sudden onset of confusion

> **Scenario**
>
> An 86-year-old man has been brought to the Emergency Department by ambulance from his warden-controlled flat. Details are scant, but the nurse asks you to assess him urgently because he seems very confused and keeps pacing around the department. His observations (BP, pulse rate, temperature, respiratory rate, oxygen saturation on air and urine dipstick) are unremarkable.

▲**Fig. 12** Comparison of the costs of hospital and residential care.

> ⚠ Don't be irritated: if he had been sent directly to a nursing home, the opportunity to treat any acute problem would have been missed. As well as the consequences for the individual, inappropriate admission to a home makes poor economic sense (Fig. 12).

Introduction

Is this delirium (acute confusion), dysphasia or dysarthria? To make a diagnosis of delirium you are looking for a disturbance of consciousness, a change in cognition (usually over hours to days with diurnal fluctuation) and evidence of a causative underlying medical condition.

History of the presenting problem

What do you do when it is difficult to get a history?

- Look at the detail on the ambulance sheet.
- If the patient can give some answers, try short direct

questions: 'Are you in pain? Show me where?' He may respond to your tone of voice and approach you. Sound encouraging and do not appear to rush him: this way you may get more out of the history and examination.

- If anyone has accompanied him to hospital then obviously speak with that person, but if not then phone whoever is appropriate to get more information, eg warden, GP or family.

- Ask for his old notes to be found urgently.

- Ask the nurses what he has been doing: if he has found his way to the toilet, then his speech is more a problem than confusion.

The most important aspects of the history of a patient presenting with confusion are described in Section 1.1.2.

Examination

General features

Vital signs are all unremarkable, but:

- note his nutritional state (reflects the previous weeks to months), hydration level (reflects the last 48 hours) and his general appearance;

- perform a full physical examination, looking particularly for evidence of infection or of stroke.

Cognitive and language assessment

Can the patient tell you his name or his age, the date or the place? Record his Abbreviated Mental Test score out of 10 (see Section 3.2). If you are not getting anywhere, check whether he can obey a one-step command that he would be able to perform physically, eg 'open your mouth'. Then check for nominal dysphasia with an available object, eg your watch. Move from the object to increasingly precise components, eg the strap, buckle or winder. He may be very deaf so use a communication aid, speak clearly with your face well lit or try writing.

Dysarthria

A defect in articulation without disturbance in language function. The patient understands you and the content of his speech is normal, if he can get anything out and you can understand it. If he has Parkinson's disease, he may also be dysphonic with abnormal voice production.

Dysphasia

A disorder of language which may affect comprehension, word finding, fluency, repetition and naming. Classification is complex: non-fluent aphasia is often due to a stroke affecting Broca's area (posterior inferior frontal lobe), while fluent aphasia with paraphasia (substitution of syllables or words) and neologisms (using nonsense words) is due to damage to Wernicke's area (posterior temporal dominant hemisphere).

> ⚠️ Fluent dysphasia in a stroke with little motor impairment often confuses the doctor.

Investigation

There is a wide range of possible causes for an acute confusional state (see Table 2). Routine investigations of a patient presenting with confusion are described in Section 1.1.2, and should be accompanied with other tests as dictated by clinical suspicion.

Management

It will not be possible to send this man home without establishing and treating the underlying cause of his confusion. Specific management will depend on the underlying problem, but consider the following in all cases.

- A well-lit room and nursing by a few attentive staff (rather than many 'popping in') will help any patient prone to confusion.

- Always seek to balance the severity of illness, the degree of confusion and what you need to achieve: a drip may be essential initially to prevent prerenal failure (choose a flat site of access and bandage carefully); alternatively you may be able to give oral ciprofloxacin (excellent absorption), encourage cups of tea and insert a drip 12 hours later when the patient's confusion is settling but he is still behind on fluids.

- Remember the age and frailty of your patient: different antibiotics may be recommended in this age group to reduce the incidence of *Clostridium difficile* (see *Infectious Diseases*, Section 2.3).

Preventive measures in hospital

Older patients often make a surprising recovery from an acute problem, only to linger in hospital with complications that could have been prevented. So make sure you assess the following.

- Is a better mattress needed to prevent pressure sores?

- Would subcutaneous heparin or compression stockings reduce the risk of deep venous thrombosis?

- If the patient is incontinent but you suspect a urinary tract infection (UTI), persuade the nurses that a catheter is not indicated until constipation and the infection have been treated because it will make any infection hard to clear and provide a route for serious nosocomial infection.

- Is he safe? Are bed rails required? If he keeps climbing over the rails, talk over options such as leaving a light on, obtaining a special low bed, enlisting the help of a relative, increasing the amount of nurse input or even putting the mattress on the floor.

- Is sedation required? This may be necessary to enable the patient to have appropriate investigations or treatment, or if he appears very distressed: give haloperidol 0.5 mg im/po (the oral dose may be repeated 2 hourly to a maximum 5 mg in 24 hours) or lorazepam 0.5 mg po if dementia with Lewy bodies is suspected (again repeated 2 hourly if needed, with a maximum of 3 mg in 24 hours).

> ⚠️ A urinary catheter makes urinary infection hard to clear.

The morning after admission

Back to the history! You need to know what the patient was like before the problem that precipitated admission: phone the warden of his flat for information about his usual capabilities (in terms of dressing, transfers, walking and continence), short- and long-term memory, orientation (does he recognise the warden or get lost about the flat?), behaviour and how he occupies his day. Ask about the following in particular.

- What changed and over what period of time?

- Before things went wrong, was the home situation adequate or have things been deteriorating for a while?

- Are there any other contacts, especially regular carers or relatives?

- What support could be offered? Schemes to avoid admission to hospital or to expedite discharge are known as 'intermediate care', and effective management of this patient may well depend on knowing, or finding out, what is available locally. Some warden schemes (sometimes called 'super-sheltered' or 'Part 2½') have on-site care, so it may be possible to arrange supervised medication and additional care without delay. A community hospital bed may be an alternative.

> ⚠ Identify key players in the community (professionals, family, friends and informal carers) at an early stage. Will distant relatives – the nephew who is an orthopaedic surgeon in New York – suddenly materialise with their own views?

A common situation

The most common diagnoses would be an acute confusional state caused by a chest infection, UTI or medication, superimposed on a background of moderate dementia (usually Alzheimer's disease; see Section 2.7). When his acute confusion is resolved, evaluate his mood. Treating an unrelated but compounding pathology, eg cataracts, can produce dramatic improvement.

Further comments

Planning discharge if the patient cannot go home

This will be time-consuming if the patient turns out to have significant dementia but is sure he can manage at home. In the UK it is exceptional for old people with dementia to be

sectioned under the Mental Health Act. Despite the risk of failure, discharge with a maximal care package is usually arranged. A home visit followed by a case conference with members from the community health team may be needed to optimise the package. If the home situation is very borderline, the patient's wishes and determination are crucial. Some members of the team and the family may feel that 'it is a disgrace to allow him to return to such squalor!' Try not to impose standards on others: the patient has survived for 86 years and is a 'nice residential home' really a better prospect for him? Phone his GP before discharge. From 2007, such patients will need an independent advocate (see Section 2.13 on the Mental Capacity Act).

> ⚠ Think ahead: patients like this get stuck in the hospital system. Minimise potential delays by early referrals to occupational therapy, physiotherapy, dietetics and social services.

1.4.2 Collapse

Scenario

An 84-year-old retired gardener presents to the Emergency Department. The previous evening he got up to pass water and slumped to the floor. His wife got him back to bed, but this morning he was drowsy, unable to speak and not moving his right side.

Introduction

Initial rapid assessment is required. While checking his vital signs, Glasgow Coma Scale score and

glucose, you notice facial asymmetry and a hemiparesis.

History of the presenting problem

Is this a stroke which should be managed as a treatable emergency (brain attack)?

In an increasing number of centres stroke is managed as a medical emergency with thrombolysis. The critical factor to establish is whether the onset of symptoms was within the last 3 hours; if so, refer to your specialist team straight away. Here, unfortunately the damage probably began on the previous evening so he is outside the time window for thrombolysis.

The history from the patient's wife

She is very likely to be upset and may need sympathetic prompting. Use a stroke proforma if one is available locally, but ask in particular about the following.

- Drugs: ask if he was taking enalapril for raised blood pressure or swollen ankles.

- Past medical history: form an impression of disease burden.

- Allergies: most patients with a severe stroke need antibiotics soon after admission, so while she is there ask about drug allergies.

- Family history: this is less relevant than in a young patient, but you may get information about her experience of stroke.

- Social history: note information about accommodation, family and other support, but if he survives this will need to be revisited in detail. Touch on his lifestyle, including smoking and drinking, and personal interests. Also find out if his wife will manage without him (he may have been her carer) or if she will need support at home.

When you talk to the patient's wife, it may be easier at this stage to broach the subject of what he would have wanted if things do not go well, when the serious nature of his problems are fresh, rather than 'cold' a couple of days later. If he has made a living will (see Section 2.13), this gives her the opportunity to mention it. In the event of cardiac arrest, resuscitation is most unlikely to succeed so explain that, although you are going to do everything for him, should he collapse unexpectedly you will just keep him comfortable.

When is a stroke not a stroke?

In every case of 'stroke', look for:

- features that raise the likelihood that this is not a stroke, eg progressive disability;
- pointers to a rare cause of stroke such as arteritis;
- any event preceding the collapse, eg chest pain or melaena (indicating hypotension), head injury (extradural or subdural) or a fit (indicating Todd's paresis).

Examination

Key features to cover include the following.

- Check the patient's vital signs, including pulse oximetry.

- Confirm your diagnosis.

- Determine the extent of the neurological impairment.

- Check for early complications, eg aspiration pneumonia and erythematous heels.

- Identify risk factors for secondary prevention: there is only limited evidence at this age, but sensible management of hypertension,

atrial fibrillation or diabetes may be required.

- Document major comorbidities.

Investigations

- FBC.

- Electrolytes and renal function.

- Biochemical profile.

- C-reactive protein.

- Glucose.

- Thyroid-stimulating hormone.

- CXR.

- ECG.

- CT brain scan.

- Other tests if clinically indicated.

Management

Immediate

There is now clear evidence that the patient would best be managed on a stroke unit but, whatever the setting, pay attention to the following.

- Pressure area care: the worst damage is often done on the Emergency Department trolley.

- Compression stockings (assuming foot pulses are palpable): subcutaneous heparin is contraindicated.

- Conveen if possible, rather than catheter.

- Antibiotics to cover aspiration if there are chest signs.

- Rectal paracetamol if febrile.

- Maintain normoglycaemia, with insulin if necessary.

- Which regular drugs need to be continued? A nasogastric (NG) tube may be needed if there is no parenteral option, eg levodopa.

- Antihypertensive drugs are not indicated for acute hypertension

unless it is so severe that it is thought to be contributing to ongoing brain damage.

- If the patient is drowsy or unable to sit, give intravenous fluids and nil by mouth; if alert and able to sit, observe drinking sips and then 50 mL water.

- Correct positioning to minimise spasticity and avoid complications such as subluxation at a flaccid shoulder.

Hypertension in acute stroke

Cerebral autoregulation is impaired in acute stroke and more harm than good will be done by treating this aggressively: most authorities would not treat pressures of up to 220/130 mmHg on a routine basis.

In the first 24 hours

Unless the patient is moribund, active management is required to prevent complications.

- Early physiotherapy: chest and passive movements.

- Aspirin: if a CT scan excludes haemorrhage.

- If there is doubt about the patient's ability to swallow safely, request speech and language therapy assessment. Thick yoghurt is usually the texture swallowed most safely, so thickening agents are often recommended; thin fluid with bits, eg minestrone soup, is the most challenging. The patient should always be sitting upright before having food. If in doubt, continue nil by mouth.

Priorities over the next few days

- Reassess the patient's swallowing daily and weigh him as soon as possible: if within a few days he still cannot swallow but is not dying, consider a fine-bore NG tube taped to the paralysed side to enable feeding and maintain hydration. If there is doubt, arrange videofluoroscopy to check for pooling or aspiration.

- Refer him to speech and language therapy for communication assessment: if he is drowsy or dysphasic, then early assessment may help the family and staff to communicate, eg he may master a picture chart.

- When his condition permits, start speech therapy and active physiotherapy: he should spend time being nursed and well positioned in a chair with adequate pressure relief (drowsiness, cognition and trunk control permitting).

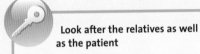

Look after the relatives as well as the patient

Help the relatives: having worried and prepared themselves for his death, this has not happened. But the situation looks grim. Encourage his wife to eat, take breaks and pace her visits. Explain that although sudden deterioration is possible (due to a further stroke, myocardial infarction or pulmonary embolism), bronchopneumonia is more likely. Provide literature from the Stroke Association about strokes and the relevant complications, eg dysphasia.

Persistent inability to swallow

If the patient still cannot swallow at 1–2 weeks after admission, but overall things are improving, consider referral for percutaneous endoscopic gastrostomy (PEG) feeding. PEG feeding permits better nutrition (NG tubes usually fall out regularly) and more dignity, although it does not remove the risk of aspiration. Paradoxically, in some situations, an advantage of NG tubes is that they do fall out: it is easier not to resite a tube than it is to remove one. If he is deteriorating or if swallowing is improving, persevere

with NG feeding. In a patient with severe dementia who reaches for food or drink despite a tendency to choke, a policy of nil by mouth and PEG is unkind, and supervised oral feeding with thickening agents is appropriate. An interim measure is a bridled NG tube, where the tube is tied around the nasal septum. It is a bedside procedure as the tube will not fall out but will need changing monthly; however, note the comments about the advantages of tubes that fall out.

A PEG tube is not always advisable and should be inserted only after a multidisciplinary discussion involving the family, especially if the patient cannot understand the procedure.

Allowing a patient to die

Patients who are going to die usually do, but death may be prolonged by medical intervention. Defer a CT brain scan rather than risk the patient dying in the scanner. In end-stage dementia, antibiotics may be inappropriate from the start. Usually, the situation is less clear and most patients who have suffered a severe stroke will receive antibiotics for their first infective complication. If there is no useful recovery and the patient is chesty 2 or 3 weeks later, is it time to let nature take its course? By now you may have a feel for what the patient wanted and his family's view, but do not place the burden of decision on the family. A medical decision is needed, taking into account the opinion of the multidisciplinary team in the interests of the patient. This should then be discussed with the family. If there is disagreement, remember that many doctors and most of the public have an inflated view of the power of antibiotics.

Given a full explanation, families usually agree with palliative care for an elderly patient with a massive stroke.

Palliative treatment

The decision about whether a patient is treated actively or palliatively is a medical one: the doctor should never ask the family to make it, or say or imply to them that they have the 'casting vote'. However, you must check that all significant family members agree. If the family is not ready to accept palliation, consider further antibiotics to give them more time. A second opinion may be useful.

If the patient is dying, ensure that symptom control is optimal as in patients dying from cancer.

Further comments

The patient who is recovering from a stroke

If the patient pulls through, treat other problems pragmatically. If he was taking an NSAID for his arthritic knees, then adequate analgesia is essential if he is to mobilise, although regular paracetamol is usually effective. If you note iron deficiency anaemia, then surgery would not be indicated so do not put him through investigations: oesophagitis or peptic ulceration is possible, so prescribe a proton pump inhibitor and recheck the FBC in 2 weeks. Look for opportunities to improve things as he progresses, eg replace lost spectacles. If he deteriorates, find out why (eg constipation, urinary tract infection and further stroke).

Is rehabilitation appropriate?

Rehabilitation after a major stroke is a long haul. The setting will depend on what is available locally. The main advantage of early supported discharge schemes is that they free-up hospital capacity. What may be achieved with a given level of neurological impairment depends on many factors: the patient's comorbidities, previous fitness, cognition and mood, and the attitude of the family.

Members of the multidisciplinary team may work with the patient, carers or both.

- Physiotherapist: works on posture, balance and functional movement. Appliances, such as a wrist or ankle splint, may be helpful.

- Occupational therapist: assesses basic activities of daily living (ADL; personal ADL), and then more sophisticated abilities (instrumental or individual ADL), to promote independence.

- Speech and language therapist: works on communication and swallowing.

- Social worker: may advise on what benefits are available and will help plan placement.

- Dietitian: gives nutritional advice, especially if tube feeding is needed.

- Chaplaincy: arranges spiritual support from the appropriate faith or pastoral care.

- Stroke Association volunteer: may come in from the community.

- Doctor: involved with ongoing and new medical problems.

- Nursing staff: these are the key people in the team. Their skill in ensuring that the patient is in a coordinated therapeutic environment all day, rather than for a couple of brief therapy sessions, is crucial.

- In rare units a psychologist and an art or music therapist may be involved.

Progress is monitored against explicit goals agreed with the patient and the family, and new goals are set at regular (often weekly) multidisciplinary case conferences. If the patient is not making the expected progress, can a barrier to rehabilitation (eg depression or the fear of being a burden) be identified? Complications of stroke, such as emotional lability, personality change or cognitive impairment, difficulties with bowels and bladder, and post stroke pain, may benefit from a team approach. The focus shifts from rehabilitation to placement once what the patient is gaining from therapy reaches a plateau: the timing depends on how much rehabilitation can be provided in the community.

> ⚠️ Plan early (eg home visit from an occupational therapist) for the likely destination; change tack later if necessary. Do not defer to see what the patient achieves because there will then be a frustrating wait while support is arranged.

What are the options for discharge if the patient does not make a full recovery?

Common options include returning home with a support package, rehousing to a warden-supervised flat, residential home or nursing home, or (in a few areas) NHS nursing care. Your assessment must take account of the carer's needs. Consider regular respite or a service such as Crossroads, which will offer a regular sitter to enable the carer to have a break.

Funding of long-term care is often problematic because of the huge cost. Patients with major disabilities can go home (usually if their accommodation needs little adaptation) to a willing and able-bodied carer, but the time required to assemble the necessary equipment, eg hospital bed, pressure mattress, standing hoist and an appropriate wheelchair, can be lengthy. The carer should work alongside therapists before discharge. A sensible spouse can manage a PEG tube: sterility is not needed but training is essential.

Reassessment should be planned because unexpected problems will arise and, after the initial elation at discharge, depression may resurface. The patient may attend the day hospital before and after discharge to provide continuity of care.

2.1 Why elderly patients are different

Many diseases in elderly people are a continuum of diseases found in middle age, so why are elderly patients different? How old is old? It depends on your perspective and where you live. Expectations of health and lifestyle are changing. In the UK now, most frail elderly people are aged over 80. Younger patients who are 'biologically old' with multisystem pathology often have arteriopathy, or are 'graduates' with chronic disability.

> 'It is not how old you are, but how you are old.' (Marie Dressler)

The effects of pathology are superimposed on the ageing process and are influenced by fitness and social factors (Fig. 13). Ageing changes are seen in most organs.

Why do ageing changes matter?
In comparison with a group of younger people, in old age there is:

- increased variability between individuals;

- impaired homeostasis, which is acceptable when individuals are at rest but significant when they are stressed (eg fasting glucose is minimally higher in elderly people, but their glucose levels are much higher after meals);

- different significance of some physical signs.

> After a post-take ward round, reflect on the different individuals you have seen of similar chronological age.

Multiple pathologies
In young adults, you try to fit all their symptoms and signs to one condition. The situation is different in elderly people, a fact recognised since antiquity, when Juvenal stated 'How incessant and great are the ills with which a prolonged old age is replete.'

Why do old people often have several diseases?
The prevalence of many diseases increases with age, eg stroke and Alzheimer's disease. There is more time for things to accrue so this may be chance, but not all occurrences will be random. Disparate conditions may have a common pathogenesis, eg failure to dispose of free radicals, which could be influenced genetically (isoenzyme activities) or environmentally (dietary antioxidant). A given genotype may be associated with several conditions. Commonly occurring risk factors (eg smoking) predispose to several diseases. Some chronic diseases have complications affecting several systems (eg diabetes) or predispose to other conditions (eg infection).

Risk factors
A parameter that is a risk factor in middle-aged individuals may not carry the same risk in old age, perhaps because an old individual may have protective factors that are less well identified. Data from trials of antihypertensives including progressively older cohorts have established that hypertension is a vascular risk factor up to around 83 years of age. HYVET (HYpertension in the Very Elderly Trial coordinated by Chris Bulpitt) is currently recruiting subjects aged over 80. The situation with high cholesterol remains unclear.

Disease susceptibility
Tuberculosis is more common in elderly people: the reasons for this may include socioeconomic factors, a cohort with prior exposure from a pretreatment era and changes in the immune system. However, ethnicity

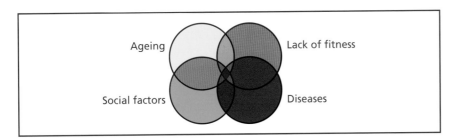

▲ **Fig. 13** The background to disease in old age.

is a much greater factor in tuberculosis. Nosocomial *Clostridium difficile* diarrhoea is more common in the frail elderly than in middle-aged people, so departments of medicine and of medicine for elderly people often have different antibiotic policies.

> ⚠ Find out about antibiotic policies in medicine and medicine for the elderly in your hospital.

Differential diagnoses

Listing the diagnostic possibilities in the probable order for a particular individual is a challenge for newly qualified doctors, and even for more experienced doctors in the heat of an examination. Ethnic background is important: the most common cause of iron deficiency anaemia worldwide is hookworm, but this is rare in East Anglia! Age is another major factor to consider before reeling off your list of probabilities (Table 10).

Altered response to disease

Illness in old age may present as it does in middle age, but not always – an intellectual challenge of the specialty. Most of the public can diagnose serious pathology in middle life (eg when the postman collapsed, nearby builders

recognised his symptoms and dialled 999 to contact the emergency services). However, spotting a heart attack or a case of pneumonia in elderly people can be trickier owing to:

- missing symptoms, eg pain may be absent in a myocardial infarction or a perforated viscus (air under the diaphragm on CXR is a surprise finding), attenuation of thirst (predisposing to dehydration);

- missing signs, eg fever may be absent despite serious infection, neck stiffness may be absent in purulent meningitis;

- non-specific or atypical presentations (eg confusion) are common.

> **Non-specific presentation of disease**
>
> The following could all be presentations of an acute problem (eg stroke), a chronic condition (eg Parkinson's disease) or *i*atrogenic disease (eg treatment with a new analgesic):
>
> - *i*nstability (falls);
> - *i*ncontinence;
> - *i*ntellectual failure (confusion);
> - *i*mmobility ('she is off her feet');
> - failure to thrive.
>
> The five '*i*'s are sometimes referred to as the 'geriatric giants'.

The presenting condition is often complicated by the consequences of immobility, particularly after a long time lying down (eg incontinence, dehydration, pressure sores, deep vein thrombosis, risk of compartment syndrome and rhabdomyolysis).

Inappropriate prescribing and polypharmacy

Contraindications to a drug, side effects, adverse events and drug interactions are all more common in old age (see Section 2.6).

Social problems

There are sadder aspects to old age medicine. Old age is a time of loss, which is not necessarily always balanced by the compensations of a fulfilling life and supportive family. Retirement is a recent phenomenon. This 'luxury' of a civilised society can leave an individual without a role and with reduced income and status, a falling standard of living and enforced membership of a group described as a 'rising tide', a 'burden' or even an 'epidemic'. Western culture now values youth and beauty above wisdom and experience. Listen, share and focus on the practical problems that result from this and how they affect the patient. What might help? Don't make assumptions, particularly across different ethnic groups.

Expectations

Things are changing (some parts of the USA are way ahead), but elderly patients may have low expectations for their health and of the system. Problems such as swollen ankles or incontinence are simply attributed to 'old age'. Elderly patients are not infrequently admitted with anasarca; ankle swelling spreads to the thighs and trunk before help is sought. In such cases it takes time to shift the fluid, but patients can often be discharged on small doses of loop

	Likely cause	
	Fits	**Jaundice**
Neonate	Birth trauma and hypoxia	Physiological
Baby/toddler	Fever	Biliary atresia
Child/teenager	Epilepsy	Hepatitis A
Young adult	Drugs, alcohol or withdrawal	Drugs and alcohol
Middle age	Brain tumour	Gallstones
Old age	Cerebrovascular disease	Carcinoma of the pancreas

TABLE 10 LIKELY CAUSES OF FITS AND JAUNDICE IN DIFFERENT AGE GROUPS

diuretic and an angiotensin-converting enzyme inhibitor. In the above scenario, the cardiac failure was not severe, just neglected. Families of elderly patients may have low expectations, but some expect miracles. Professionals in all disciplines may have ageist attitudes: 'Well, my dear, what do you expect at your age?' Where resources are short, the old are frequently at the end of the queue. Ageism should be as unacceptable as racism, but common sense is required.

Differences in health and social services within the UK

Since the advent of the Scottish parliament, there are increasing differences between Scotland and England and Wales in terms of health service organisation, social services, charges and access to drug treatment. Age Concern Scotland provides clear online information about some aspects which differ in Scotland. Recommendations from the National Institute for Health and Clinical Excellence (NICE) may be altered by National Health Service Quality Improvement Scotland.

FURTHER READING

Bowker LK, Price JD and Smith SC, eds. *Oxford Handbook of Geriatric Medicine*. Oxford: Oxford University Press, 2006.

Bracewell C, Gray R and Rai G. *Essential Facts in Geriatric Medicine*. Abingdon: Radcliffe, 2004.

Bulpitt CJ, Beckett NS, Cooke J, *et al.* Results of the pilot study for the Hypertension in the Very Elderly Trial. *J. Hypertens*. 2003; 21: 2409–17.

Copeland JRM, Abou-Saleh MT and Blazer DG, eds. *Principles and Practice of Geriatric Psychiatry*, 2nd edn. Chichester: John Wiley & Sons, 2002.

Cristian A, ed. Geriatric rehabilitation. *Clin. Geriatr. Med.* 2006; 22: 221–498

(reviews of many aspects of rehabilitation for older people).

Evans JG, Williams TF, Beattie BL, Michel J-P and Wilcock GK, eds. *Oxford Textbook of Geriatric Medicine*, 2nd edn. Oxford: Oxford University Press, 2003.

Nicholl C, Webster S and Wilson KJ. *Lecture Notes in Medicine for the Elderly*, 7th edn. Oxford: Blackwell Science, 2007.

Pathy MSJ, Sinclair AJ and Morley JE, eds. *Principles and Practice of Geriatric Medicine*, 4th edn. Chichester: John Wiley & Sons, 2005.

Tallis R and Fillit HM, eds. *Brocklehurst's Textbook of Geriatric Medicine and Gerontology*, 6th edn. Edinburgh: Churchill Livingstone, 2002.

Websites
Age Concern England: excellent statistics and practical information fact sheets (may be very helpful for grandparents). Available at http://www.ageconcern.org.uk/

Age Concern Scotland. Available at http://www.ageconcernscotland.org.uk

American Geriatrics Society: the transatlantic view. Available at http://www.americangeriatrics.org/

British Geriatrics Society trainees' section: information about careers, training and practice, including areas poorly covered in textbooks. Available at http://www.bgs.org.uk/

Carers UK: source of information for carers. Available at http://www.carersuk.org/

Counsel and Care: information about residential care. Available at http://www.counselandcare.org.uk

National Institute of Aging (USA): links to research in progress and trials, especially concerning Alzheimer's. Available at http://www.nia.nih.gov

National Institute for Health and Clinical Excellence (NICE): issues guidelines on cost-effectiveness of licensed drugs and produces technology reviews. Available at http://www.nice.org.uk

NHS Quality Improvement Scotland: the body that aims to improve quality of healthcare in Scotland. Available at http://www.nhshealthquality.org

2.2 General approach to management

History

Obtaining an accurate history may require detective work and the history needs to extend beyond the presenting problem. Make sure that your investigations cover:

- several informants, eg phone the home help/GP;
- social history, especially what a patient could manage before they were ill;
- medication (prescribed and over the counter).

Examination

In many other specialties the examination, especially when done by a consultant in outpatients, is very focused, but in a frail older patient remember the following.

- Examination is usually comprehensive rather than targeted to one system.
- Rushing is counterproductive.
- Beware of short cuts: take the patient's socks off and look under any bandages.
- Remember the breast examination in women and the rectal

examination (especially in problems with bladder or bowel, gynaecological symptoms, neurology affecting the legs, anaemia and back pain).

- Assess cognition, function and mood.

Investigations

> Remember why you are doing investigations, ie to confirm diagnoses, look for complications and as a baseline for therapy. In a stressful situation (examinations) or when you feel overwhelmed (you have identified seven different problems), it helps to think of tests in groups and work from the basic to the complex.

Most geriatricians use a mix of specific and 'screening' tests when a patient is admitted to hospital because of the prevalence of non-specific presentations and unexpected pathologies.

- Urine tests.
- Blood tests (think by laboratory: haematology and biochemistry, etc.).
- Other specimens for bacteriology.
- CXR.
- ECG.
- Other tests: echocardiography, 24-hour tape, tilt testing, lung function, endoscopy, electroencephalography and electromyography.
- Imaging: plain radiographs, ultrasonography, contrast studies, CT and MRI scans, positron emission tomography, etc.
- Histology? With the expansion in imaging, tissue diagnosis may be delayed.

> Once the results of the basic investigations are available, it is important to take stock.
>
> - What am I dealing with?
> - What is treatable?
> - What is important? (To the patient and carer as well as to the doctor.)
>
> Don't lose sight of the wood for the trees!

Management

Summarise the situation and decide on a plan of action. Management almost always involves the multidisciplinary team and the process of rehabilitation to maximise the function (physical, mental and social) of the individual patient (see Section 1.4.2). Consider the following:

- education (patients' societies can be very useful);
- physiotherapy, speech and language therapy, occupational therapy, dietetic support and podiatry;
- social services;
- improving general health (remember eyes and ears, and nutrition);
- treating other treatable conditions;
- specific drug treatment;
- controlling any remaining symptoms;
- supporting the carer;
- legal aspects (check if the patient is still driving).

End of life decisions

For these, see the General Medical Council and British Medical Association guidelines. Each decision about when to move from cure to care is unique, but there are some general principles. It may be hard for doctors to accept the inevitable, particularly if there is no clear diagnosis (it is easier in cases of cancer) and if earlier management was suboptimal. Issues around food and fluid intake are becoming harder to manage with increasing pressure for feeding tubes and drips. There is less and less experience of the natural process of dying and relatives can become fixed on ideas like 'they mustn't die hungry or thirsty'. Discussion with a patient's family can become time-consuming and may become more complex in 2007 when attorneys, deputies, advocates and the Court of Protection will have legal rights to contribute to health decisions if a patient is no longer competent.

> 'In the name of Hippocrates, doctors have invented the most exquisite form of torture ever known to man: survival.' (Luis Buñuel)

The decision to stop 'curative' treatment should not be placed on the family and legally responsibility remains with the consultant, although it would be foolish to ignore the views of the multidisciplinary team. Good communication with the patient, family and the team is essential. Do not take away hope from the patient or family, but reassure them that symptom control is paramount.

Do not attempt resuscitation orders

The decision not to perform cardiopulmonary resuscitation is not the same as the decision to withhold active treatment, but the two are sometimes confused. Many patients who would not be resuscitated in the event of a cardiorespiratory arrest receive a whole range of other treatments.

It has been recommended that all do not attempt resuscitation (DNAR) decisions should be discussed with the patient and the family. However, this discussion is not an easy one. On admission, elderly patients who are ill but not expecting to die may be distressed by the concept, however well it is handled. Later in their stay, patients may interpret this discussion as evidence that things are much worse than you have let on. The family view is important, but relatives may not be available and may disagree among themselves, and your primary duty is to the patient. Doctors are not obliged to discuss futile treatments with patients and the results of resuscitation in non-cardiac care unit settings are very poor. Chronological age itself is not a reason for a DNAR decision. However, the burden of pathology in many elderly patients often makes resuscitation inappropriate because they are so unlikely to survive the procedure or a stay in an intensive therapy unit and the return home. As a junior doctor, find out your consultant's policy, be aware of the guidelines of your hospital and always discuss a DNAR decision with the nursing staff. If a decision needs to be made, draw this to your specialist registrar or consultant's attention. If a patient's death is likely, plan to talk things over with the family (suggested timing is discussed in Section 1.4.2).

> ⚠️ Poor communication with colleagues results in poor medicine and many complaints. Try to plan ahead and record your decisions clearly in the patient's notes so that covering teams know the plan if your patient deteriorates. Different levels of intervention may be appropriate, eg 'intravenous antibiotics, but not a central line or ventilation'.

FURTHER READING

British Medical Association. *Withholding and Withdrawing Life-prolonging Medical Treatment: Guidance for Decision Making*, 3nd edn. Oxford: Blackwell, 2007.

British Medical Association. *Decisions Relating to Cardiopulmonary Resuscitation: A Joint Statement from the British Medical Association, the Resuscitation Council (UK) and the Royal College of Nursing.* London: BMA, 2002. Available at http://web.bma.org.uk

Cervo FA, Bryan L and Farber S. To PEG or not to PEG: a review of evidence for placing feeding tubes in advanced dementia and the decision-making process. *Geriatrics* 2006; 61: 30–5.

Driver and Vehicle Licensing Agency (Drivers Medical Group). *At a Glance Guide to the Current Medical Standards of Fitness to Drive: For Medical Practitioners.* Swansea: DVLA, 2003. Available at http://www.dvla.gov.uk/medical

General Medical Council. *Withholding and Withdrawing Life-prolonging Treatments: Good Practice in Decision-making.* London: GMC, 2006. Available at http://www.gmc-uk.org/guidance

2.3 Falls

> **Falls**
> • Very common with increasing age.
> • Significant cause of morbidity and mortality.
> • A cause of older people being institutionalised.
> • Often preventable.
> • A marker of failing function.

Epidemiology

Almost one-third of those aged over 65 years have at least one fall per year. Furthermore:

- the incidence increases with age so that 50% of those aged over 85 years fall every year;

- women fall more often than men (increased body sway and longer lifespan);

- falls may be a marker of acute illness, such as myocardial infarction (MI), pulmonary embolus, pneumonia or urinary tract infection (UTI);

- falls may be a sign of chronic illness, including anaemia, myxoedema and dementia.

Aetiology

Falls are usually multifactorial, so all contributing factors need to be identified (Table 11). People with dementia are at particular risk of falls, but remediable causes must still be sought, especially the side effects of psychotropic medication.

Clinical presentation

The history may point to the systems involved. Make sure you carry out the following.

- Examine the relevant systems.

- Always check vision, hearing, gait, feet and shoes, and postural BP.

- Check for any injuries.

- Review drugs: hepatic drug extraction and metabolism, and most significantly glomerular filtration rate (GFR; estimated GFR is readily available online), all decrease with age, so elderly people are more susceptible to adverse effects when taking drugs.

TABLE 11 CAUSES, INVESTIGATION AND MANAGEMENT OF FALLS

System	Associated symptoms	Signs	Investigations	Causes	Treatment
Cardiovascular	Transient loss of consciousness with rapid recovery, but may have retrograde amnesia	Slow pulse	ECG, Holter monitor	Bradyarrhythmia/complete heart block	Permanent pacing
	Palpitations	Fast AF	ECG, Holter monitor	Symptomatic tachyarrhythmia, eg paroxysmal AF	Antiarrhythmic therapy
	None/angina/breathlessness	Ejection systolic murmur	Echocardiography	Aortic stenosis	Aortic valve replacement
	Dizziness on standing	Drop in BP of >20 mmHg systolic or >10 mmHg diastolic after standing for 3 min	Consider tilt table and Synacthen test	Postural hypotension secondary to drugs, Addison's disease, autonomic neuropathy (eg diabetes)	Stop diuretics and antihypertensives. Try TED stockings, fludrocortisone and midodrine
	Acute nausea and vomiting followed by transient loss of consciousness with rapid recovery	Pale and clammy, may be bradycardic		Vasovagal episode	Reassurance only
	Recurrent syncope		Tilt	Cardioinhibitory syncope Vasodepressor syncope	Pacemaker Consider beta-blockers and paroxetine
				Long QT syndrome	Review drugs
Neurological	Unilateral weakness	Hemiplegia, carotid bruit	CT brain scan	Stroke	Secondary prevention
	Loss of consciousness with incontinence, tongue biting and postictal drowsiness or confusion	Tonic–clonic movements, bilateral upgoing plantars	EEG, CT brain scan	Epilepsy	Antiepileptic therapy
	Difficulty turning over in bed, tremor, poverty of movement, freezing in doorways and drooling	Mask-like facies, pill-rolling tremor, cogwheel rigidity, flexed posture, festinant gait	CT brain scan to exclude atherosclerotic pseudo-PD	Idiopathic PD	Levodopa therapy, dopamine agonists, COMT inhibitors
	Confusion and incontinence Difficulty getting out of a chair	Broad-based gait Weakness of proximal muscles	CT brain scan TSH	Normal-pressure hydrocephalus Proximal myopathy	VP shunt Thyroid replacement
Psychiatrics	Low mood	Flat affect	Geriatric Depression Scale	Depression	Antidepressants
	Poor memory and confusion	May be signs of previous strokes	CT brain scan, TSH, vitamin B$_{12}$, folate	Vascular dementia, Alzheimer's disease, Lewy body dementia	Review drugs
Decreased sensory input and balance disturbance	Poor vision	Visual acuity fields, fundoscopy	Ophthalmology review	Presbyopia, glaucoma, macular degeneration, cataracts, diabetic retinopathy	Spectacles of correct prescription. Treatment for glaucoma. Cataract extraction. Laser therapy if indicated
	Deafness	Ear wax, perforated drum	Audiometry, CT brain scan	Presbyacusis, wax, otosclerosis, acoustic neuroma	Remove wax. Hearing aid (check batteries)
	Dizziness Short recurrent episodes of vertigo	Low BP, ear wax, anaemia Positive Hallpike manoeuvre	FBC, CT brain scan	Drugs or CVA BPPV	Stop drugs and treat cause Vestibular rehabilitation

AF, atrial fibrillation; BPPV, benign paroxysmal positional vertigo; COMT, catechol-*O*-methyltransferase; CVA, cerebrovascular accident; EEG, electroencephalography; PD, Parkinson's disease; TED, thromboembolic device; TSH, thyroid-stimulating hormone; VP, ventriculoperitoneal.

> ⚠ Taking four or more different medications correlates most strongly with a high risk of falling (Table 12).

Examination

Is the patient ill, suggesting an acute condition such as a silent MI, pneumonia, a UTI or hyponatraemia? Are there chronic, unrecognised problems, eg anaemia, hypothyroidism/hyperthyroidism and cataracts? Also consider the following.

- Has the patient been lying on the ground? (This would cause bruising, pressure sores and hypothermia.)

- Are there any injuries?

Signs of neglect, such as poor personal hygiene or overgrown toenails, may point to dementia. In particular, check the following.

- General state, temperature, nutrition and Abbreviated Mental Test score.

- Bones and joints, especially knees and hips, neck, 'spring' rib cage and pelvis.

- Careful cardiological examination, including lying and standing BP, and carotid sinus massage.

- Full neurological assessment looking for evidence of stroke, PD, myopathy or neuropathy.

- Visual acuity.

- Hearing, and look for wax in the ears. If the patient has true vertigo, perform the Hallpike manoeuvre to exclude benign paroxysmal positional vertigo.

- Watch the patient walk. Look for a classic shuffling parkinsonian gait, a hemiplegic gait or the scissoring gait of a fixed arthritic pelvis. Watch the patient turn to assess balance.

- Do not forget to look at her feet and shoes.

Investigations

General investigations depend on what was found in the history and examination. Carotid sinus massage and tilt-table testing are useful in diagnosing carotid hypersensitivity, cardioinhibitory syncope and vasodepressor syncope.

TABLE 12 DRUGS ASSOCIATED WITH INCREASED RISK OF FALLING

Class	Effect	Example	Possible solution
Antipsychotic medication	Sedation Extrapyramidal effects Postural hypotension	Chlorpromazine Haloperidol Chlorpromazine	Try an atypical such as risperidone As above, or lorazepam Avoid coprescribing with diuretics
Tricyclic antidepressants	Postural hypotension Arrhythmias	Lofepramine, amitriptyline	SSRIs are less likely to cause dysrhythmias and *may* cause less hypotension
Analgesics	Sedation	Opiates	Try a non-opiate, eg paracetamol, given regularly
Antiepileptic drugs	Overdosage causes cerebellar side effects	Phenytoin, carbamazepine	Monitor levels
Alcohol	Acute intoxication causes reduced level of consciousness		Education
	Chronic abuse causes cerebellar damage		Thiamine therapy
	Sudden withdrawal causes acute confusion		High index of suspicion, protect with reducing doses of chlordiazepoxide on admission
Benzodiazepines	Sedation. Sudden withdrawal can cause confusion and falls	Diazepam, nitrazepam	Avoid if possible. If withdrawal symptoms are suspected, slowly reduce the dose
Cardiovascular medications	Low BP	Diuretics, nitrates, other vasodilators	Use lowest therapeutic dose
Parkinson's disease medication	Postural hypotension	Levodopa preparations: Madopar and Sinemet Dopamine agonists: pergolide	Coprescribe fludrocortisone and TED stockings

SSRI, selective serotonin reuptake inhibitor; TED, thromboembolic device.

Treatment

> 🔑 The best strategy for preventing falls is by multiple interventions.

Review all medications. Are they necessary? Are they causing interactions? Are they causing postural hypotension? Treat all contributing factors.

Refer patients to an occupational therapist, who will:

- assess the patient's home for accessibility and adequate lighting, as well as advising on the removal of potential hazards (eg mats on shiny floors, loose wires, clutter and pets);

- arrange for provision of appropriate aids such as a toilet raise, a trolley for transporting drinks and food from room to room, and perching stools for tasks such as washing and cooking;

- assess patients' ability to look after themselves.

Also refer patients to a physiotherapist, who will:

- advise whether walking aids will help patients mobilise more safely and, if so, assess each individual for the appropriate aid (see Table 9 for more details regarding walking aids);

- teach people how to get up once they have fallen;

- encourage balance training exercises such as Tai Chi.

Social workers will arrange a package of care to meet the needs of the individual. Also, there is frequently a need for investment by local government, eg good lighting and early gritting of icy pavements around older people's housing.

For sticks and most frames, the top of the aid should come up to the crease in the wrist or radial styloid of the patient when the arm is hanging straight down at the side. All walking aids make the upper limbs weight bearing, thereby increasing osteoarthritis (OA) at the shoulder, so you may suspect severe OA in the hip or knee from the CXR.

Complications

Falls result in significant morbidity and mortality. Complications include the following.

- Decreased mobility, which leads to the potential for pressure sores, deep vein thromboses, incontinence and even contractures in severe cases.

- Minor injury in 20% of those who fall.

- Loss of confidence, which may deter people from leaving their homes (or concerned relatives may encourage them not to); this can be addressed by encouraging exercise and attendance at a day centre.

- Low mood.

- Decreased quality of life.

- A significant proportion of elderly people who present to the Emergency Department after a fall are admitted.

- Of the elderly who fall, 5% sustain a fracture; therefore consider prevention of osteoporosis with bisphosphonates, calcium and vitamin D, or the use of hip protector pads (though the evidence base for this is poor).

- Recurrent falls may eventually lead to people being institutionalised prematurely.

Information for patients

Refer patients to suitable sources of information.

FURTHER READING

Age Concern and Royal Society for the Prevention of Accidents. *Falls: How to Avoid Them and How to Cope. A Practical Guide for Older People and Their Carers.* Newton Abbot: Age Concern, 2004. Available at http://www.natpact.nhs.uk/uploads/2004_Sep/Falls_leaflet.pdf

American Geriatrics Society. Guidelines for the prevention of falls in older persons. *J. Am. Geriatr. Soc.* 2001; 49: 664–72.

Chang JT, Morton SC, Rubenstien LZ, *et al.* Interventions for the prevention of falls in older people: systematic review and meta-analysis of randomised clinical trials. *BMJ* 2004; 328: 680.

Close J, Ellis E, Hooper R, *et al.* Prevention of Falls in the Elderly Trial (PROFET). *Lancet* 1999; 353: 93–7.

National Collaborating Centre for Nursing and Supportive Care. *Falls: The Assessment and Prevention of Falls in Older People.* London: National Institute for Clinical Excellence, 2004. Available at http://www.nice.org.uk

Parry SW and Kenny RA. Tilt table testing in the diagnosis of unexplained syncope. *Q. J. Med.* 1999; 92: 623–9.

Royal Society for the Prevention of Accidents. *Growing Older Safely.* Edinburgh: ROSPA, 1989.

Tinetti ME, Baker DI, McAvey G, *et al.* A multifactorial intervention to reduce the risk of falling among elderly people living in the community. *N. Engl. J. Med.* 1994; 331: 821–7.

Wilkinson TJ and Sainsbury R. Hip protectors. *Age Ageing* 1998; 27: 89–90.

2.4 Urinary and faecal incontinence

2.4.1 Urinary incontinence

Urinary incontinence is defined as the involuntary loss of urine sufficient in volume or frequency to be a social or a health problem.

> **Urinary incontinence**
>
> - Very common.
> - Often concealed by the patient.
> - A major cause of poor quality of life.
> - An important factor contributing to institutionalisation.
> - An enormous burden both to the individual and to society.
> - Treatable.

Aetiology and pathophysiology

There are four main types of urinary incontinence: stress, urge, mixed and retention with overflow. Their features and management are listed in Table 13. Overactive bladder syndrome is defined as urgency that occurs with or without urge incontinence, and usually with frequency and nocturia. Several factors predispose to urinary incontinence.

General age-related changes

- Reduced bladder capacity.

- Increase in residual volume of bladder.

- Increased number of bladder spasms (detrusor contractions).

- Change in the normal diurnal production of antidiuretic hormone so that less is produced at night, leading to nocturia.

- Decreased mobility.

Factors associated with female gender

- Anatomy: the longer urethra and presence of the prostate gland enhance continence in men; the short urethra in women increases the risk of urinary tract infection (UTI).

- Multiparity: vaginal delivery of large babies, with stretching and perineal tears and particularly inadequate pelvic floor exercises afterwards, leads to weakness of the pelvic floor and hypermobility of the neck of the bladder.

- Postmenopausally: the fall in oestrogen leads to reduced smooth

TABLE 13 CAUSES AND MANAGEMENT OF DIFFERENT TYPES OF INCONTINENCE

Type	Symptoms	Examination findings	Investigations	Causes	Treatments
Stress incontinence	Involuntary leaking of small amounts of urine on coughing, laughing and exercising	Vaginal examination: cystocele, vaginal prolapse	MSU, stable bladder on cystoscopy, leakage on stress testing	Multiparity, pelvic surgery in women, prostate surgery in men, collagen disorders	Pelvic floor exercises Ring pessary Surgical procedures
Urge incontinence	Overwhelming and instant urge to pass urine with involuntary emptying of the bladder	No specific findings	MSU, unstable detrusor contractions during cystometry	Detrusor instability caused by ageing or hyperreflexia in neurological disease, eg MS, CVA, PD	Anticholinergic drugs: tolterodine, oxybutynin, trospium DDAVP
Mixed	Symptoms of both stress and urge incontinence	Signs as above	Mixture of above	Mixture of above	Treat for urge incontinence first, then stress
Overflow incontinence	Constant dribbling of urine, sensation that the bladder is not empty	Palpable bladder and faecal loading in either sex, enlarged prostate in men, cystocele in women	Ultrasound demonstrates an enlarged bladder with large residual volume	Prostatism, urethral stricture, bladder overdistension, faecal loading. Also drugs	Surgical relief of obstruction (eg TURP or urethral dilatation) Cholinomimetics such as bethanechol Catheters
Functional and iatrogenic	Inability to reach the toilet secondary to reduced mobility; also confusion	Signs of underlying disease	Normal ultrasonography and urodynamics	Arthritis, PD, CVA, acute confusion, dementia, plaster cast, drugs, etc.	Treat the underlying problem. Change drugs. Commode, toilet raise, pad and pants, conveen, catheter

CVA, cerebrovascular accident; DDAVP, desmopressin acetate; PD, Parkinson's disease; MS, multiple sclerosis; MSU, midstream urine sample; TURP, transurethral prostatectomy.

muscle tone in the urethra, a higher pH permits pathogens to flourish and dryness causes the sensation of urgency, as well as dyspareunia.

Other risk factors

- Concurrent drug treatments: review and stop diuretics if possible, and check that drugs are not causing constipation and that analgesia, eg for arthritis, is adequate.

- Acute and chronic confusional states.

- Comorbid diseases, eg diabetes.

Epidemiology

Urinary incontinence is very common and not just confined to elderly people:

- affects 10% of the general population;

- affects 20% of those aged over 70 years (although this is probably an underestimate);

- is twice as common in women;

- is very common in people living in nursing homes;

- is frequently concealed, with only 25% of affected women consulting a doctor.

Clinical presentation

See Section 1.1.3. If patients are able, they should keep a diary for 3 days to give a clear idea of the pattern.

Examination

The examination focuses on the abdomen, but the legs must also be examined neurologically. Check the following.

- Abdomen: is the bladder palpable? Are there any pelvic masses, eg ovarian tumours pressing on the bladder?

- Rectal examination: look for faecal loading, anal tone and perineal sensation, and prostatic size and nature in men.

- Vaginal examination: look for prolapse and cystocele.

- Stress test: does patient leak urine on coughing?

Investigation

If incontinence persists despite simple measures, further investigation is indicated.

- Urodynamic investigation: measures free flow rate and residual volume.

- Cystometry: the bladder is filled at a steady rate while the difference between intra-abdominal and intravesical pressures is recorded. This is the detrusor pressure, which will be increased if there are uninhibited detrusor contractions, leading to urgency.

- Cystoscopy will reveal causes of bladder irritation and haematuria, such as bladder stones, interstitial cystitis and transitional cell carcinoma.

> Establish the cause of the incontinence. Although general measures (eg treating constipation) are the same, the exercise regimens and drug management depend on the type of incontinence. Drugs for the treatment of urge incontinence are contraindicated in prostatic outflow obstruction.

Treatment

General principles that should be applied to most patients include the following.

- Look for and treat any UTI in all cases.

- Constipation must be sought and treated (rectal examination is essential).

- Exclude diabetes.

- Advise weight loss if BMI is >30.

- Limit or increase fluid intake to 1.5 L per day, but ensure intake is no less than this as concentrated urine is more irritant to the bladder wall.

- Avoid bladder irritants, eg caffeine, alcohol and aspartame.

- Oestrogen topically for atrophic vaginitis.

- Improve mobility where possible.

- Increase accessibility of toilets: toilet raise, rails, wide doors and a large sign on the door.

- Consider a commode, or a urine bottle for men and various designs of slipper pans for women.

- Choose sensible clothes, eg with Velcro fastenings.

- Regular toileting, initially voiding every 1–1.5 hours.

- Bladder retraining: patient gradually increases the time between voiding.

Stress incontinence

Non-surgical measures

- Exercises, eg Kegel's exercises (concentrate on contracting the pelvic floor as if to interrupt the flow of urine), do work but require the patient to be cognitively intact, motivated and only work while the patient continues to exercise. First digitally assess that the patient can contract the pelvic floor. Aim for eight contractions three times a day for a minimum of 3 months.

- Duloxetine, a serotonin and noradrenaline reuptake inhibitor, may increase pudendal nerve stimulation, tightening the urethral sphincter.

- Consider electrical stimulation and/or biofeedback in women who cannot contract their pelvic floor.

Surgical measures

- Periurethral bulking agent (collagen or synthetic polymer) injections: this can be done using local anaesthesia and oral sedation. It is suitable for frail patients, but is limited in effectiveness and duration.

- Retropubic mid-urethral tape procedures using a 'bottom-up' approach with macroporous polypropylene meshes (tension-free vaginal tape); a day-case or short-stay procedure.

- Repositioning of the bladder neck: anterior repair (less effective) or Burch colposuspension (best results, but requires major surgery).

Urge incontinence

Several groups of drugs may be tried, but this should always be in addition to the general measures.

Oxybutynin and tolterodine

The drugs most often prescribed, although newer ones are becoming available all the time, eg trospium and solifenacin. These are antimuscarinic agents and block M_2 and M_3 receptors on the detrusor muscle, reducing contractions and making the bladder more stable. They have little effect on cardiac function, but can cause drowsiness and confusion in elderly people; other side effects include dry mouth, constipation and blurred vision. Also note the following.

- Tolterodine has less effect on salivary gland receptors, so a dry mouth is less common. The side-effect profile may be reduced further with modified-release

preparations, which also improve adherence.

- There is increasing evidence that trospium has the advantage of not crossing the blood–brain barrier and is therefore less likely to cause confusion.

Desmopressin This is a vasopressin analogue. Taken intranasally at night it reduces nocturia by up to 50%, but this use is not licensed and this must be explained. It is contraindicated in heart failure.

Persistent incontinence

If the incontinence cannot be eliminated, good containment is essential.

- Pads and pants: these are expensive and problems can arise over the delivery of supplies and the disposal of soiled pads.

- Intermittent self-catheterisation: the patient must be motivated and dexterous.

- Indwelling catheters may seem ideal, but they predispose to chronic UTIs, get blocked, cause trauma to local tissue and limit the patient's sex life.

- Early liaison with local continence adviser, and also advise the patient to join self-help groups.

Complications

Complications of recurrent incontinence are associated with a marked reduction in quality of life.

- Unpleasant smell and discomfort.

- Skin irritation and maceration, leading to pressure sores.

- Loss of self-esteem and reluctance to go out, leading to social isolation, loss of fitness, depression and sexual problems: all contribute to a marked decrease in the quality of life.

- Increased burden on carers (such as extra washing), making it more difficult for affected people to remain in their own home.

Information for patients

Patients can be referred to the Continence Society.

2.4.2 Faecal incontinence

> **Faecal incontinence**
>
> - **Common with advancing age.**
> - **Very common in the setting of a residential or nursing home.**
> - **A frequent reason for institutionalisation.**

Aetiology

In frail elderly people common causes include:

- overflow diarrhoea secondary to high constipation;

- sudden severe diarrhoea of any cause in an immobile patient;

- dementia.

In the general population common causes include the following.

- Damage to the anal sphincters during vaginal delivery, especially if the baby was large, the mother was aged 35 years or older when she gave birth or forceps were used (stretching of the pudendal nerve).

- Structural causes, including rectal prolapse and anal fistula.

- Damage to the sphincters during anal surgery (eg repair of a chronic anal fissure) or rarely haemorrhoidectomy.

- Neurological causes such as stroke, multiple sclerosis and spinal cord lesions, and the loss of sensation secondary to diabetes.

- Laxative abuse and taking large volumes of indigestion remedies containing magnesium.

Epidemiology

Faecal incontinence affects:

- 2% of the general population;

- 15% of those aged over 85 years who are living at home;

- 10–60% of residents in care homes.

Physical signs

Perform a general examination, a rectal examination to exclude a mass, assess the presence of a hard impacted stool and assess anal tone, and a neurological and cognitive assessment if appropriate.

Investigations

Basic blood tests including thyroid function are needed (to exclude hypothyroidism as a cause of constipation). Specific tests include:

- abdominal film to exclude high constipation;

- manometry to assess rectal compliance and sensation;

- anal endosonography for imaging the anal canal (can detect anal tears postpartum that are not detected clinically).

Treatment

The following options may be helpful.

- Treat overflow diarrhoea. Explain! If it is the first time the patient and family have encountered this problem, they will be very puzzled by your prescription of laxatives.

- Trial of regular toileting.

- Enema every 3 days, using codeine or loperamide in between if necessary to prevent leakage.

- Behavioural therapy (not evidence based).

- Biofeedback.

- Rarely, there is a case for colostomy in a patient with intractable incontinence who wants to have more freedom.

- Sacral nerve stimulation for patients with a structurally intact sphincter: electrodes are implanted via the sacral foramina and connected to the bowels and anal sphincters. These produce a continuous signal maintaining continence. The patient interrupts the signal with a magnet to open the bowels.

Complications

- Social isolation, low mood and embarrassment.

- Macerated skin and risk of pressure sores.

- Risk of institutionalisation.

- Risk of transmission of intestinal infections, such as *Clostridium difficile*.

FURTHER READING

Burgio KL, Mathew KA and Engel BT. Prevalence, incidence and correlates of urinary incontinence in healthy, middle-aged women. *J. Urol.* 1991; 146: 1255–9.

Dawson C and Whitfield H. ABC of urology: urinary incontinence and urinary infection. *BMJ* 1996; 312: 961–4.

National Collaborating Centre for Women's and Children's Health. *Urinary Incontinence: The Management of Urinary Incontinence in Women.* London: National Institute for Clinical Excellence, 2006. Available at http://www.nice.org.uk/guidance/CG40/?c=91526

Norton C, Thomas L and Hill J. Management of faecal incontinence in adults: summary of NICE guidence. *BMJ* 2007; 334: 1370–1.

Peet SM, Castleden CM and McGrowther CW. Prevalence of urinary and faecal incontinence in hospitals and residential and nursing homes for older people. *BMJ* 1995; 311: 1063–4.

Royal College of Physicians of London. Incontinence: causes, management and provision of services. *J. R. Coll. Physicians Lond.* 1995; 29: 272–4.

Saint S and Lipsky BA. Preventing catheter-related bacteriuria: should we? Can we? How? *Arch. Intern. Med.* 1999; 159: 800–8.

Staskin DR. Overactive bladder in the elderly: a guide to pharmacological management. *Drugs Aging* 2005; 22: 1013–28.

UK Continence Foundation. Available at http://www.continence-foundation.org.uk/

Wall PG and Ryan MJ. Faecal incontinence in hospitals and residential and nursing homes for elderly people. *BMJ* 1996; 312: 378.

Wise BG and Cardozo LD. Urinary urgency in women. *Br. J. Hosp. Med.* 1993; 50: 243–50.

2.5 Hypothermia

Hypothermia occurs, by definition, when the core temperature of the body falls below 35°C.

Hypothermia can be classified into mild (32–35°C), moderate (30–32°C) and severe (<30°C). The literature on management is confusing because hypothermia occurs in two very different populations.

- People with normal thermoregulation who are exposed to extreme cold or immersion in cold water (often young fit individuals following outdoor accidents).

- People with impaired thermoregulation (usually frail older people). In this group hypothermia can occur at any time of year and at any ambient temperature but is commoner in winter, particularly a couple of days into a spell of very cold weather.

Aetiology

If a low core temperature cannot be attributed to direct exposure to the cold, it should alert the physician to an occult pathology. Except in cases of cold exposure, hypothermia is usually multifactorial, with an interaction between ageing changes, disease processes and social factors. Risk factors include:

- old age;

- living alone;

- sarcopenia due to malnutrition or chronic illness;

- autonomic dysfunction, eg diabetes mellitus;

- immobility as a result of Parkinson's disease or rheumatoid arthritis;

- falls;

- hypothyroidism (reduced metabolic rate, drowsiness, poor mobility and apathy);

- underlying sepsis, eg chest infection;

- drugs that cause vasodilatation, eg phenothiazines, calcium antagonists and alcohol;

- cerebrovascular disease (this may affect hypothalamic regulation);

- cognitive impairment (Alzheimer's disease and multi-infarct dementia both cause damage to central thermoregulation and thus the normal behavioural adjustments to cold are absent);

- poor socioeconomic conditions, eg no central heating/insulation and poor clothing.

Pathophysiology

There is impairment of thermoregulation with ageing. The hypothalamus is thought to act in a similar fashion to a thermostat. In response to cold, the hypothalamus triggers mechanisms of peripheral vasoconstriction, shivering and piloerection via the autonomic nervous system. Changes in the autonomic nervous system with ageing, chiefly a reduction in receptor sensitivity, result in a reduced response to sympathetic and parasympathetic nerve stimulation. The metabolic rate is also reduced in old age which reduces heat generation. These changes reduce the homeostatic response to cold.

As the temperature falls below 35°C, hypothermic patients become lethargic and confused. Consciousness is lost at a lower, but variable, temperature of 26–33°C. After an initial rise in cardiac output, associated with shivering, cardiac output falls with bradycardia due to the depressant effect of cold on the cardiac muscle. A variety of arrhythmias may then ensue and between 17 and 26°C the cardiac output becomes insufficient to maintain life. The failure of haemoglobin to release normal amounts of oxygen, due to a left shift in the oxyhaemoglobin dissociation curve, contributes to anoxia. Glucose metabolism is depressed and levels of both glucose and potassium rise as the body temperature falls. Blood volume falls initially due to cold diuresis, and then later because of loss of fluid into the extravascular tissue. Shivering may compound the lactic acidosis that typically accompanies hypovolaemia. There is increased coagulopathy and increased incidence of wound infection.

Epidemiology

Studies estimate that 10% of people living at home who are aged over 75 years have a core body temperature of less than 35°C and 1–3% of all patients admitted to hospital in the winter are hypothermic.

Clinical presentation

Patients are often found at home alone on the floor following a fall. Confusion, hallucinations and paranoid features can occur.

Physical signs

Patients are pale, cold to the touch and consciousness is impaired. The core body temperature, taken rectally with a low-range thermometer, is <35°C (oral readings are inaccurate); measurements should be continued for monitoring purposes. There is bradycardia and hypotension. There may be evidence of pneumonia or pulmonary oedema (caused by cardiac depression and bradycardia). Muscles are generally rigid and speech may be slurred. There may be signs of a stroke that could have precipitated hypothermia. Be alert for signs of hypothyroidism, which may be a precipitating cause.

Investigations

Baseline investigations include FBC, urea and electrolytes, blood glucose, arterial blood gases, thyroid function tests, C-reactive protein, amylase, serum calcium, drug screen if indicated, CXR and ECG.

The ECG may show a variety of abnormalities. Hypothermia is associated with bradycardia and prolongation of the PR and QT intervals. As the core temperature

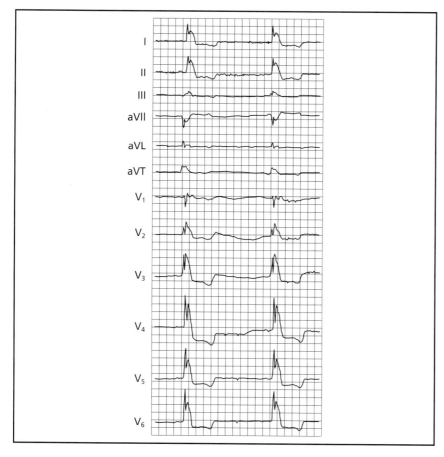

▲ **Fig. 14** ECG changes in hypothermia: sinus bradycardia and PR interval of 0.2 seconds. Broad slurred J waves are seen adjacent to the initial QRS deflection in all leads, but most obviously in leads I, II and V2–V6. There is pronounced ST-segment depression and T-wave inversion. (ECG kindly provided by Dr Derek J. Rowlands, Consultant Cardiologist, from his text *Understanding the Electrocardiogram*, Section 2, morphological abnormalities. Copyright ICI plc 1982.)

falls, sinus bradycardia tends to give way to atrial fibrillation followed by ventricular fibrillation (VF) and finally asystole. Development of an extra deflection occurring at the end of the QRS complex, called a J wave, is characteristic of the ECG in patients with severe hypothermia (Fig. 14); the J wave increases in size as the temperature falls. Pronounced ST-segment depression and T-wave inversion occur. The changes usually reverse as the patient is warmed up.

Treatment

Most elderly patients are treated with passive or active external warming. The patient should be rewarmed slowly (0.5–1°C per hour) in a warm room and covered with a blanket or 'Bair hugger', a device through which warm air is blown. Foil blankets are outdated – they keep the cold in! Oxygen should be humidified. Rapid rewarming increases mortality as a result of sudden hypotension from vasodilatation and cardiac arrhythmias. Cardiac monitoring is advisable. Intravenous fluids should be used with caution; avoid overload while the patient is cold but give enough to minimise hypotension as the patient warms up and vasodilates. Watch for hyperkalaemia in this phase. A urinary catheter is needed for accurate measurement of urine output. Antibiotics are often indicated, because chest infections are common. Both prophylactic heparin and a proton pump

inhibitor may be given in the early phase of recovery as, anecdotally, both gastric bleeds and deep vein thrombosis may occur. Any underlying disease, eg hypothyroidism, should be treated.

The hypothermic patient may be unresponsive to cardioactive drugs, pacemaker stimulation and attempted defibrillation. The metabolism and efficacy of drugs is impaired in hypothermia and as a consequence drugs are often withheld until the patient has been warmed up. Arrhythmias other than VF tend to revert spontaneously as the core temperature rises. VF may not respond to defibrillation until the core temperature rises above 30°C.

Active internal warming is usually reserved for young cold exposure victims in an intensive therapy unit setting. Measures may include warm oxygen (40–46°C); gastric, peritoneal, pleural and bladder lavage with warm fluids (40°C) and cardiopulmonary bypass; continuous veno-venous haemofiltration with warm replacement fluids, or even cardiopulmonary bypass in some centres.

Complications

An important complication of hypothermia is pancreatitis: epigastric pain, shock and the consequences of hypocalcaemia.

Prognosis

A full recovery without any neurological deficit is possible after a prolonged hypothermic cardiac arrest as hypothermia confers a degree of protection to the brain. An extremely low core temperature and significant comorbidity are predictors of a poor outcome. The mortality rate varies from 30 to 80%, reflecting the diverse nature of hypothermic patients.

Prevention

Prevention is better than cure. Campaigns are now run to increase public awareness; elderly people are encouraged to have good home heating and insulation, electric blankets and sufficient clothing. Also, grants are available (eg winter fuel payment) and those at risk need regular visits (eg to provide hot food).

Hyperthermia

Impaired thermoregulation also predisposes to hyperthermia in heat waves. Again, ageing physiology (eg impaired thirst and poor renal water conservation) interacts with social factors (eg lack of air conditioning) and drugs to increase the risk of death in older people, both at home and in hospital. In a heat wave, persuade the nurses to do an extra cold drinks round.

FURTHER READING

Adult Advanced Life Support, Resuscitation Council Guidelines 2005. Available at http://www.resus.org.uk/pages/als.pdf

- - - - - - - - - - - - -

Age Concern England. *Help with Heating*. Newton Abbot: Age Concern, 2006. Available at http://www.ageconcern.org.uk

- - - - - - - - - - - - -

Epstein E and Anna K. Accidental hypothermia. *BMJ* 2006; 332: 706–9.

2.6 Drugs in elderly people

General points

Elderly people consume most medications (remember prescribed and over-the-counter drugs). Older people:

- are more sensitive to drugs (often have low weight, reduced renal clearance and decreased hepatic blood flow, etc.);

- are more susceptible to side effects and adverse effects;

- experience side effects that are more likely to have serious sequelae.

Nellie Smith does not get out much because of her arthritic knees (think vitamin D deficiency and lack of fitness). She is prescribed an NSAID and gets indigestion, but decides this is normal at her age (expectation and acceptance of symptoms). She has a haematemesis. Blood loss that would be tolerated in a younger person causes collapse (diminished homeostatic reserve). She fractures her hip (osteoporosis). She lives alone, so she is not found until the next day (social factors). She is admitted, but has renal failure (blood loss, unable to obtain water, poor renal-concentrating ability, the NSAID and her furosemide) and must be 'stabilised' before surgery. Pressure sores worsen, antibiotics are prescribed and she develops *Clostridium difficile* diarrhoea. You can predict the outcome. Was the NSAID indicated initially?

Multiple pathology means a greater likelihood that a drug will be contraindicated. It also necessitates multiple medications. Older people on several drugs are likely to:

- experience drug interactions (the number of drugs and increased sensitivity to each);

- have problems with adherence, especially if confused.

Writing up or reviewing a drug chart

Review your patient's problem list and prioritise those that are treatable. The patient is usually on many drugs already. Always check that the list of drugs reflects the clinical diagnoses.

Drug considerations

- Is a drug still indicated? (Would a non-drug alternative be as effective? Find out if the situation has changed, eg stop tolterodine if the patient has a long-term catheter.)

- Is the drug still effective? (Low-dose sulphonylureas that have been given for years may be stopped with little deterioration in glycaemic control.)

- Do likely benefits outweigh the risks? (If the patient is only 71 but has dementia, is prone to falls and is admitted with an INR of 7.2, then replace warfarin for atrial fibrillation with aspirin.)

- Is it the 'nicest' drug for the job? (Clarithromycin instead of erythromycin.)

- Cheapest? (If there are equivalents, eg statins and proton pump inhibitors, then choose the drug that costs less in the community.)

- Is a drug causing the symptoms? (Nausea or confusion occur as a result of codeine.)

- Could a single agent replace two? (Angiotensin-converting enzyme inhibitor for hypertension with heart failure.)

- Is the formulation/route of administration the best? (Syrups and patches may help.)

- Are the timings appropriate? (Once or twice daily options aid adherence, especially if drugs are given by visiting carers).

- Could there be any aids to administration? (Spacer for inhalers and avoidance of childproof tops.)

- Could there be any aids to adherence? (Dosette box.)

- Should drugs be regular or 'as required'? (Analgesics for chronic pain are usually best given on a regular basis.)

- Does the patient understand the medications and any precautions? (Provide written information and record advice given, eg for a sore throat on carbimazole, in the notes.)

Should a new drug be started?

A drug may be considered for cure or disease modification, symptom control or primary or secondary prevention.

- • When prescribing start low and go slow, but increase the dose up to the therapeutic range or until limiting side effects develop.
- • Give a drug for long enough before deciding it is ineffective (eg antidepressants).
- • If problems arise and a drug is stopped, record why (eg angiotensin-converting enzyme inhibitor led to hypotension).
- • In prevention, consider the overall burden of pathology and drugs, but avoid therapeutic nihilism.

Overall picture

- If there are multiple drugs, is everything essential?

- Try to avoid prescribing a drug to treat the side effects of another (eg furosemide and fludrocortisone).

- Look for potential interactions.

- If the patient has renal or hepatic failure, do not rely on memory: check every drug against the lists in the *British National Formulary* (BNF). Check if your hospital subscribes to BNF online.

- Use generic names unless bioavailability is crucial or when using a slow-release preparation.

- The patient will change. Always review medication.

⚠ Never write up drugs from a GP letter when you are not sure what they are!

FURTHER READING

British National Formulary (section on prescribing for the elderly). London: BMJ Publishing Group and the Royal Pharmaceutical Society of Great Britain.

2.7 Dementia

'Perhaps being old is having lighted rooms inside your head, and people in them, acting. People you know, yet can't quite name.' (Philip Larkin)

Dementia is a syndrome (with lots of causes) of acquired (not congenital), chronic (lasts months to years) and global (not just memory or just language problems) impairment of higher brain function in an alert patient (not drowsy) that interferes with the ability to cope with daily living.

It does not usually matter if an elderly woman doesn't know it's Tuesday, but if she doesn't know it's winter and 4 am she might freeze. Presentation depends on familiarity with, and complexity of, the patient's environment, as well as on cognition.

Aetiology

The common primary dementias (ie disease mainly affects the brain) in old age are Alzheimer's disease, dementia in Parkinson's disease (PD) and Lewy body disease. The most common secondary dementia is vascular dementia, which includes multiple small infarcts and white matter ischaemia. It is increasingly recognised that symptoms are often due to a primary process exacerbated by vascular change. Reversible secondary dementias are becoming rarer in hospital practice as they are detected early in primary care more often.

Normal-pressure hydrocephalus (NPH) classically presents with dementia, abnormal gait and incontinence. The ventricles are disproportionately large for the degree of sulcal atrophy. There is evidence of abnormal cerebrospinal fluid circulation, although the exact pathogenesis is still disputed. NPH is a difficult diagnosis in the elderly. This CT appearance is relatively common, but even after specialist assessment the results of shunting are often disappointing. It is worth considering if the incontinence and gait problems (often apraxia) are very marked for the degree of cognitive impairment.

DEMENTIA: an acronym for those with poor memories!

Drugs and alcohol
Eyes and ears
Metabolic (thyroid)
Emotional (often are really psychiatric problems)
Nutritional (vitamin B_{12} and other vitamin deficiencies) and NPH
Trauma and tumours
Infections (syphilis and HIV)
Atheroma (vascular dementia)

Epidemiology

Dementia is rare in those below 55 years of age, but its prevalence increases dramatically with age to about 2% in the over-65s and 20% in the over-80s. In elderly people, Alzheimer's disease probably accounts for around two-thirds of dementia cases. Demographic changes are resulting in marked increases in the number of people who are very old and dementia is a major cause of dependency and institutional care. In a recent study for the Alzheimer's Society, the total costs of dementia were estimated at £17 billion a year in the UK (£25,000 per person, per year). This is greater than for stroke, heart disease or cancer.

Clinical presentation

> **Remember:**
> *My* (memory)
> *old* (orientation)
> *grandmother* (grasp)
> *converses* (communication)
> *pretty* (personality change)
> *badly* (behaviour disorder)
> (Brice Pitt, Emeritus Professor of Old Age Psychiatry, St Mary's, London)

Postoperative or acute confusion may reflect 'decreased brain reserve' and may predict later dementia. Delirium is divided into hypoactive, hyperactive and mixed subtypes; everyone is familiar with the agitated hyperactive presentation but the apathy and reduced movement of the hypoactive form carries a worse prognosis. The onset of dementia is usually insidious, with gradual changes in memory, thinking processes, language use, personality, behaviour and orientation. Families report that it can be difficult to obtain a diagnosis. If the patient lives alone, there may be no third party to give a history and, unless cognition is tested, it is easy to be misled by 'a good social front'. The condition progresses to obvious problems with short-term memory and basic activities of daily living, increasing disorientation and sometimes difficult or distressing behaviour. Eventually, the patient ceases to communicate and becomes totally dependent. Dementia may present acutely, eg with the death of the caring spouse in a couple.

There is no ante-mortem diagnostic test for most of the primary dementias, so the likely cause is determined by the clinical features and investigations. Progressive deterioration is common in Alzheimer's disease, whereas stepwise deterioration is characteristic of vascular dementia. Neuropsychiatric phenomena such as delusions and hallucinations, an early tendency to falls and extreme sensitivity to major tranquillisers are a feature of Lewy body disease. Parkinsonian features on examination suggest vascular dementia or Lewy body disease. Common conditions such as vascular dementia and Alzheimer's disease may coexist.

Physical signs

A mental state examination is essential (including mood). Record a recognised score, eg Mini-Mental State Examination (MMSE). The general state of the patient (check for signs of neglect) reflects the severity of the management problem. Focus on the neurological and cardiovascular systems, but physical signs may be absent and another unreported pathology may be found.

Investigations

Investigations typically include blood tests to exclude reversible causes or other major pathologies (FBC, biochemical profile, erythrocyte sedimentation rate, thyroid function, vitamin B_{12} and folate), CXR, ECG and CT brain scan.

Differential diagnosis

Many old people are slightly forgetful and it can be difficult to distinguish ageing changes from early dementia. The differential diagnosis includes acute confusion (delirium), depression, communication difficulties caused by deafness, poor vision or language deficits, PD, schizophrenia and mania. In an acute confusional state consciousness is impaired. A person can become delirious at any age, but frail older people often become confused when they are ill. The confusion may resolve with the illness, or merely improve if there is underlying dementia as well as the illness. Depression may be overlooked or missed in elderly people, may mimic dementia (pseudo-dementia) and may be more common in patients with dementia for pathological and psychological reasons.

Treatment

> **Management** depends on severity of the dementia and whether the patient lives alone. It requires a multidisciplinary, multiagency package of care, which is coordinated and evolves as the needs of the patient and carer change.

Management options include the following.

- Coping strategies and psychological techniques.

- Optimise hearing and vision, and improve general health.

- Treat other conditions that may impair cognition (eg anaemia and heart failure).

- Education and support for carers is essential (see below).

- Genetic counselling (not indicated for patients or their families in cases of dementia in old age).

- Legal advice, eg an Enduring Power of Attorney may obviate the need for the Court of Protection at a later date (see Section 2.13), advice about driving, and advance directives.

- Therapy assessments: occupational therapy, speech and language therapy to aid swallowing and communication, and physiotherapy. The aim is usually assessment to plan care and advise the carers rather than to treat the patient.

- Assistive technology: technological solutions to various problems, eg automatic bath-tap cut-off and light sensors. May be run by social services or the occupational therapy department.

- Assessment by social services: financial entitlements, especially Attendance Allowance, and the provision of services such as home help and access to 'care management', the process by which frail old people are assessed for substantial packages of care at home or residential care.

- District nurse/community psychiatric nurse support.

- Sitting services (Crossroads), day hospital and respite care.

- Proper provision of long-term care.

Drugs

- For secondary prevention (eg aspirin and antihypertensives to try to slow progression in vascular dementia).

- To treat specific symptoms and behaviours (major tranquillisers, unfortunately, are often the only option).

- To enhance cholinergic transmission in Alzheimer's disease in which cholinergic neurons bear the brunt of the damage. Acetylcholinesterase inhibitors (eg donepezil, rivastigmine and galantamine) enhance the effect of endogenous acetylcholine in the brain. They have some efficacy, but there is debate about their cost-effectiveness. In 2006, the National Institute for Health and Clinical Excellence (NICE) restricted their use to moderate Alzheimer's disease (defined as an MMSE of 10–20) with a shared care protocol between primary care and old-age psychiatry or geriatrics. Debate continues as to whether this is reasonable 'rationing': many feel that to limit prescribing to within a range of scores is arbitrary as the impact of dementia depends not only on the cognitive score but also the complexity of the environment.

- To modify other transmitter pathways: memantine is an uncompetitive N-methyl-D-aspartate receptor antagonist that blocks the effects of pathologically elevated tonic levels of glutamate that may lead to neuronal dysfunction. Although licensed, it is not currently approved by NICE: check their website for the current situation (http://www.nice.org.uk/).

Complications
Dementia is devastating for the patient and the family. In the late stages the patient is debilitated, doubly incontinent and bed-bound.

Prognosis
In addition to the considerable morbidity, Alzheimer's disease is the fourth leading cause of death in Western nations. The prognosis in cases of dementia depends on the pathology, age and support that the patient receives.

Prevention
Nothing has been proven to prevent Alzheimer's disease. Possibilities include keeping the brain active, anti-inflammatory agents and antioxidants; certainly avoid head injuries and risk factors for vascular disease. Earlier reports that oestrogen (hormone-replacement therapy, HRT) may be beneficial were not confirmed in randomised trials and probably reflected the healthier non-random group who elected to use HRT.

Disease associations
Other illnesses may not be reported and the carer may also become depressed and neglect his or her own physical illnesses.

Important information for patients/carers
Carers need considerable support. The Alzheimer's Society deals with other dementias besides Alzheimer's and produces excellent literature for carers and professionals, especially their wide range of up-to-date online factsheets. The Carers' National Association supports carers in all settings.

FURTHER READING

Bertram L and Tanzi RE. The genetic epidemiology of neurodegenerative disease. *J. Clin. Invest.* 2005; 115: 1449–57. Available at http://www.jci.org/cgi/content/full/115/6/1449

Birks J. Cholinesterase inhibitors for Alzheimer's disease. *Cochrane Database Syst. Rev.* 2006; 25(1): CD005593.

Breen DA, Breen DP, Moore JW, Breen PA and O'Neill D. Driving and dementia. *BMJ* 2007; 334: 1365–9.

Knapp M, Prince M, *et al. Dementia UK; the Full Report* (A report to the Alzheimer's Society on the prevalence and economic cost of dementia in the UK produced by King's College London and London School of Economics). London: Alzheimer's Society, 2007. Available at http://www.alzheimers .org.uk

Knopman DS. Dementia and cerebrovascular disease. *Mayo Clin. Proc.* 2006; 81: 223–30.

Lowin A, Knapp M and McCrone P. Alzheimer's disease in the UK: comparative evidence on cost of illness and volume of health services research funding. *Int. J. Geriatr. Psychiatry* 2001; 16: 1143–8.

National Institute for Health and Clinical Excellence. *Donepezil, Galantamine, Rivastigmine (Review) and Memantine for the Treatment of Alzheimer's Disease (Includes a Review of NICE Technology Appraisal Guidance 19).* London: NICE, 2006. Available at http://www.nice.org.uk

Potter J and George J. The prevention, diagnosis and management of delirium in older people: concise guidelines. *Clin. Med.* 2006; 6; 303–8.

Scottish Intercollegiate Guidelines Network. *Management of Patients With Dementia: A National Guideline.* Edinburgh: SIGN, 2006. Available at http://www.sign.ac.uk

Websites
Alzheimer Research Forum: an excellent scientific website. Available at http://www.alzforum.org/

Alzheimer's Society: a source for practical information. Available at http://www.alzheimers.org.uk

2.8 Rehabilitation

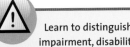

Learn to distinguish between impairment, disability and handicap.

Definitions

- Rehabilitation: the process by which an individual attains his or her maximum physical, mental and social capability.
- Impairment: an objective reduction in physical or mental ability of an individual caused by disease or disorder and which may be temporary or permanent.
- Disability: the effect that the impairment has on daily function.
- Handicap: the disadvantage within society that results from impairment or disability.
- Activities of daily living (ADL): functional abilities that a person needs to live independently, eg washing, dressing, shopping and cooking.

A 76-year-old man has a hemiplegia following a stroke. The grade 3–4 weakness affecting his left side is the impairment. This results in disability, eg he is unable to walk independently. The handicap he experiences will depend on his previous lifestyle, but would include not being able to go to the pub or take his wife dancing.

Epidemiology

The number of disabled people is increasing as the population is ageing. This reflects the increased prevalence of disabling conditions in old age, eg stroke, cardiorespiratory disease, blindness and arthritis. About 4.3 million people aged over 60 years in the UK are disabled and 90% of these live in their own homes.

Rehabilitation

The team
Rehabilitation is an active and energetic process and involves a team, the patient being a member of the team and at its centre. The other members of this multidisciplinary team include the doctor (usually a geriatrician), nurses, physiotherapists, occupational therapists, speech and language therapists, and a medical social worker. Other members who may be approached as appropriate include a podiatrist (chiropodist), psychologist, continence adviser and dietitian.

The setting
Rehabilitation can be performed anywhere, but it is usual to have a dedicated unit or ward where staff with the appropriate skills are concentrated. Purpose-built units have adequate space around beds and in bathrooms to encourage independence. Patients need space to store their belongings because they will usually be out of bed and dressed in their own clothes. There is usually a large day room and dining area for social activities. The physiotherapy gym and occupational therapy department (with bedroom and kitchen) are part of the unit. The doctor's role is to determine pathology and impairments, ie diagnosis, and often to coordinate the team.

The process
The process of rehabilitation is usually focused on setting appropriate short- and longer-term goals. The goals must be realistic, so it is essential to know what the patient could do before the current episode and what the patient wants. Case conferences are usually held weekly to monitor each patient's progress.

Discharge planning

Various ADL scales are used to monitor the patient's progress, eg the Barthel Index (see Section 3.2). Discharge planning begins at the time of admission. The process is fine-tuned as the patient progresses. An independent flatlet within the unit may be used to monitor a patient's capabilities as the time for discharge approaches. If functional impairment remains, which is often the case, the patient has a 'needs assessment' before discharge. If it is thought that he or she can live in the community, a home visit is carried out by the occupational therapist with his or her spouse/relatives present. This helps determine whether aids and appliances at home would be needed to lessen disability and whether the living environment needs alteration, such as the widening of doorways for wheelchair access, or the removal of obstacles such as worn carpets. A social worker is involved in the process to assess the need for social care, eg home helps for shopping or a meals-on-wheels service. The social worker will also assess whether the patient is eligible for benefits, eg Attendance Allowance (see Section 2.12).

Specialist units

There are also specialised rehabilitation units (eg stroke units and orthogeriatric units) that usually have specific protocols for admission. Admission to stroke units has been shown to result in a better outcome for stroke patients in terms of mortality and functional recovery (see Section 1.4.2). Orthogeriatric units, in which elderly patients with a fractured neck of femur are under the joint care of an orthopaedic surgeon and a geriatrician, enable better provision of perioperative care. There is also early rehabilitation assessment and, if necessary, transfer to the general rehabilitation unit.

Day rehabilitation

Geriatric day hospitals are day rehabilitation units that are within the hospital and run by geriatricians. Patients usually attend 1 or 2 days a week on an outpatient basis. They attend for rehabilitation, maintenance treatment or medical and nursing investigations. In some areas of the UK the day hospital has been replaced by 'outreach rehabilitation teams', where rehabilitation is provided in the patient's own home but is coordinated in the hospital by a geriatrician.

If after the process of rehabilitation it is apparent that the patient cannot continue to live in his or her own home, residential or nursing home accommodation has to be considered (see Section 1.4).

> **FURTHER READING**
>
> Pathy MSJ, Sinclair AJ and Morley JE, eds. *Principles and Practice of Geriatric Medicine*, 4th edn. Chichester: John Wiley & Sons, 2005.
>
> - - - - - - - - - - - - - - - -
>
> Young J. Rehabilitation and older people. *BMJ* 1996; 313: 677–81.

2.9 Aids, appliances and assistive technology

Aids, appliances and assistive technology can reduce a patient's disability, increase independence and safety, and may lessen handicap.

A huge range of aids and appliances is available, ranging in price from pence (rubber non-slip mats for plates) to thousands of pounds (stair lifts). Many families buy aids privately, and if these are costly they should always be encouraged to obtain professional advice before parting with their cash. Information and catalogues about aids for specific conditions are usually most helpful from specialist societies, eg the Royal National Institute for the Blind, the Stroke Association and the Parkinson's Disease Society. Occupational therapists assess patients for most of these products, with the exception of walking aids for which patients are assessed by a physiotherapist. A brief summary of some of the most common aids is given below.

Kitchen aids

- Tap turner (Fig. 15): easier to turn taps for those with limb weakness or arthritis.

- Kettle tipper (Fig. 16): useful for those with tremor, weakness or poor vision.

- Cutlery (Fig. 17): antispill device for the plate for those who only have the use of one hand, and easy to hold cutlery for those who have weak or arthritic hands.

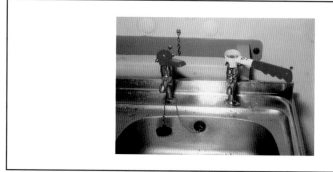

▲**Fig. 15** Tap turner.

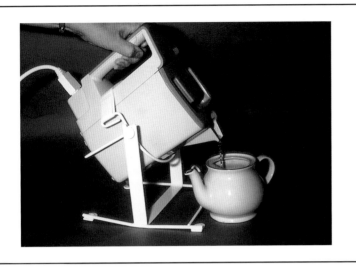

▲ **Fig. 16** Kettle tipper.

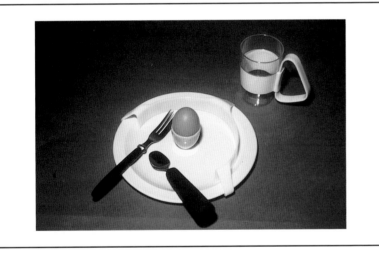

▲ **Fig. 17** Cutlery.

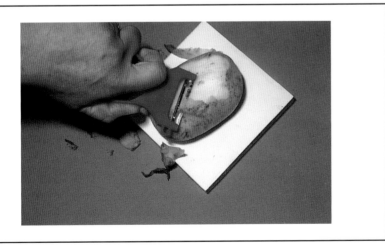

▲ **Fig. 18** Potato peeler.

- Potato peeler (Fig. 18): for a hemiplegic patient.

Dressing aids

- Long-handled shoehorn.

- Much can be achieved by altering the style of dress, eg opt for a V-necked sweater rather than a cardigan or slip-on shoes rather than lace-ups, or replace fastenings with Velcro.

Mobility aids

- Walking sticks: these relieve pain by giving support and aid balance by widening the base. One or two sticks may be required. Many types exist, eg single rod, tripods and tetrapods (the latter two are useful as they remain 'standing' if put down temporarily). Assessment and accurate length measurement of these aids is essential. Most walking aids are measured from the floor to the wrist crease (radial styloid) with the patient's arm hanging down at the side.

- Zimmer frames/rollators: consider the home as well as the person; individuals may need a frame both upstairs and downstairs.

- Wheelchairs: these are expensive. Correct size, wheel style (push or self-propel) and padding are essential.

Others

- Helping hand.

- Key holder (Fig. 19).

- Pendant alarm: to call for help, alerting family/neighbours by remote control.

- High seat chairs.

- Extra stair rails (both sides of a steep flight and adjacent to steps between rooms).

- Raised toilet seat.

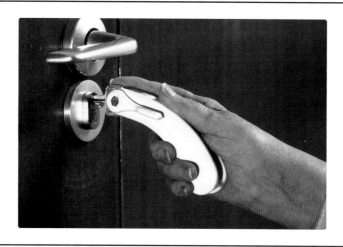

▲ **Fig. 19** Key holder.

Assistive technology

Telecare is the use of electronic technology to monitor people and assist them to maintain independence in their own environment. A telecare service can comprise three components: monitoring safety and security, physiological parameters, and activity. Devices include:

- video monitoring;

- fall detectors;

- sensors to monitor activity (eg a pressure mat activated as the person gets out of bed can turn on the light, detectors monitoring the fridge and front door can be used to monitor feeding and wandering);

- wet bed alerts to summon a night carer;

- automatic taps to prevent floods;

- everyone should have smoke alarms.

Check what is available locally to help in discharge planning. Disabled Living Centres are in the telephone directory.

FURTHER READING

Audit Commission. *Implementing Telecare: Strategic Analysis and Guidelines for Policy Makers, Commissioners and Providers.* London: Audit Commission, 2004. Available at http://www.audit-commission. gov.uk/olderpeople/

— — — — — — — — — — —

Mulley G, Penn N and Burns E, eds. *Older People at Home: Practical Issues.* London: BMJ Books, 1998.

2.10 Hearing impairment

- Deafness is very common in elderly people (about 60% of those over 70 years old).
- Presbyacusis is the most common cause in the over-70s.
- Always examine the eardrums of any patient with deafness.
- Use a communicator.
- Beware unilateral deafness; think of acoustic neuroma and cholesteatoma.

Aetiology

Conductive deafness may be caused by the following.

- Wax.

- Foreign body.

- Postinfective mastoiditis.

- Chronic suppurative otitis media.

- Paget's disease of the skull.

- Tumours: glomus tumour or cholesteatoma.

- Otosclerosis: a congenital disease caused by (usually) bilateral replacement of the stapes with spongy non-conducting bone; it is twice as common in women and 50% of sufferers have a family history. Management involves stapedectomy with an artificial implant.

Sensorineural deafness is caused by the following.

- Presbyacusis: the loss of high-frequency hearing with age.

- Noise-induced damage.

- Neurological conditions: acoustic neuroma, Ménière's disease (usually middle-aged people), meningioma, multiple sclerosis, stroke.

- Ototoxic drugs: aminoglycosides (especially gentamicin), loop diuretics, cisplatin, aspirin.

- Infections: measles, mumps, meningitis, influenza, herpes, syphilis.

- Congenital.

Congenital sensorineural deafness may be isolated or part of a syndrome.

- Alport's syndrome: sensorineural deafness and glomerulonephritis.

- Apert's syndrome: sensorineural deafness and acrocephalosyndactyly.

- Usher's syndrome: sensorineural deafness and retinitis pigmentosa.

Epidemiology

Hearing impairment occurs in 60% of those aged over 70 years; of this age group, 25% would benefit from a hearing aid.

Clinical presentation

Usually this is obvious, but deafness may be overlooked as a contributory factor in depression, paranoia, acute confusion and dementia. Coexisting tinnitus may be troublesome.

Physical signs

Always look in the ear canal, mainly for wax but also for cholesteatoma (a cystic lesion associated with a perforated eardrum in 90% of cases, but it may be masked by granulation tissue). Tuning fork tests will discriminate between conductive and sensory deafness.

- Rinne's test: normally air conduction is better than bone conduction, so in a positive (normal) Rinne's test sound is heard better with the prongs of the tuning fork held near the ear than when the base is placed on the mastoid process.

- Weber's test: the tuning fork is placed on the top of the forehead and the test is normal when the sound is detected equally well in both ears.

In unilateral deafness look for signs of a cerebellopontine angle lesion.

Investigations

Refer to the audiology service where a pure-tone audiogram and speech audiogram will be performed. In hearing loss associated with old age the pure-tone audiogram shows that high frequencies are particularly impaired. To record a speech audiogram, a list of sentences is presented under controlled conditions; this gives the best indication of whether a hearing aid will be helpful.

Treatment

General measures

- When talking with people with hearing impairment, make sure that they can see your face and also try to reduce background noise or use a communication device.

- To remove wax, first prescribe ear drops to soften it (sodium bicarbonate or olive oil) and then refer the patient for syringing.

- Refer the patient to audiology for an assessment for a hearing aid or masker for tinnitus.

- Educate about environmental aids: warning light on telephones, door bells and smoke alarms, vibrating pillows as alarm clocks, subtitles on television and the 'closed caption' system on videos.

- Hospitals must flag patients' notes so that clinic staff are aware of those with hearing impairment.

- An older person may be greatly helped by a hearing dog (see below).

Hearing aids

Many elderly people do not wear their hearing aids. This may be because the aids do not restore normal hearing (all noises are amplified so that speech especially is difficult to hear), because of feedback problems (the loud whistling associated with hearing aids) and because of the attached stigma.

To get the best from a hearing aid:

- encourage the new wearer to use it regularly so as to become accustomed to it;
- ensure that the ear mould fits well and is comfortable;
- make sure that the patient is able to fit it independently;
- batteries should be live and the aid should be switched on;
- avoid wax build-up in the ear canals;
- arrange regular follow-up and support;
- ensure that the switch is in the 'M' position for 'most of the time';
- explain use of the 'T' position (induction loop) with adapted telephones, ticket offices and theatres, etc. (Fig. 20).

Advantages of digital hearing aids:

- can be programmed to suit the individual, eg speech frequencies can be amplified and background noise reduced for most people, or a wider range of frequencies can be programmed for people who enjoy listening to classical music for example.
- reduced feedback.

For the future

Implantable hearing aids also reduce feedback and improve speech clarity. Centres in the USA are offering cochlear implants to elderly people and these have excellent outcomes.

Complications

Deafness is more disabling than it appears and can cause:

Fig. 20 Symbol that indicates loop induction system is available for people with hearing aids.

- social isolation because of reduced ability to communicate;

- impaired sense of balance and increased falls;

- increased risk of accidents because of lack of audible cues (car horns and warning shouts);

- potential for confusion (and paranoia) when admitted to hospital.

Patient information

Make the patient aware of the following.

- Hearing Concern (http://www.hearingconcern.org.uk).

- Royal National Institute for Deaf People (http://www.rnid.org.uk/).

- Hearing dogs: identified by their burgundy jackets, these dogs highlight their owners' hearing problems and improve their independence (http://www.hearing-dogs.co.uk).

FURTHER READING

Mills R. The auditory system. In: Pathy MSJ, Sinclair AJ and Morley JE, eds. *Principles and Practice of Geriatric Medicine*, 4th edn. Chichester: John Wiley & Sons, 2005: 1093–104.

2.11 Nutrition

'Thousands are annually starved in the midst of plenty for want alone of the means to take food.' (Florence Nightingale)

Although Florence Nightingale's patients were considerably younger, many older people today are poorly nourished both at home and (particularly) in institutions.

Introduction

Nutrition is essential for good health; both malnutrition and obesity have an adverse impact on morbidity and mortality in patients of all ages. In the UK approximately 5% of the adult population have a BMI <20 and up to 40% of older hospital patients admitted acutely are undernourished on admission. People with either acute or chronic weight loss are also at risk of vitamin and trace element deficiencies. Individuals in long-term care are at particular risk, especially of vitamin D, iron, folate and vitamin C deficiency. Before you investigate weight loss, try to verify it by finding a definite record.

Obesity is defined as a BMI >30 and is of such importance that it should be considered as a disease in its own right.

Many elderly patients investigated for 'weight loss' weighed more in middle age, but have been a stable weight for several years.

Epidemiology

Undernutrition is common in elderly people and causes substantial morbidity and mortality. The National Diet and Nutrition Survey, commissioned by the Ministry of Agriculture, Fisheries and Food and the Department of Health in 1995, assessed people aged over 65 years (1275 living at home and 412 in institutions). Some of its conclusions are as follows:

- There is a strong correlation between diet, nutritional status and oral health.

- Energy intakes for those living at home were lower than estimated average requirements.

- Average fibre intake was below the average recommended levels in both groups.

- Average intakes of vitamins A, B_6 and D and folate were below the recommended level.

- Those of low socioeconomic status had lower intakes of energy, protein, carbohydrate, fibre and vitamins (especially vitamin C).

Low body weight, defined as a BMI of 20 kg/m^2 or less, was particularly common in those in institutions, occurring in 3% of men and 6% of women who lived at home, but in 16% of men and 15% of women who lived in institutions.

Although the most concern is focused on childhood obesity, a health survey in 1998 in England and Wales showed that 17% of men and 21% of women were obese and unfortunately this trend has continued to rise. Most hospital departments of geriatric medicine need special beds, chairs and wheelchairs for very obese patients.

Aetiology

Malnutrition is usually multifactorial, with contributions from the consequences of ageing, social factors and pathology.

Groups at risk of malnutrition include those with the following problems/circumstances.

- Difficulty in eating: poor dentition, sore mouth, difficulty with mastication or swallowing disorders.

- Vulnerable psychosocial situation: the elderly living alone, those in poverty, residents of nursing or residential homes.

- Mental illness: depression causes anorexia and apathy, and in severe cases food refusal. Bereavement may remove the social aspects of eating. Undernutrition in Alzheimer's disease is not fully understood, but decreased food intake and increased energy expenditure as a result of agitation are contributory factors. Behavioural eating disorders are uncommon in older patients but can occur.

- Physical illness: a number of conditions make food preparation difficult. Illness may cause anorexia and nausea, resulting in reduced energy intake. There may be swallowing problems, eg stroke, or malabsorption, for which there are many causes (eg inflammatory bowel disease, coeliac disease, small bowel bacterial overgrowth), all of which are not uncommon in elderly people. Protein may be lost via the kidney, gut or skin, and energy expenditure may be increased, eg in infection. Any severe illness may be associated with undernutrition, including malignant disease.

- Hospital admission: people may be malnourished before or after hospital admission and in the convalescent period after major surgery or severe illness.

- Iatrogenic: drugs causing anorexia (eg digoxin), altered taste (eg angiotensin-converting enzyme inhibitors), dry mouth and nausea (eg selective serotonin reuptake inhibitors), and constipation (eg opiates).

- Special diets or food textures (eg low-salt diets or thickened foods) are often unpalatable.

Causes are often multiple. For example, cardiac cachexia (Fig. 21) is defined as undernutrition occurring as a consequence of congestive heart failure. Its aetiology is multifactorial and includes decreased intake as a result of anorexia caused by breathlessness, drugs, gastric and liver congestion, increased metabolic rate and malabsorption. A similar situation occurs in end-stage chronic obstructive pulmonary disease and many cancers.

There are two types of energy depletion:

- chronic protein energy deficiency shown by a low BMI;

- acute undernutrition evidenced by recent unintended weight loss.

Complications of undernutrition

- Apathy.

- Impaired immune response with increased susceptibility to infection.

- Impaired wound healing.

- Reduced muscle strength with increased susceptibility to falls.

- Impaired thermoregulation leading to hypothermia.

- Reduced respiratory muscle strength with poor cough pressure predisposing to chest infection and delayed recovery from chest infection.

- Inactivity predisposing to thromboembolic disease and pressure sores.

- Increased length of stay in hospital.

Physical signs
Clinical features vary but may include the following.

- Protein undernutrition: muscle wasting, peripheral oedema and leuconychia.

- Anaemia: pallor, angular stomatitis, glossitis and koilonychia.

- Vitamin K deficiency: superficial bruises, oral haemorrhages.

- Vitamin D deficiency: proximal myopathy, bone pain, pathological fracture, tetany.

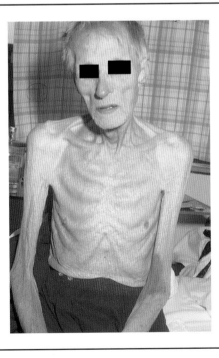

▲ **Fig. 21** Severe cachexia with loss of body fat and lean body mass in a patient with cardiac cachexia resulting from mitral valve disease.

- Vitamin C deficiency: petechial, perifollicular and mucosal haemorrhages, corkscrew hairs, gum hypertrophy, haemarthroses.

- Vitamin B_{12} deficiency: peripheral neuropathy, subacute combined degeneration of the cord, dementia, optic atrophy.

Remember: the obese woman who lives on tea and toast or even sweet sherry may have severe protein and vitamin deficiencies.

Signs of underlying cause

There may be signs of a specific underlying cause, eg a mass or organomegaly from a cancer (check breasts and thyroid), lymphadenopathy or chronic heart, lung or abdominal disease. Figure 22 shows ascites secondary to cirrhosis of the liver.

Investigations

Document the patient's weight (surprisingly difficult in hospital), noting whether this is distorted by oedema. Refer to the dietitian who will calculate BMI (weight in kg divided by height in m², or calculated from the demi-span if the patient cannot stand), assess previous diet and recommend treatment. Refer for speech and language therapy if dysphagia is a problem. Conducting other investigations will depend on the clinical picture.

Check for hypercalcaemia in nauseated patients with cancer.

Treatment

Provision of nutritional support for undernourished patients reduces mortality, complications and length of stay. A multidisciplinary, multifaceted approach is most likely to be successful.

- Work with nursing staff, relatives, hospital catering and dietetics to try to provide nutritious appetising food, making sure that it is served in such a way that patients eat as much as they are able. Snacks should be available.

- Treat the underlying causes of poor nutrition.

- Review the drug chart.

- Improve symptom control, especially for a sore mouth, nausea, reflux, pain control, constipation or diarrhoea.

- Consider a little alcohol; low-dose steroids may help in some cancers.

- Dietary supplements, eg Fortisip, Ensure or specific vitamins.

- Consider non-oral feeding if indicated, eg nasogastric or percutaneous endoscopic gastrostomy feeding or parenteral nutrition if the gut is not functioning but is expected to recover.

- When the patient is at home, liaise with social services to arrange a luncheon club, provision of meals on wheels or frozen meals, etc.

Complications

Malnutrition is associated with considerable morbidity and has been estimated to cost the NHS in the UK millions of pounds. Consequences include:

- falls and their sequelae, eg fractured neck of femur;

- reduced immunity resulting in recurrent infections, eg oral candidiasis (Fig. 23);

- pressure sores and slow wound healing;

- loss of independence;

- depression and a vicious circle of anorexia and poor nutrition.

Obesity

Chronic conditions associated with obesity include:

- metabolic disorders (diabetes and dyslipidaemia);

- cardiovascular disease and hypertension;

- respiratory problems (sleep apnoea syndrome);

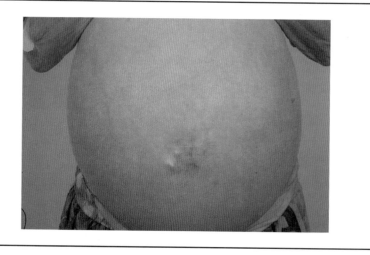

▲ **Fig. 22** Gross abdominal distension caused by ascites. There are also caput medusae and the patient has had the umbilicus removed after surgery for an umbilical hernia. The cause is portal hypertension resulting from hepatic cirrhosis.

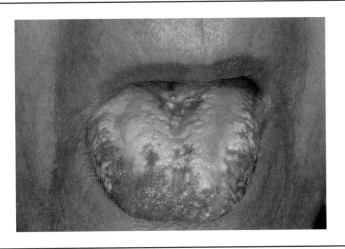

▲ **Fig. 23** Oral candidiasis.

- certain cancers (breast);

- musculoskeletal problems;

- psychological disorders;

- reproductive disorders (including infertility);

- gastrointestinal disorders (gastro-oesophageal reflux and gallstones).

Health benefits achievable from a 5–10% weight loss in an obese patient include:

- reduction in the symptoms of angina by up to 90%;

- 33% increase in exercise tolerance;

- fall of 30–50% in plasma glucose;

- fall of 10 mmHg in systolic and diastolic BP;

- fall by 15% in low-density lipoprotein and increase by 8% in high-density lipoprotein cholesterol;

- reduced snoring with improvement in quality of sleep.

Prognosis

In old age, a low BMI is associated with a poor prognosis. Obesity may increase morbidity, eg from angina or osteoarthritic knees, and mortality from the metabolic syndrome and other associated conditions.

Prevention

Identify at-risk patients on the post-take round and take immediate action.

Osteomalacia

This results from lack of vitamin D or a disturbance of its metabolism. The main histological feature is defective mineralisation of the bone matrix. The predominant source of vitamin D is from ultraviolet irradiation of the skin by sunlight of a wavelength that occurs in the UK between May and September. In the absence of cutaneous synthesis an intake of 5–10 µg/day is required (from foods such as oily fish and egg yolk). It is then hydroxylated in the liver and kidney to form active 1,25-dihydroxyvitamin D. Vitamin D deficiency impairs intestinal absorption of calcium, resulting in a lower serum and urinary calcium than normal. Absorption of phosphate is also defective. A low serum calcium stimulates the secretion of parathyroid hormone (PTH), which tends to correct the calcium but exaggerates the low phosphate (PTH increases calcium and phosphate reabsorption from bone but decreases phosphate reabsorption by the kidney). Osteoblastic activity is increased and, as a consequence, plasma alkaline phosphatase is increased.

Causes

The elderly are at increased risk of osteomalacia for several reasons.

- Reduced exposure to sunlight: elderly people often get out infrequently or are housebound; they also tend to cover their arms.

- Low dietary intake of vitamin D (poor diet) and impaired absorption (conditions such as coeliac disease, biliary disease and previous partial gastrectomy or intestinal resection).

- Reduced renal function with age (makes 1,25-dihydroxylation of vitamin D less efficient).

- More commonly occurs if elderly peple are taking first-generation anticonvulsants (eg phenytoin, valproate, carbamazepine), which interfere with vitamin D metabolism.

Clinical features

- Bone pain and tenderness.

- Skeletal deformity.

- Weakness of proximal muscles.

Radiology

The hallmark of active osteomalacia is the finding of Looser's zones. These are ribbon-like areas of demineralisation which may be found in almost any bone, especially the long bones, pelvis and ribs.

Treatment

Vitamin D, usually with calcium for nutritional deficiencies, eg Adcal-D3/Calcichew D3 Forte; alfacalcidol for renal bone disease

Thiamine deficiency

Thiamine (vitamin B_1) deficiency is not just confined to patients with alcohol dependence but can occur in the elderly due to dietary deficiency. Thiamine deficiency causes selective cellular necrosis in the mammillary bodies, resulting in Wernicke's encephalopathy. The onset may be sudden, causing clinical confusion with a brainstem stroke.

Clinical features

- Ophthalmoplegia (nystagmus and paralysis of abduction of the eye).

- Cerebellar ataxia.

- Confusion (may be that of delirium tremens or mild confusion/drowsiness).

The most serious associated mental disorder is Korsakoff's psychosis in which the patient is alert but has anterograde amnesia (cannot transfer new information to memory stores) and retrograde amnesia, and often confabulates as well. Thiamine deficiency also causes wet and dry beriberi (symptoms of which include cardiac failure and neuropathy).

Diagnostic test

Erythrocyte transketolase levels.

Treatment

Wernicke's encephalopathy is an emergency. If the diagnosis is suspected, thiamine should be given intravenously for 7 days.

Prognosis

If left untreated, patients may die; if treated most of the signs usually resolve.

Vitamin C deficiency

Normal collagen synthesis depends on the hydroxylation of proline and lysine residues. The hydroxylases require vitamin C, so in those suffering from scurvy poor-quality collagen is formed. Elderly bachelors and widowers who live alone are at risk.

Clinical features

- Weakness and aching in joints and muscles.

- Keratosis of the hair follicles and surrounding haemorrhage.

- Ecchymoses: haemorrhage may occur into muscles, joints and under the nails.

- Gum changes occur in relation to natural teeth.

- Old scars break down and new wounds fail to heal.

Diagnostic test

Look for vitamin C of <0.1 mg/dL in leucocyte–platelet layer.

Treatment

Vitamin C 250 mg qds.

FURTHER READING

Bates CJ, Prentice A, Cole TJ, *et al.* Micronutrients: highlights and research challenges from the 1994–5 National Diet and Nutrition Survey of people aged 65 years and over. *Br. J. Nutr.* 1999; 82: 7–15. (References other papers from this survey.)

Erens B and Primatesta P, eds. *Health Survey for England: Cardiovascular Disease '98.* London: Stationery Office, 1999.

Lesourd B and Mazari L. Nutrition and immunity in the elderly. *Proc. Nutr. Soc.* 1999; 58: 685–95.

McWhirter JP and Pennington CR. Incidence and recognition of malnutrition in hospital. *BMJ* 1994; 308: 945–8.

Royal College of Physicians of London. *Nutrition and Patients: A Doctor's Responsibility. Report of a Working Party of the Royal College of Physicians.* London: RCP, 2002.

Vetta F, Ronzoni S, Taglieri G and Bollea MR. The impact of malnutrition on the quality of life in the elderly. *Clin. Nutr.* 1999; 18: 259–67.

2.12 Benefits

In general, elderly people have low incomes and being poor correlates strongly with ill-health. As a doctor, you are not expected to know all the benefits available, but it is your responsibility to inform patients that there is help available and to direct them to sources of information such as the Citizens Advice Bureau or Age Concern. However, your patients (and possibly even your family) will benefit if you know about the key benefits listed here.

The benefits described here apply across the UK. However, some aspects of the benefit system differ in Scotland (see Age Concern Scotland for details).

- Older people tend to have low incomes.
- Attendance Allowance is tax free and not means tested.
- People who get Attendance Allowance can claim other benefits such as the Warm Front Scheme.
- Remember that the Special Rules apply to patients dying of end-stage heart failure and lung disease as well as of cancer.

Disability Living Allowance

This is paid to people under the age of 65 who need help with mobility and personal hygiene because of physical or mental health disability. The key points about the allowance are as follows.

- There are two different components: a care component

that has three levels and a mobility component that has two levels.

- It is not taxable and is not means tested.

- There is no requirement on how the money is used.

Attendance Allowance

This is paid to individuals aged 65 years and over who are physically or mentally ill or disabled and who need frequent help with activities of daily living, especially washing, dressing and personal care. It is available whether or not they live alone, and depends on their needs irrespective of whether they are already getting help. The key points about the allowance are as follows.

- It is not means tested and is tax free.

- It is paid at two rates. The lower rate is given to people requiring regular supervision through the day or night, and the higher rate to those needing supervision all the time.

- People getting Attendance Allowance may also be eligible for higher rates of Pension Credit, Housing Benefit or Council Tax Benefit.

Attendance Allowance under the Special Rules

This is money set aside for people who have a terminal illness with an estimated prognosis of 6 months or less, even if they are completely independent. It can be applied for on the patient's behalf on a very simple form without telling the patient the prognosis. The money does not have to be used to pay for care, but to improve the quality of life for the last few months, eg to pay for heating, microwave food or taxis to the hospital.

Carer's Allowance

This is available to the carers of people already claiming Attendance Allowance. Carers must spend at least 35 hours a week looking after the elderly. Carers should apply for the allowance before they reach 65 years of age. It is not income related, but is not paid if the carer is earning more than £84 (2006) a week from employment after allowable expenses and it may affect other benefits. The sum is not large, but the carer will usually be credited with National Insurance contributions, which protect the basic retirement pension. Carers over 65 may be eligible for some help but the rules are very complex so carers should seek advice.

FURTHER READING

Age Concern England. *Attendance Allowance and Disability Living Allowance (Factsheet 34)*. London: Age Concern England, 2006. Available at http://www.ageconcern.org.uk

- - - - - - - - - - - - - - - - - - -

Age Concern England. *Carer's Allowance (Factsheet 15)*. London: Age Concern England, 2006. Available at http://www.ageconcern.org.uk

- - - - - - - - - - - - - - - - - - -

Websites
Age Concern Scotland factsheets. Available at http://www. ageconcernscotland.org.uk

- - - - - - - - - - - - - - - - - - -

UK Government website. http://www.direct.gov.uk

2.13 Legal aspects of elderly care

Although the ethical principles are similar in many developed countries, there are differences in both what is ethically acceptable and the legal

background. This account applies to England and Wales. For information about Scotland and other countries see the relevant literature.

Mental capacity

A lack of mental capacity may arise because someone is unable to make a legally acceptable decision because of his or her mental state, because he or she cannot communicate that decision, or a combination of the two. A person's capacity may vary depending on the nature of the decision or fluctuate from day to day. If a person has communication problems, an attempt must be made to overcome the difficulties before concluding that the person does not have mental capacity.

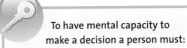

To have mental capacity to make a decision a person must:

- understand the information relevant to the decision;
- retain that information;
- be able to use or weigh that information as part of the process of making a decision;
- communicate that decision by any means.

The question that needs to be asked is: 'Does the person understand the nature and likely consequence of the decision that needs to be made, and can he or she communicate this?'

Testamentary capacity

People who are confused or have mental health problems may still have testamentary capacity (be able to make a valid will). They must be aware that a will is being made; have a reasonable grasp of the nature and extent of their assets, and the relationship they have with the possible beneficiaries; and be able to communicate their wishes. Any assessment of a patient's testamentary capacity should include standard tests of cognitive function (eg Mini-Mental State Examination) but it is often more helpful to ask directly about their family members and whether they own their house, where it is, and so on.

Power of Attorney

This is a legal document where a person (the donor) enables another (known as the attorney, but who is usually a family member and not a solicitor) to act on his or her behalf. It is restricted to financial matters. The donor must have capacity (as described above) to make it valid. The donor directs the attorney. If the donor becomes mentally incompetent, a Power of Attorney ceases and the Court of Protection has to be contacted to take over the donor's financial affairs.

Enduring Power of Attorney

This is a Power of Attorney that endures, ie is still legally effective even if the donor becomes mentally incompetent (at which point the power must be registered with the Court of Protection). It was introduced in England and Wales in 1985.

If you suspect that a patient has a dementing illness, raise the subject of an Enduring (or Lasting) Power of Attorney at an early stage with the spouse or children. It is a simple and cheap procedure. If it is not applied for there will be no alternative but direct application to the Court of Protection once the patient loses capacity, which is (and is likely to remain) expensive and cumbersome.

The Court of Protection

Currently, this exists to supervise the management of the financial affairs of those who are mentally incapable. It can write or change a will as appropriate for a patient. Referral to the Court of Protection can be made by a relative, friend or doctor. A doctor (the patient's GP or consultant) is asked to complete a medical certificate stating that the patient is incapable of managing his or her affairs as a result of mental disorder as defined in the Mental Health Act. The Court appoints a receiver (often a relative) to manage the patient's affairs.

Living Wills or Advance Directives

A person of sound mind can state that if certain circumstances arise in the future and he or she becomes mentally and/or physically incapacitated from a serious illness, certain treatments should not occur. Advance directives have force in common law. There must be evidence that they were completed and witnessed when the subject was in sound mind and not depressed, and that he or she fully understood the nature of the directions. Advance directives can only direct the refusal of treatment and not direct the treatment that is to be given.

The legislation in this area in England and Wales has just changed: Enduring Powers of Attorney have been replaced by Lasting Powers of Attorney (LPA) with provisions extending to health decisions, Advance Directives have been replaced by Advance Decisions (with clear legal status) and a new Court of Protection (which also has jurisdiction over health decisions) has been set up.

The Mental Capacity Act 2005

The Act, which came into force in 2007 in England and Wales, states that everyone should be treated as able to take their own decisions until it is shown that they cannot. The Act intends to strengthen the protection of people who lose the capacity to make their own decisions.

- The Act will enable individuals, while still able, to appoint someone (eg a trusted relative or friend) to make decisions on their behalf once they lose the ability to do so. A major change is that this person (the Attorney) can make decisions on the individual's health and personal welfare. Previously, the law only covered financial matters.

- The Act will also ensure that decisions made on behalf of individuals are in their best interests. The Act provides a check-list of things that decision-makers must work through.

- The Act introduces a Code of Practice for people such as healthcare workers who support people who have lost the capacity to make their own decisions.

- The Act provides strict guidance for research in patient groups without capacity.

The New Court of Protection has powers to direct all aspects of the person's care, including healthcare. If a one-off decision is not appropriate, it will appoint a deputy to manage the person's affairs. The Public Guardian will oversee the functioning of deputies. There will be a new criminal offence of neglect or ill-treatment of a person who lacks capacity.

People with no one to act for them will be able to leave instructions for their care under the new provisions. If such people lack capacity, they will be supported and represented by an Independent Mental Capacity Advocate service.

Mental Capacity Act

The key changes to the law resulting from this act include the following.

- LPA: Attorney can make health decisions.
- New Court of Protection: appointed Deputy can make health decisions.
- Office of the Public Guardian: registers LPAs and oversees Deputies.
- It is a criminal offence to mistreat a person lacking capacity.
- Independent Mental Capacity Advocate service.

- general neglect (eg deprivation of food, clothing and warmth);
- financial;
- sexual;
- misuse of medication (eg withholding antianginal drugs, oversedation);
- institutional (moving frail old patients around the hospital at night for the benefit of others).

relevant inspection body has to be informed immediately. If there is fraud or identifiable injury, the police should be informed with the agreement of the patient, if he or she is mentally competent.

Elder abuse

Elder abuse was first described in the UK in 1975. In the USA there is a legal requirement to notify the authorities of suspected cases, but this is not so at present in the UK. However, hospitals now have elder abuse policies and police stations have officers with special responsibility for elder abuse.Studies show that 5% of elderly people experience abuse from their carers.

There are several forms of elder abuse:

- physical (hitting, restraining an individual against his or her will);
- psychological;
- verbal;

The abuser is often the immediate carer. Abuse is more likely if the patient is immobile, incontinent or mentally impaired, or if there were poor family relationships before the caring became necessary. Awareness of elder abuse is the first step to the management of it. Suspicion should be aroused if there are unexplained bruises or falls, or if there is excessive alcohol consumption by the carer. The patient will often appear frightened and the carer may exhibit anger or despair. If abuse is suspected, the patient and carer must be interviewed alone. The carer must be told of the concerns and the case referred to a social worker for continued monitoring. If abuse is taking place in a residential or nursing home, the

FURTHER READING

Age Concern England. *Legal Arrangements for Managing Financial Affairs (Factsheet 22)*. London: Age Concern England, 2006. Available at http://www.ageconcern.org.uk

Age Concern Scotland. *Legal Arrangements for Managing Financial Affairs (Factsheet 22S)*. Edinburgh: Age Concern Scotland 2004. Available at http://www.ageconcernscotland.org.uk

Miller SS and Marin DB. Assessing capacity. *Emerg. Med. Clin. North Am.* 2000; 18: 233–42.

Websites
Department of Constitutional Affairs (UK Government), Mental Capacity Act 2005 and related documents. Available at http://www.dca.gov.uk/menincap/legis.htm

Action on Elder Abuse. Available at http://www.elderabuse.org.uk

3.1 Diagnosis vs common sense

Will it be helpful to investigate the problem?

Not all symptoms, abnormal physical findings or results should be investigated. The overall likelihood of doing some good must be considered. However, the decision *not* to investigate should be active, not an oversight and be recorded (eg 'erythrocyte sedimentation rate 85 mm/hour and myeloma screen negative – decision taken not to investigate further').

Which investigation?

If investigation is appropriate, which investigation should be chosen? For example, a barium swallow and oesophago-gastroduodenoscopy can both be used to investigate dysphagia, but have different risks and advantages. Balance diagnostic yield with acceptability to the patient, risk of the procedure and availability in your hospital. Be aware of costs, but most costs are insignificant compared with those caused by delays in discharge.

Is investigation justified?

A diagnostic test may be justified if it helps social management, even if immediate medical management will not change, eg an elderly man with confusion, iron deficiency and a change in bowel habit is a poor candidate for surgery, so why pursue a diagnosis? An abdominal CT scan is usually well tolerated (unlike a

barium enema) and if it is highly suggestive of cancer it may enable the family to struggle on for another few months without seeking institutional care, knowing that the end is in sight. Support can be arranged from palliative care services and, if a chest infection or acute obstruction supervenes, the GP can arrange terminal care without having to go through the process of urgent admission. Conversely, investigation of risk factors when treatment would not be appropriate is unhelpful and may increase a patient's anxiety. Carotid endarterectomy would not be carried out in a 91-year-old person who has recovered well from a stroke, so do not arrange Doppler carotid studies. Patients' views about how far they wish to be investigated must be respected.

3.2 Assessment of cognition, mood and function

Management of an older patient requires more than a medical diagnosis; a holistic approach, which includes evaluation of the person's cognition, mood and functional ability, is essential.

> Aspects of mental state and function are best recorded using standardised instruments that have been shown to be valid and repeatable. Without such scores, dementia and depression are often overlooked and typical medical notes give little idea of what the patient can actually do.

Abbreviated Mental Test score

The Abbreviated Mental Test (AMT) is the most common and quick on-ward test to identify patients who may have cognitive problems. Although it is still widely used, two of the questions are not ideal in a multicultural population and one question is outdated – knowledge of the year World War I began is fading, even in people born in the UK. Therefore, it has been proposed that the AMT should be 'retired', but there is no generally accepted alternative.

> **Abbreviated Mental Test score**
>
> Each question scores 1 mark and the test is marked out of 10. No half marks are allowed. A score of 6 or below is likely to indicate impaired cognition.
>
> 1. Age?
> 2. Time (to nearest hour)?
> 3. Address for recall at end of test (eg 42 West Street).
> 4. What year is it?
> 5. Name of institution?
> 6. Recognition of two persons' identities (can the patient identify your job and that of a nurse?).
> 7. Date of birth (day and month)?
> 8. In what year did World War I begin?
> 9. Name of the present monarch?
> 10. Count backwards from 20 to 1.

> A low score on a cognitive test indicates that further assessment is needed. It is often the result of acute or chronic confusion (delirium or dementia), but patients also have a low score if they are deaf, dysphasic, depressed, do not speak English or refuse to answer!

Mini-Mental State Examination

If more time is available, the Mini-Mental State Examination (MMSE), devised by Folstein, is more comprehensive. Cognitive domains tested include orientation, registration of information, attention and calculation, recall, language (naming and repeating), reading, writing, the ability to follow a three-stage command, and construction (copying two overlapping pentagons). The MMSE is widely used as a screening tool in population studies and may be used to monitor mental change and the response to treatment in Alzheimer's disease. Education does affect the score. The maximum is 30, but a score of 30 (or 10 on the AMT) does not rule out dementia (eg a barrister may score 30 but have problems at work). A score of 28–30 does not support the diagnosis of dementia, 25–27 is borderline and <25 suggests confusion. Of over-75s in the general population, 13% have scores of <25.

Assessment of delirium using the Confusion Assessment Method

Having identified impaired cognition using the AMT or MMSE, the Confusion Assessment Method (CAM) can be used if delirium is suspected. The measure is scored based on ratings of four key features of delirium:

1. acute onset and fluctuating course;

2. inattention;

3. disorganised thinking;

4. altered level of consciousness.

The diagnosis of delirium by CAM requires the presence of features 1, 2 and either 3 or 4.

For further information and to view the CAM Training Manual, see http://elderlife.med.yale.edu/pdf/The%20Confusion%20Assessment%20Method.pdf

Geriatric Depression Scale

Depression is common in elderly people. The 15-point Geriatric Depression Scale is a useful screening tool for this.

Geriatric Depression Scale

A score indicating depression includes positive and negative answers but, unless you are very stressed, you will be able to work this out! A patient scoring 0–4 is not depressed; a patient scoring 5–15 requires further assessment.

Score 1 point for the following responses: No to questions 1, 5, 7, 11 and 13; Yes to questions 2, 3, 4, 6, 8, 9, 10, 12, 14 and 15.

1. Are you basically satisfied with your life?
2. Have you dropped many of your activities and interests?
3. Do you feel that your life is empty?
4. Do you often get bored?
5. Are you in good spirits most of the time?
6. Are you afraid that something bad is going to happen to you?
7. Do you feel happy most of the time?
8. Do you often feel helpless?
9. Do you prefer to stay at home, rather than going out and doing new things?
10. Do you feel that you have more problems with memory than most?
11. Do you think it is wonderful to be alive?
12. Do you feel pretty worthless the way you are now?
13. Do you feel full of energy?
14. Do you feel that your situation is hopeless?
15. Do you think that most people are better off than you are?

Barthel Activities of Daily Living Index

This score, devised by the physiotherapist Barthel, is the most common basic activities of daily living scale. It has limitations – there is a marked ceiling effect (a person could score 100 despite considerable handicap) – but it can be scored by a nurse and the score correlates with discharge destination, so it is widely used in elderly people.

Barthel Index

Range 0–100, with 100 the most able.

Feeding

10 = independent and at a reasonable speed
5 = needs help, eg with cutting and spreading
0 = unable

Bathing

5 = independent
0 = dependent
0 = unable

Grooming

5 = takes care of face/hair/teeth/shaving all alone
0 = dependent

Dressing

10 = independent, ties shoes and copes with zips, etc.
5 = needs help, but does half the process in reasonable time
0 = dependent

Bowels

10 = no accidents
5 = occasional accidents/needs help with enemas
0 = incontinent

Bladder

10 = no accidents; manages catheter alone (if used)
5 = occasional accidents or needs help with catheter
0 = incontinent

Toilet

10 = independent
5 = needs help
0 = unable

Bed/chair

15 = totally independent transfer
10 = minimal help needed either verbally or physically
5 = is able to sit up, but needs major help beyond that and for transfer
0 = is unable/has to be lifted bodily

Ambulation

15 = independent for 50 m but may use aid
10 = can manage 50 m but with verbal/physical assistance
5 = requires a wheelchair, but is independent over 50 m
0 = immobile

Stairs

10 = independent
5 = needs verbal/physical help
0 = unable

The timed 'Up & Go' test

This is a test of basic functional mobility for frail elderly persons that does not require any special equipment. The patient is observed and timed while rising from an armchair, walking 3 m, turning, walking back and sitting down again. The time score is reliable, correlates well with a balance scale, gait speed and Barthel Index, and appears to predict the patient's ability to go outside alone safely, although it does not predict falls in a hospital setting.

STRATIFY risk assessment

This is a simple 5-point score that predicts the likelihood of the patient falling in hospital, but it does not perform well in all settings. The factors recorded are previous falls, agitation, visual impairment, the need for frequent toileting and poor transfers or mobility.

FURTHER READING

Hodkinson HM. Evaluation of a mental test score for assessment of mental impairment in the elderly. *Age Ageing* 1972; 1: 233–8.

Inouye SK, van Dyck CH, Alessi CA, *et al.* Clarifying confusion: the confusion assessment method. A new method for detection of delirium. *Ann. Intern. Med.* 1990; 113: 941–8.

Longmore M, Wilkinson IB, Turemezei T and Cheung C-K. *Oxford Handbook of Clinical Medicine*, 7th edn. Oxford: Oxford University Press, 2007.

Nicholl C, Webster S and Wilson KJ. Lecture Notes in Medicine for the Elderly, 7th edn. Oxford: Blackwell Science, 2007.

Oliver D, Britton M, Seed P, Martin FC and Hopper AH. Development and evaluation of evidence based risk assessment tool (STRATIFY) to predict which elderly inpatients will fall: case–control and cohort studies. *BMJ* 1997; 25: 1049–53.

Podsiadlo D and Richardson S. The timed 'Up & Go': a test of basic functional mobility for frail elderly persons. *J. Am. Geriatr. Soc.* 1991; 39: 142–8.

Sheikh JI, Yesavage JA, Brooks JO III, *et al.* Proposed factor structure of the Geriatric Depression Scale. *Int. Psychogeriatr.* 1991; 3: 23–8.

4.1 Self-assessment questions

Question 1

Clinical scenario

A 74-year-old man is admitted with a history of poor mobility and an increasing number of falls over the last week. He has had low back pain for the last 6 weeks. He complains of bilateral leg weakness and numbness. He has noticed some urinary hesitancy but is adamant that he has no other urinary symptoms. He has bilateral extensor plantar responses on examination.

Question

Which of the following do you think would be the most important investigation to organise?

Answers

A Spinal radiographs
B CT scan of the brain
C MRI scan of the spine
D Bone scan
E Lumbar myelogram

Question 2

Clinical scenario

An 84-year-old man who has been admitted to a medical ward develops urinary retention. A junior doctor is called to review the patient, confirms a palpable bladder and arranges urinary catheterisation. The patient complains bitterly about lumbar back pain that has gradually come on over the last 2–3 weeks. Examination reveals bilateral leg weakness and loss of pinprick,

position and vibration sense. The patient's reflexes are brisk and plantars extensor.

Question

Which of the following statements concerning pain from spinal cord compression are correct?

Answers

A The pain is always radicular and never localised
B The onset of pain is always acute and never insidious
C Valsalva manoeuvres have no effect on radicular pain
D Pain from vertebral metastases may worsen in a recumbent position
E Once symptoms other than pain appear, they progress slowly

Question 3

Clinical scenario

A 69-year-old man with known prostatic carcinoma is admitted via his GP with a history of falls and increasingly unsteady gait. He has had low back pain intermittently for the last 20 years, but has noted a gradual worsening in his back pain that has been persistent for the last 72 hours. He denies any new urinary symptoms but has noted increasing constipation. Examination reveals bilateral weakness of his lower limbs at 4/5. Sensation is intact, tendon reflexes are hypoactive and plantars flexor. The admitting doctor believes the patient may have spinal cord compression and wants to discuss urgent investigation with the radiologists.

Question

Which one of the following statements in relation to spinal cord compression is *not* correct?

Answers

A Lax rectal sphincter is an early sign of spinal cord compression
B Physical examination corresponds to the location of the tumour, the degree of spinal cord compression and the duration of compression
C Deep tendon reflexes may initially be hypoactive or absent
D Plantar responses may be flexor initially
E Leg weakness, sensory loss, bilateral extensor plantar responses and hyperreflexia are late signs of spinal cord compression

Question 4

Clinical scenario

An 81-year-old man is admitted as an emergency with intermittent right upper quadrant (RUQ) pain, jaundice and rigors. His family are also concerned that during the last week he has been very confused. According to the family he is 'normally bright as a button'. An abdominal ultrasound shows a shrunken gallbladder and dilated common bile duct.

Question

Which two of the following statements are correct in relation to this clinical scenario?

Answers

A Charcot's triad includes jaundice, RUQ pain and a palpable gallbladder

B His confusion is unlikely to be associated with his pain, jaundice and rigors

C Cholangitis does not usually involve bacterial infection

D Charcot's triad occurs in all patients with cholangitis

E Approximately 1% of patients after cholecystectomy have retained common bile duct stones

F Porta hepatis tumours or metastases may cause cholangitis

G Pancreatic carcinoma never causes cholangitis

H Endoscopic retrograde cholangiopancreatography (ERCP) is a rare cause of cholangitis

I Most patients with cholangitis present with septic shock

J Hepatomegaly never occurs in cholangitis

Question 5

Clinical scenario

A 78-year-old woman is admitted as an emergency with jaundice, rigors and intermittent right upper quadrant (RUQ) pain. Six weeks previously she had undergone a cholecystectomy but has felt generally unwell since, and has complained bitterly about pruritus for the last 2 weeks. The admitting doctor requests an ultrasound and takes blood cultures in addition to other blood tests.

Question

Which two of the following statements are correct in relation to this clinical scenario?

Answers

A The history of a recent cholecystectomy does not increase her risk of cholangitis

B Pruritus does not occur in cholangitis

C Blood cultures are positive in 90% of patients with cholangitis

D *Escherichia coli*, *Klebsiella*, *Enterobacter* and enteroccoci are common bacteria found in cholangitis on blood culture

E Cholangitis always responds to antibiotic therapy

F Charcot's triad of fever, RUQ pain and jaundice is found in 70% of patients with cholangitis

G Patients with cholangitis always have a raised white cell count

H Urinalysis is never helpful in jaundiced patients

I Amylase is always normal in patients with cholangitis

J Anaerobes may be cultured in 50% cases

Question 6

Clinical scenario

An 86-year-old man is referred to a medical outpatient clinic with a history of generalised muscle weakness. He has noted increasing difficulty in standing up from a seated position. A radiograph of his pelvis shows a Looser's zone.

Question

Which of the following is the most likely biochemical finding?

Answers

A Elevated serum calcium

B Elevated phosphate

C A low serum alkaline phosphatase

D A normal serum calcium

E An elevated albumin

Question 7

Clinical scenario

An 82-year-old woman who is housebound is referred to clinic because of an abnormal waddling gait. She has a poor diet and lives on tea, biscuits and chapattis. She has severe varicose leg ulcers. Biochemistry is consistent with a diagnosis of osteomalacia. Her daughter wants to know how her mother developed this condition.

Question

Which of the following is *not* related to the development of osteomalacia?

Answers

A Being housebound

B Venous ulceration

C Her age

D Poor nutrition

E Eating chapattis

Question 8

Clinical scenario

A 74-year-old type 2 diabetic woman is reviewed in clinic. She has always been overweight but has gained 10 kg in 12 months, giving her a BMI of >30. She is very upset with her GP who has advised a diet. She wants to know why she should lose weight when she diligently takes all her tablets.

Question

Which of the following benefits is *least* likely if she manages a 5–10% reduction in weight?

Answers

A Reduced snoring

B Improved quality of sleep

C An increase of 50% in high-density lipoprotein cholesterol

D Improved exercise tolerance

E Fall of 10 mmHg systolic BP

Question 9

Clinical scenario

An 84-year-old woman is admitted with a history of general malaise. She has been suffering from depression following the death of her son. She has a single pension and finds it difficult to get to the shops due to generalised osteoarthritis. Examination shows a BMI of <18.

Question

Which of the following is correct?

Answers

A She has a normal immune response

B She is not at increased risk of falls

C She is not at increased risk of chest infections

D Wound healing may be impaired

E Thermoregulation is likely to be normal

Question 10

Clinical scenario

A 76-year-old man is admitted as an emergency with a history of confusion and ataxia. He is malnourished with a BMI of <18, lives alone and is adamant that he is a teetotaler. Examination shows nystagmus and a lesion of cranial nerve VI. He is referred from the Emergency Department as a brainstem stroke, but he may have another condition.

Question

Which of the following statements is correct?

Answers

A He is unlikely to have thiamine deficiency if he does not drink

B The ataxia is cerebellar in type

C He is not at risk of dying

D No immediate treatment is indicated

E His ophthalmoplegia is irreversible

Question 11

Clinical scenario

An 83-year-old man presents to the outpatient clinic with a history of increasing falls. On examination he is generally well, but has past pointing more marked on his left than right arm. Power in all limbs is normal. His gait is wide-based and unsteady. Romberg's sign is negative.

Question

What is the most likely explanation of his falls?

Answers

A Cerebellar disease

B Peripheral neuropathy

C Lacunar infarcts

D Parkinson's disease

E Multi-infarct dementia

Question 12

Clinical scenario

A 70-year-old man, who is known to have ischaemic heart disease and has had short-lived episodes of atrial fibrillation (AF) in the past, presents with 48 hours of fatigue and breathlessness. He is not very ill, but his pulse is 150/minute in AF.

Question

Which two drugs would be most appropriate to achieve 'chemical cardioversion'?

Answers

A Digoxin

B Quinidine

C Procainamide

D Disopyramide

E Sotalol

F Atenolol

G Propranolol

H Verapamil

I Amiodarone

J Diltiazem

Question 13

Clinical scenario

A 75-year-old man is assessed in the Emergency Department following a fall and is found to have a serum sodium of 118 mmol/L.

Question

Which of these drugs is *least* likely to be the cause of his hyponatraemia?

Answers

A Glipizide

B Citalopram

C Bendroflumethiazide

D Tolterodine

E Venlafaxine

Question 14

Clinical scenario

An 82-year-old retired architect needs help with the basic activities of daily living following a right middle cerebral infarct. He returns home to live with his daughter. An application for Attendance Allowance is made.

Question

Which of the following statements about Attendance Allowance is *not* correct?

Answers

A It is tax-free

B It is not means tested

C It is paid to the carer

D It is available at two rates depending on whether care is needed at night as well as by day

E It could still be paid if the architect lived alone and had no help

Question 15

Clinical scenario

An 82-year-old retired publican is found to have a haemoglobin of 8.9 g/dL with a mean corpuscular volume of 104.3 fL.

Question

Which of the following blood tests is *least* likely to help in identifying a cause for his anaemia?

Answers

A Vitamin B_{12}

B Red cell folate

C Thyroid-stimulating hormone

D Serum urate

E γ-Glutamyl transpeptidase

Question 16

Clinical scenario

An 82-year-old woman with type 2 diabetes has been managed on diet alone, but her recent HbA_{1c} was found to be 9.8%. She has a background of ischaemic heart disease with controlled cardiac failure and a serum creatinine of 165 µmol/L.

Question

Which antidiabetic agent would be most suitable?

Answers

A Glibenclamide
B Metformin
C Gliclazide
D Rosiglitazone
E Nateglinide

Question 17

Clinical scenario

An 88-year-old former builder has become more confused since his medication was altered.

Question

Which of the following drugs that he is taking will *not* be responsible for his confusion?

Answers

A Zopiclone
B Paroxetine
C Ranitidine
D Paracetamol
E Codeine

Question 18

Clinical scenario

The daughter of your patient with Alzheimer's disease wants some more information about donepezil, which you are proposing as treatment for her mother.

Question

Which of the following statements is *not* correct?

Answers

A Donepezil is a cholinesterase inhibitor, so it reduces the breakdown of the endogenous acetylcholine of the brain

B The most troublesome side effect is usually dizziness due to postural hypotension
C Donepezil is given once a day, so as the daughter visits daily it will be possible for her to supervise her mother's medication
D Caution is advised if the patient has sick sinus syndrome
E Treatment will be initiated in the specialist clinic and will be continued by her GP under a shared care protocol

Question 19

Clinical scenario

A 78-year-old woman is brought to the Emergency Department by ambulance following a witnessed fit in a supermarket. Her husband confirms that, apart from treated hypertension and a right total knee replacement last year for which she still takes ibuprofen, she has no significant past medical history. On examination she has a Glasgow Coma Scale score of 10 and appears to have a left hemiparesis. She is pyrexial (38.2°C) and dipstick of her urine is positive for nitrites and blood.

Question

Which of the following statements is *not* correct?

Answers

A The commonest cause of a first fit at this age is cerebrovascular disease
B She must not drive for 12 months following this episode
C Focal neurological signs that resolve within 24 hours could be either a transient ischaemic attack or Todd's paresis
D Ciprofloxacin is a good choice for the presumed urinary sepsis that may have precipitated her fit
E Her chest should be examined carefully because she may develop an aspiration pneumonia

Question 20

Clinical scenario

An 81-year-old man is referred to the Outpatients Department with progressive decline in his short-term memory. He has had several small strokes in the past. You suspect he has a vascular dementia and examine him carefully.

Question

Which two of these physical findings would make you concerned that your diagnosis is *not* correct?

Answers

A BP of 118/87 mmHg
B Atrial fibrillation
C Brisk reflexes in the right arm
D Impaired down-gaze
E Increased tone in the legs
F Impaired joint position and vibration sense
G Shuffling gait
H Right homonymous hemianopia
I Mini-Mental State Examination score of 28/30
J Dressing dyspraxia

Question 21

Clinical scenario

An 85-year-old man with metastatic carcinoma of the prostate has had a pathological hip fracture successfully treated with a total hip replacement. He is referred to you for rehabilitation. He is keen to return to his warden-supervised flat where he previously had morning care 5 days a week.

Question

Which two statements are *not* correct?

Answers

A Palliative care would be more appropriate than rehabilitation
B Rehabilitation goals should be discussed with the patient
C He may benefit from a blood transfusion if his haemoglobin is below 8 g/dL

D Care should be taken with his dose of morphine tablets to avoid the development of tolerance

E His mild dementia is not a barrier to rehabilitation

F His opiate dose may need adjusting to minimise nausea and constipation

G Depression should be identified and may respond to drug treatment

H His motivation to return home to his spaniel may improve the outcome

I Paracetamol provides useful background analgesia

J A chair of the correct height, with arms, will improve his transfers

Question 22

Clinical scenario

A 74-year-old woman is admitted with a dense right hemiparesis, right homonymous, hemianopia and drowsiness. There is concern that she cannot swallow safely.

Question

Which two statements about the management of her dysphagia are correct?

Answers

A Thin fluid is more easily aspirated than thickened fluids

B A percutaneous endoscopic gastrostomy (PEG) feeding tube should be inserted in the first week

C A ward swallow test should be carried out when she is well positioned and as alert as possible

D Bridled nasogastric tubes must be inserted in the endoscopy suite

E If you give her 50 mL of water and she does not cough, then it is safe to give oral fluids

F The occupational therapist will help evaluate her swallow

G Until she is drinking adequately she will require at least 2 L of intravenous fluid per day

H Once tube feeding has been started it cannot be discontinued on ethical grounds

I One advantage of a PEG tube is that it prevents aspiration

J The FOOD trial showed that once this patient can swallow safely she should be offered nutritional supplements

4.2 Self-assessment answers

Answer to Question 1

C

An urgent MRI scan would be the most important investigation to organise. If MRI is not available, then a CT myelogram can be used. Spinal radiographs are often abnormal but are non-specific

Answer to Question 2

D

The pain may be radicular, localised or both. The onset of pain is often insidious. Valsalva manoeuvres may exacerbate radicular pain. Pain from vertebral metastases may worsen on recumbency, in contrast to degenerative back pain which is often relieved on recumbency. Once symptoms other than pain appear, they progress rapidly.

Answer to Question 3

A

Lax rectal sphincter is not an early sign of spinal cord compression.

Answer to Question 4

E and F

Charcot's triad is RUQ pain, jaundice and fever, and occurs in 70% of patients with cholangitis. Reynold's pentad adds confusion and hypotension to the triad and suggests septicaemia. Confusion does occur in cholangitis, especially in older patients. Cholangitis results from bacterial infection, with *Escherichia coli*, *Klebsiella*, *Enterobacter* and enteroccoci common organisms. Approximately 1% of patients with cholecystectomy have retained common bile duct stones. Porta hepatis tumours, metastases or pancreatic cancer can cause cholangitis, but common bile duct stones and ERCP are the most common causes. Approximately 5% of patients with cholangitis present with septic shock. Mild hepatomegaly can be present in cholangitis.

Answer to Question 5

D and F

Having a recent cholecystectomy increases the risk of cholangitis. Pruritus can occur in cholangitis. Blood cultures are positive in 20–30% of cases; *Escherichia coli*, *Klebsiella*, *Enterobacter* and enteroccoci are the commonest bacteria found in cholangitis on blood culture. Anaerobes may be cultured in 15%. Cholangitis does not always respond to antibiotic therapy. Charcot's triad of fever, RUQ pain and jaundice is found in 70% of patients with cholangitis. Patients may not always have a raised white cell count in cholangitis: leucopenia may occur, especially in older patients with severe sepsis. Urinalysis may be helpful in confirming that jaundice is obstructive in nature with positive bilirubin but negative urobilinogen. Amylase may be elevated if there is involvement of the lower common bile duct.

Answer to Question 6

D

The Looser's zone (named after a Swiss surgeon) suggests a diagnosis of osteomalacia. A proximal myopathy would explain his difficulty on standing. In osteomalacia the biochemistry classically would be expected to show low serum calcium, low phosphate and elevated alkaline phosphatase. However, the serum calcium can return to normal with development of secondary hyperparathyroidism. His albumin is likely to be low or normal.

Answer to Question 7

B

Being housebound will reduce cutaneous synthesis of vitamin D. Poor nutrition will reduce oral vitamin D intake. Eating chapattis impairs absorption of calcium because of the phytate content.

Answer to Question 8

C

A 5–10% weight loss in an obese patient will reduce snoring, improve quality of sleep and improve exercise tolerance. It will also reduce systolic BP by 10 mmHg. There will probably be an increase in high-density lipoprotein, but of less than 10%.

Answer to Question 9

D

Patients who are malnourished have impaired immune response, predisposing them to infection. Reduced muscle strength predisposes to falls and chest infections. Wound healing may be impaired. Thermoregulation is impaired, predisposing to hypothermia.

Answer to Question 10

B

He has confusion, ataxia and ocular signs consistent with Wernicke's encephalopathy. Although the commonest cause is alcoholism, thiamine deficiency can also occur in patients who are malnourished. The ataxia is cerebellar in type. He is at increased risk of death and should receive intravenous thiamine for 7 days. The ophthalmoplegia is likely to recover.

Answer to Question 11

A

Peripheral neuropathy would not cause past pointing, and Romberg's sign would be positive. Features of Parkinson's disease would include tremor and shuffling gait.

Answer to Question 12

E and I

Digoxin could be used to achieve rate control but would not be expected to achieve chemical cardioversion.

Answer to Question 13

D

Diuretics, selective serotonin reuptake inhibitors and venlafaxine (a serotonin/norepinephrine reuptake inhibitor) are all relatively commonly associated with hyponatraemia. Some sulphonylureas enhance antidiuretic hormone secretion and may also cause hyponatraemia.

Answer to Question 14

C

It is paid to the patient.

Answer to Question 15

D

All the other tests would suggest a cause for macrocytosis.

Answer to Question 16

C

Glibenclamide is too long-acting in older people, metformin is contraindicated in even mild renal impairment and rosiglitazone is contraindicated in heart failure. Nateglinide is licensed in combination with metformin. Gliclazide would be suitable, but the initial dose should be low because of the renal impairment.

Answer to Question 17

D

It should be easy to remember that A, B and E all cause confusion. Histamine H_2 blockers also have this side effect.

Answer to Question 18

B

Donepezil can cause dizziness, but the commonest side effects (often dose-limiting) are gastrointestinal: nausea, vomiting and diarrhoea.

Answer to Question 19

D

Although ciprofloxacin may be given for urinary sepsis, it is epileptogenic, particularly in combination with an NSAID.

Answer to Question 20

D and F

D would suggest progressive supranuclear palsy and F vitamin B_{12} deficiency as causes for his memory impairment.

Answer to Question 21

A and D

Just because a patient has metastatic cancer does not mean that he needs palliative care. Many patients rehabilitate well after a pathological fracture has been pinned. In this setting, dependence on opiate analgesics is not a problem: the patient should receive adequate analgesia to make him pain-free if possible (balancing this with side effects).

Answer to Question 22

A and C

In neurological dysphagia thin fluid is more easily aspirated than thickened fluids, which is why thickening agents are used. To give the patient the best chance of swallowing, a ward swallow test should be carried out when she is well positioned and alert. It is difficult for anyone to swallow lying down! Early PEG feeding has not been shown to improve outcome. Bridled nasogastric tubes can be inserted at the bedside. If you give her 50 mL of water and she does not cough, she may be aspirating silently. The speech and language therapist will help evaluate her swallow. Unless she is febrile, 1 L of fluid a day may meet her needs.

THE MEDICAL MASTERCLASS SERIES

Scientific Background to Medicine 1

GENETICS AND MOLECULAR MEDICINE

Nucleic Acids and Chromosomes 3

Techniques in Molecular Biology 11

Molecular Basis of Simple Genetic Traits 17

More Complex Issues 23

Self-assessment 30

BIOCHEMISTRY AND METABOLISM

Requirement for Energy 35

Carbohydrates 41

Fatty Acids and Lipids 45

3.1 Fatty acids 45
3.2 Lipids 48

Cholesterol and Steroid Hormones 51

Amino Acids and Proteins 53

5.1 Amino acids 53
5.2 Proteins 56

Haem 59

Nucleotides 61

Self-assessment 66

CELL BIOLOGY

Ion Transport 71

1.1 Ion channels 72
1.2 Ion carriers 79

Receptors and Intracellular Signalling 82

Cell Cycle and Apoptosis 88

Haematopoiesis 94

Self-assessment 97

IMMUNOLOGY AND IMMUNOSUPPRESSION

Overview of the Immune System 103

The Major Histocompatibility Complex, Antigen Presentation and Transplantation 106

T Cells 109

B Cells 112

Tolerance and Autoimmunity 115

Complement 117

Inflammation 120

Immunosuppressive Therapy 125

Self-assessment 130

ANATOMY

Heart and Major Vessels 135

Lungs 138

Liver and Biliary Tract 140

Spleen 142

Kidney 143

Endocrine Glands 144

Gastrointestinal Tract 147

Eye 150

Nervous System 152

Self-assessment 167

PHYSIOLOGY

Cardiovascular System 171

1.1 The heart as a pump 171
1.2 The systemic and pulmonary circulations 176
1.3 Blood vessels 177
1.4 Endocrine function of the heart 180

Respiratory System 182

2.1 The lungs 182

Gastrointestinal System 187

3.1 The gut 187
3.2 The liver 190
3.3 The exocrine pancreas 193

Brain and Nerves 194

4.1 The action potential 194
4.2 Synaptic transmission 196
4.3 Neuromuscular transmission 199

Endocrine Physiology 200

5.1 The growth hormone–insulin-like growth factor 1 axis 200
5.2 The hypothalamic–pituitary–adrenal axis 200
5.3 Thyroid hormones 201
5.4 The endocrine pancreas 203
5.5 The ovary and testis 204
5.6 The breast 206
5.7 The posterior pituitary 207

Renal Physiology 209

6.1 Blood flow and glomerular filtration 209
6.2 Function of the renal tubules 211
6.3 Endocrine function of the kidney 217

Self-assessment 220

Scientific Background to Medicine 2

CLINICAL PHARMACOLOGY

Introducing Clinical Pharmacology 3

1.1 Risks versus benefits 4
1.2 Safe prescribing 4
1.3 Rational prescribing 5
1.4 The role of clinical pharmacology 5

Pharmacokinetics 7

2.1 Introduction 7
2.2 Drug absorption 7
2.3 Drug distribution 11
2.4 Drug metabolism 12
2.5 Drug elimination 17
2.6 Plasma half-life and steady-state plasma concentrations 19
2.7 Drug monitoring 20

Pharmacodynamics 22

3.1 How drugs exert their effects 22
3.2 Selectivity is the key to the therapeutic utility of an agent 25
3.3 Basic aspects of the interaction of a drug with its target 27
3.4 Heterogeneity of drug responses, pharmacogenetics and pharmacogenomics 31

Prescribing in Special Circumstances 33

4.1 Introduction 33
4.2 Prescribing and liver disease 33
4.3 Prescribing in pregnancy 36
4.4 Prescribing for women of childbearing potential 39
4.5 Prescribing to lactating mothers 39
4.6 Prescribing in renal disease 41
4.7 Prescribing in the elderly 44

Adverse Drug Reactions 46

5.1 Introduction and definition 46
5.2 Classification of adverse drug reactions 46
5.3 Clinical approach to adverse drug reactions 47
5.4 Dose-related adverse drug reactions (type A) 48
5.5 Non-dose-related adverse drug reactions (type B) 51
5.6 Adverse reactions caused by long-term effects of drugs (type C) 56
5.7 Adverse reactions caused by delayed effects of drugs (type D) 57
5.8 Withdrawal reactions (type E) 58
5.9 Drugs in overdose and use of illicit drugs 59

Drug Development and Rational Prescribing 60

6.1 Drug development 60
6.2 Rational prescribing 65
6.3 Clinical governance and rational prescribing 66
6.4 Rational prescribing: evaluating the evidence for yourself 68
6.5 Rational prescribing, irrational patients 68

Self-assessment 70

STATISTICS, EPIDEMIOLOGY, CLINICAL TRIALS AND META-ANALYSES

Statistics 79

Epidemiology 86

2.1 Observational studies 87

Clinical Trials and Meta-Analyses 92

Self-assessment 103

Clinical Skills

CLINICAL SKILLS FOR PACES

Introduction 3

History-taking for PACES (Station 2) 6

Communication Skills and Ethics for PACES (Station 4) 10

Examination for PACES Stations 1, 3 and 5: General Considerations 12

Station 1: Respiratory System 15

Station 1: Abdominal System 20

Station 3: Cardiovascular System 26

Station 3: Central Nervous System 35

Station 5: Brief Clinical Consulations 53

PAIN RELIEF AND PALLIATIVE CARE

PACES Stations and Acute Scenarios 61

1.1 History-taking 61
   1.1.1 Pain 61
   1.1.2 Constipation/bowel obstruction 63
1.2 Communication skills and ethics 65
   1.2.1 Pain 65
   1.2.2 Breathlessness 66
   1.2.3 Nausea and vomiting 67
   1.2.4 Bowel obstruction 69
   1.2.5 End of life 70
1.3 Acute scenarios 71
   1.3.1 Pain 71
   1.3.2 Breathlessness 74
   1.3.3 Nausea and vomiting 76
   1.3.4 Bowel obstruction 79

Diseases and Treatments 82

2.1 Pain 82
2.2 Breathlessness 87
2.3 Nausea and vomiting 88
2.4 Constipation 89
2.5 Bowel obstruction 90
2.6 Anxiety and depression 91
2.7 Confusion 93
2.8 End-of-life care: the dying patient 94
2.9 Specialist palliative care services 96

Self-assessment 98

MEDICINE FOR THE ELDERLY

PACES Stations and Acute Scenarios 107

1.1 History-taking 107
   1.1.1 Frequent falls 107
   1.1.2 Recent onset of confusion 110
   1.1.3 Urinary incontinence and immobility 114
   1.1.4 Collapse 116
   1.1.5 Vague aches and pains 119
   1.1.6 Swollen legs and back pain 121
   1.1.7 Failure to thrive: gradual decline and weight loss 127
1.2 Clinical examination 129
   1.2.1 Confusion (respiratory) 129
   1.2.2 Confusion (abdominal) 130
   1.2.3 Failure to thrive (abdominal) 131
   1.2.4 Frequent falls (cardiovascular) 131
   1.2.5 Confusion (cardiovascular) 132
   1.2.6 Frequent falls (neurological) 132
   1.2.7 Confusion (neurological) 134
   1.2.8 Impaired mobility (neurological) 135
   1.2.9 Confusion (skin) 135
   1.2.10 Frequent falls (locomotor) 136
   1.2.11 Confusion (endocrine) 136
   1.2.12 Confusion (eye) 136
1.3 Communication skills and ethics 137
   1.3.1 Frequent falls 137
   1.3.2 Confusion 138
   1.3.3 Collapse 139
1.4 Acute scenarios 141
   1.4.1 Sudden onset of confusion 141
   1.4.2 Collapse 143

Diseases and Treatments 147

2.1 Why elderly patients are different 147
2.2 General approach to management 149
2.3 Falls 151
2.4 Urinary and faecal incontinence 155
   2.4.1 Urinary incontinence 155
   2.4.2 Faecal incontinence 157
2.5 Hypothermia 158
2.6 Drugs in elderly people 161
2.7 Dementia 162
2.8 Rehabilitation 165
2.9 Aids, appliances and assistive technology 166
2.10 Hearing impairment 168
2.11 Nutrition 170

2.12 **Benefits 174**

2.13 **Legal aspects of elderly care 175**

Investigations and Practical Procedures 178

3.1 **Diagnosis vs common sense 178**

3.2 **Assessment of cognition, mood and function 178**

Self-assessment 181

Acute Medicine

ACUTE MEDICINE

PACES Stations and Acute Scenarios 3

1.1 **Communication skills and ethics 3**
  1.1.1 Cardiac arrest 3
  1.1.2 Stroke 4
  1.1.3 Congestive cardiac failure 5
  1.1.4 Lumbar back pain 6
  1.1.5 Community-acquired pneumonia 7
  1.1.6 Acute pneumothorax 7

1.2 **Acute scenarios 8**
  1.2.1 Cardiac arrest 8
  1.2.2 Chest pain and hypotension 12
  1.2.3 Should he be thrombolysed? 15
  1.2.4 Hypotension in acute coronary syndrome 20
  1.2.5 Postoperative breathlessness 21
  1.2.6 Two patients with tachyarrhythmia 23
  1.2.7 Bradyarrhythmia 27
  1.2.8 Collapse of unknown cause 30
  1.2.9 Asthma 33
  1.2.10 Pleurisy 36
  1.2.11 Chest infection/pneumonia 39
  1.2.12 Acute-on-chronic airways obstruction 42
  1.2.13 Stridor 44
  1.2.14 Pneumothorax 46
  1.2.15 Upper gastrointestinal haemorrhage 48
  1.2.16 Bloody diarrhoea 51
  1.2.17 Abdominal pain 54
  1.2.18 Hepatic encephalopathy/alcohol withdrawal 56
  1.2.19 Renal failure, fluid overload and hyperkalaemia 59
  1.2.20 Diabetic ketoacidosis 62
  1.2.21 Hypoglycaemia 65
  1.2.22 Hypercalcaemia 67
  1.2.23 Hyponatraemia 69
  1.2.24 Addisonian crisis 71
  1.2.25 Thyrotoxic crisis 74
  1.2.26 Sudden onset of severe headache 75
  1.2.27 Severe headache with fever 77
  1.2.28 Acute spastic paraparesis 79
  1.2.29 Status epilepticus 81
  1.2.30 Stroke 83
  1.2.31 Coma 86
  1.2.32 Fever in a returning traveller 89
  1.2.33 Anaphylaxis 90
  1.2.34 A painful joint 91
  1.2.35 Back pain 94
  1.2.36 Self-harm 96
  1.2.37 Violence and aggression 97

Diseases and Treatments 100

2.1 **Overdoses 100**
  2.1.1 Prevention of drug absorption from the gut 100
  2.1.2 Management of overdoses of specific drugs 100

Investigations and Practical Procedures 103

3.1 **Central venous lines 103**
  3.1.1 Indications, contraindications, consent and preparation 103
  3.1.2 Specific techniques for insertion of central lines 104
  3.1.3 Interpretation of central venous pressure measurements 106

3.2 **Lumbar puncture 106**

3.3 **Cardiac pacing 107**

3.4 **Elective DC cardioversion 109**

3.5 **Intercostal chest drain insertion 109**

3.6 **Arterial blood gases 112**
  3.6.1 Measurement of arterial blood gases 112
  3.6.2 Interpretation of arterial blood gases 113

3.7 **Airway management 113**
  3.7.1 Basic airway management 113
  3.7.2 Tracheostomy 116

3.8 **Ventilatory support 117**
  3.8.1 Controlled oxygen therapy 117
  3.8.2 Continuous positive airway pressure 117
  3.8.3 Non-invasive ventilation 118
  3.8.4 Invasive ventilation 118

Self-assessment 120

Infectious Diseases and Dermatology

INFECTIOUS DISEASES

PACES Stations and Acute Scenarios 3

1.1 **History-taking 3**
  1.1.1 A cavitating lung lesion 3
  1.1.2 Fever and lymphadenopathy 5
  1.1.3 Still feverish after 6 weeks 7
  1.1.4 Chronic fatigue 10

1.1.5 A spot on the penis 12
1.1.6 Penile discharge 15
1.1.7 Woman with a genital sore 17
1.2 Communication skills and ethics 20
1.2.1 Fever, hypotension and confusion 20
1.2.2 A swollen red foot 21
1.2.3 Still feverish after 6 weeks 22
1.2.4 Chronic fatigue 23
1.2.5 Malaise, mouth ulcers and fever 24
1.2.6 Don't tell my wife 25
1.3 Acute scenarios 27
1.3.1 Fever 27
1.3.2 Fever, hypotension and confusion 30
1.3.3 A swollen red foot 33
1.3.4 Fever and cough 34
1.3.5 Fever, back pain and weak legs 37
1.3.6 Drug user with fever and a murmur 40
1.3.7 Fever and heart failure 44
1.3.8 Persistent fever in the intensive care unit 47
1.3.9 Pyelonephritis 49
1.3.10 A sore throat 52
1.3.11 Fever and headache 55
1.3.12 Fever with reduced conscious level 60
1.3.13 Fever in the neutropenic patient 62
1.3.14 Fever after renal transplant 65
1.3.15 Varicella in pregnancy 68
1.3.16 Imported fever 70
1.3.17 Eosinophilia 74
1.3.18 Jaundice and fever after travelling 76
1.3.19 A traveller with diarrhoea 78
1.3.20 Malaise, mouth ulcers and fever 81
1.3.21 Breathlessness in a HIV-positive patient 83
1.3.22 HIV positive and blurred vision 86

1.3.23 Abdominal pain and vaginal discharge 88
1.3.24 Penicillin allergy 91

Pathogens and Management 94

2.1 Antimicrobial prophylaxis 94
2.2 Immunisation 95
2.3 Infection control 97
2.4 Travel advice 99
2.5 Bacteria 100
2.5.1 Gram-positive bacteria 101
2.5.2 Gram-negative bacteria 104
2.6 Mycobacteria 108
2.6.1 Mycobacterium tuberculosis 108
2.6.2 Mycobacterium leprae 113
2.6.3 Opportunistic mycobacteria 114
2.7 Spirochaetes 115
2.7.1 Syphilis 115
2.7.2 Lyme disease 117
2.7.3 Relapsing fever 118
2.7.4 Leptospirosis 118
2.8 Miscellaneous bacteria 119
2.8.1 *Mycoplasma* and *Ureaplasma* 119
2.8.2 Rickettsiae 120
2.8.3 *Coxiella burnetii* (Q fever) 120
2.8.4 Chlamydiae 121
2.9 Fungi 121
2.9.1 *Candida* spp. 121
2.9.2 *Aspergillus* 123
2.9.3 *Cryptococcus neoformans* 124
2.9.4 Dimorphic fungi 125
2.9.5 Miscellaneous fungi 126
2.10 Viruses 126
2.10.1 Herpes simplex viruses 127
2.10.2 Varicella-zoster virus 128
2.10.3 Cytomegalovirus 130
2.10.4 Epstein–Barr virus 130
2.10.5 Human herpesviruses 6 and 7 130

2.10.6 Human herpesvirus 8 131
2.10.7 Parvovirus 131
2.10.8 Hepatitis viruses 132
2.10.9 Influenza virus 133
2.10.10 Paramyxoviruses 134
2.10.11 Enteroviruses 134
2.10.12 Coronaviruses and SARS 135
2.11 Human immunodeficiency virus 135
2.11.1 Prevention following sharps injury 140
2.12 Travel-related viruses 142
2.12.1 Rabies 142
2.12.2 Dengue 143
2.12.3 Arbovirus infections 143
2.13 Protozoan parasites 144
2.13.1 Malaria 144
2.13.2 Leishmaniasis 145
2.13.3 Amoebiasis 146
2.13.4 Toxoplasmosis 147
2.14 Metazoan parasites 148
2.14.1 Schistosomiasis 148
2.14.2 Strongyloidiasis 149
2.14.3 Cysticercosis 150
2.14.4 Filariasis 151
2.14.5 Trichinosis 151
2.14.6 Toxocariasis 152
2.14.7 Hydatid disease 152

Investigations and Practical Procedures 154

3.1 Getting the best from the laboratory 154
3.2 Specific investigations 154

Self-assessment 159

DERMATOLOGY

PACES Stations and Acute Scenarios 175

1.1 History taking 175
1.1.1 Blistering disorders 175
1.1.2 Chronic red facial rash 177

1.1.3 Pruritus 178
1.1.4 Alopecia 180
1.1.5 Hyperpigmentation 181
1.1.6 Hypopigmentation 183
1.1.7 Red legs 185
1.1.8 Leg ulcers 187
1.2 **Clinical examination 189**
1.2.1 Blistering disorder 189
1.2.2 A chronic red facial rash 193
1.2.3 Pruritus 198
1.2.4 Alopecia 200
1.2.5 Hyperpigmentation 202
1.2.6 Hypopigmentation 205
1.2.7 Red legs 207
1.2.8 Lumps and bumps 210
1.2.9 Telangiectases 212
1.2.10 Purpura 214
1.2.11 Lesion on the shin 216
1.2.12 Non-pigmented lesion on the face 217
1.2.13 A pigmented lesion on the face 219
1.2.14 Leg ulcers 221
1.2.15 Examine these hands 223
1.3 **Communication skills and ethics 225**
1.3.1 Consenting a patient to enter a dermatological trial 225
1.3.2 A steroid-phobic patient 227
1.3.3 An anxious woman with a family history of melanoma who wants all her moles removed 228
1.3.4 Prescribing isotretinoin to a woman of reproductive age 229
1.4 **Acute scenarios 231**
1.4.1 Acute generalised rashes 231
1.4.2 Erythroderma 238

Diseases and Treatments 243

2.1 **Acne vulgaris 243**
2.2 **Acanthosis nigricans 245**
2.3 **Alopecia areata 245**
2.4 **Bullous pemphigoid 246**
2.5 **Dermatomyositis 248**
2.6 **Dermatitis herpetiformis 249**
2.7 **Drug eruptions 249**
2.8 **Atopic eczema 251**
2.9 **Contact dermatitis 252**
2.10 **Erythema multiforme, Stevens–Johnson syndrome and toxic epidermal necrolysis 253**
2.11 **Erythema nodosum 254**
2.12 **Fungal infections of skin, hair and nails (superficial fungal infections) 255**
2.13 **HIV and the skin 257**
2.14 **Lichen planus 258**
2.15 **Lymphoma of the skin: mycosis fungoides and Sézary syndrome 260**
2.16 **Pemphigus vulgaris 261**
2.17 **Psoriasis 263**
2.18 **Pyoderma gangrenosum 265**
2.19 **Scabies 266**
2.20 **Basal cell carcinoma 268**
2.21 **Squamous cell carcinoma 270**
2.22 **Malignant melanoma 271**
2.23 **Urticaria and angio-oedema 274**
2.24 **Vitiligo 275**
2.25 **Cutaneous vasculitis 276**
2.26 **Topical therapy: corticosteroids and immunosuppressants 277**
2.27 **Phototherapy 278**
2.28 **Retinoids 279**

Investigations and Practical Procedures 281

3.1 **Skin biopsy 281**
3.2 **Direct and indirect immunofluorescence 282**
3.3 **Patch tests 282**
3.4 **Obtaining specimens for mycological analysis 284**

Self-assessment 285

Haematology and Oncology

HAEMATOLOGY

PACES Stations and Acute Scenarios 1

1.1 **History-taking 3**
1.1.1 Microcytic hypochromic anaemia 3
1.1.2 Macrocytic anaemia 5
1.1.3 Lymphocytosis and anaemia 8
1.1.4 Thromboembolism and fetal loss 11
1.1.5 Weight loss and thrombocytosis 12
1.2 **Clinical examination 14**
1.2.1 Normocytic anaemia 14
1.2.2 Thrombocytopenia and purpura 14
1.2.3 Jaundice and anaemia 16
1.2.4 Polycythaemia 17
1.2.5 Splenomegaly 18
1.3 **Communication skills and ethics 19**
1.3.1 Persuading a patient to accept HIV testing 19
1.3.2 Talking to a distressed relative 20
1.3.3 Explaining a medical error 22
1.3.4 Breaking bad news 23
1.4 **Acute scenarios 25**
1.4.1 Chest syndrome in sickle cell disease 25
1.4.2 Neutropenia 27
1.4.3 Leucocytosis 29
1.4.4 Spontaneous bleeding and weight loss 31
1.4.5 Cervical lymphadenopathy and difficulty breathing 32
1.4.6 Swelling of the leg 35

Diseases and Treatments 37

2.1 **Causes of anaemia 37**
  2.1.1 Thalassaemia syndromes 38
  2.1.2 Sickle cell syndromes 39
  2.1.3 Enzyme defects 41
  2.1.4 Membrane defects 41
  2.1.5 Iron metabolism and iron-deficiency anaemia 43
  2.1.6 Vitamin B_{12} and folate metabolism and deficiency 44
  2.1.7 Acquired haemolytic anaemia 44
  2.1.8 Bone-marrow failure and infiltration 46

2.2 **Haematological malignancy 46**
  2.2.1 Multiple myeloma 46
  2.2.2 Acute leukaemia: acute lymphoblastic leukaemia and acute myeloid leukaemia 49
  2.2.3 Chronic lymphocytic leukaemia 52
  2.2.4 Chronic myeloid leukaemia 54
  2.2.5 Malignant lymphomas: non-Hodgkin's lymphoma and Hodgkin's lymphoma 55
  2.2.6 Myelodysplastic syndromes 58
  2.2.7 Non-leukaemic myeloproliferative disorders (including polycythaemia vera, essential thrombocythaemia and myelofibrosis) 60
  2.2.8 Amyloidosis 62

2.3 **Bleeding disorders 64**
  2.3.1 Inherited bleeding disorders 64
  2.3.2 Aquired bleeding disorders 67
  2.3.3 Idiopathic throbocytopenic purpura 68

2.4 **Thrombotic disorders 69**
  2.4.1 Inherited thrombotic disease 69
  2.4.2 Acquired thrombotic disease 72

2.5 **Clinical use of blood products 74**

2.6 **Haematological features of systemic disease 76**

2.7 **Haematology of pregnancy 79**

2.8 **Iron overload 80**

2.9 **Chemotherapy and related therapies 82**

2.10 **Principles of bone-marrow and peripheral blood stem-cell transplantation 85**

Investigations and Practical Procedures 87

3.1 **The full blood count and film 87**

3.2 **Bone-marrow examination 89**

3.3 **Clotting screen 91**

3.4 **Coombs' test (direct antiglobulin test) 91**

3.5 **Erythrocyte sedimentation rate versus plasma viscosity 92**

3.6 **Therapeutic anticoagulation 92**

Self-assessment 94

ONCOLOGY

PACES Stations and Acute Scenarios 109

1.1 **History-taking 109**
  1.1.1 A dark spot 109

1.2 **Clinical examination 110**
  1.2.1 A lump in the neck 110

1.3 **Communication skills and ethics 111**
  1.3.1 Am I at risk of cancer? 111
  1.3.2 Consent for chemotherapy (1) 113
  1.3.3 Consent for chemotherapy (2) 114
  1.3.4 Don't tell him the diagnosis 116

1.4 **Acute scenarios 117**
  1.4.1 Acute deterioration after starting chemotherapy 117
  1.4.2 Back pain and weak legs 119
  1.4.3 Breathless, hoarse, dizzy and swollen 121

Diseases and Treatments 124

2.1 **Breast cancer 124**

2.2 **Central nervous system cancers 126**

2.3 **Digestive tract cancers 129**

2.4 **Genitourinary cancer 132**

2.5 **Gynaecological cancer 136**

2.6 **Head and neck cancer 139**

2.7 **Skin tumours 140**

2.8 **Paediatric solid tumours 144**

2.9 **Lung cancer 146**

2.10 **Liver and biliary tree cancer 149**

2.11 **Bone cancer and sarcoma 151**

2.12 **Endocrine tumours 157**

2.13 **The causes of cancer 159**

2.14 **Paraneoplastic conditions 162**

Investigations and Practical Procedures 167

3.1 **Investigation of unknown primary cancers 167**

3.2 **Investigation and management of metastatic disease 169**

3.3 **Tumour markers 171**

3.4 **Screening 173**

3.5 **Radiotherapy 175**

3.6 **Chemotherapy 176**

3.7 **Immunotherapy 179**

3.8 **Stem-cell transplantation 180**

3.9 **Oncological emergencies 180**

Self-assessment 185

Cardiology and Respiratory Medicine

CARDIOLOGY

PACES Stations and Acute Scenarios 3

1.1 History-taking 3
- **1.1.1** Paroxysmal palpitations 3
- **1.1.2** Palpitations with dizziness 6
- **1.1.3** Breathlessness and ankle swelling 9
- **1.1.4** Breathlessness and exertional presyncope 12
- **1.1.5** Dyspnoea, ankle oedema and cyanosis 14
- **1.1.6** Chest pain and recurrent syncope 16
- **1.1.7** Hypertension found at routine screening 19
- **1.1.8** Murmur in pregnancy 23

1.2 Clinical examination 25
- **1.2.1** Irregular pulse 25
- **1.2.2** Congestive heart failure 27
- **1.2.3** Hypertension 29
- **1.2.4** Mechanical valve 29
- **1.2.5** Pansystolic murmur 30
- **1.2.6** Mitral stenosis 31
- **1.2.7** Aortic stenosis 32
- **1.2.8** Aortic regurgitation 33
- **1.2.9** Tricuspid regurgitation 34
- **1.2.10** Eisenmenger's syndrome 35
- **1.2.11** Dextrocardia 36

1.3 Communication skills and ethics 37
- **1.3.1** Advising a patient against unnecessary investigations 37
- **1.3.2** Explanation of uncertainty of diagnosis 38
- **1.3.3** Discussion of the need to screen relatives for an inherited condition 38
- **1.3.4** Communicating news of a patient's death to a spouse 39
- **1.3.5** Explanation to a patient of the need for investigations 40
- **1.3.6** Explanation to a patient who is reluctant to receive treatment 41

1.4 Acute scenarios 42
- **1.4.1** Syncope 42
- **1.4.2** Stroke and a murmur 46
- **1.4.3** Acute chest pain 49
- **1.4.4** Hypotension following acute myocardial infarction 52
- **1.4.5** Breathlessness and collapse 54
- **1.4.6** Pleuritic chest pain 57
- **1.4.7** Fever, weight loss and a murmur 60
- **1.4.8** Chest pain following a 'flu-like illness 64

Diseases and Treatments 69

2.1 Coronary artery disease 69
- **2.1.1** Stable angina 69
- **2.1.2** Unstable angina and non-ST-elevation myocardial infarction 71
- **2.1.3** ST-elevation myocardial infarction 72

2.2 Cardiac arrhythmia 76
- **2.2.1** Bradycardia 76
- **2.2.2** Tachycardia 78

2.3 Cardiac failure 82

2.4 Diseases of heart muscle 86
- **2.4.1** Hypertrophic cardiomyopathy 86
- **2.4.2** Dilated cardiomyopathy 89
- **2.4.3** Restrictive cardiomyopathy 89
- **2.4.4** Arrhythmogenic right ventricular cardiomyopathy 90
- **2.4.5** Left ventricular non-compaction 90

2.5 Valvular heart disease 90
- **2.5.1** Aortic stenosis 90
- **2.5.2** Aortic regurgitation 92
- **2.5.3** Mitral stenosis 93
- **2.5.4** Mitral regurgitation 95
- **2.5.5** Tricuspid valve disease 97
- **2.5.6** Pulmonary valve disease 98

2.6 Pericardial disease 98
- **2.6.1** Acute pericarditis 98
- **2.6.2** Pericardial effusion 100
- **2.6.3** Constrictive pericarditis 102

2.7 Congenital heart disease 104
- **2.7.1** Acyanotic congenital heart disease 105
  - **2.7.1.1** Atrial septal defect 105
  - **2.7.1.2** Isolated ventricular septal defect 107
  - **2.7.1.3** Patent ductus arteriosus 107
  - **2.7.1.4** Coarctation of the aorta 108
- **2.7.2** Cyanotic congenital heart disease 109
  - **2.7.2.1** Tetralogy of Fallot 109
  - **2.7.2.2** Complete transposition of great arteries 111
  - **2.7.2.3** Ebstein's anomaly 112
- **2.7.3** Eisenmenger's syndrome 113

2.8 Infective diseases of the heart 114
- **2.8.1** Infective endocarditis 114
- **2.8.2** Rheumatic fever 119

2.9 Cardiac tumours 120

2.10 Traumatic heart disease 122

2.11 Disease of systemic arteries 124
  2.11.1 Aortic dissection 124
2.12 Diseases of pulmonary arteries 126
  2.12.1 Primary pulmonary hypertension 126
  2.12.2 Secondary pulmonary hypertension 129
2.13 Cardiac complications of systemic disease 130
  2.13.1 Thyroid disease 130
  2.13.2 Diabetes 131
  2.13.3 Autoimmune rheumatic diseases 131
  2.13.4 Renal disease 132
2.14 Systemic complications of cardiac disease 133
  2.14.1 Stroke 133
2.15 Pregnancy and the heart 134
2.16 General anaesthesia in heart disease 136
2.17 Hypertension 136
  2.17.1 Hypertensive emergencies 140
2.18 Venous thromboembolism 141
  2.18.1 Pulmonary embolism 141
2.19 Driving restrictions in cardiology 145

Investigations and Practical Procedures 147

3.1 ECG 147
  3.1.1 Exercise ECGs 151
3.2 Basic electrophysiology studies 152
3.3 Ambulatory monitoring 154
3.4 Radiofrequency ablation and implantable cardioverter defibrillators 156
  3.4.1 Radiofrequency ablation 156
  3.4.2 Implantable cardioverter defibrillator 157
  3.4.3 Cardiac resynchronisation therapy 158
3.5 Pacemakers 159

3.6 Chest radiograph in cardiac disease 161
3.7 Cardiac biochemical markers 163
3.8 CT and MRI 164
  3.8.1 Multislice spiral CT 164
  3.8.2 MRI 165
3.9 Ventilation–perfusion imaging 166
3.10 Echocardiography 167
3.11 Nuclear cardiology 170
  3.11.1 Myocardial perfusion imaging 170
  3.11.2 Radionuclide ventriculography 170
  3.11.3 Positron emission tomography 171
3.12 Cardiac catheterisation 171
  3.12.1 Percutaneous coronary intervention 172
  3.12.2 Percutaneous valvuloplasty 173**

Self-assessment 176

RESPIRATORY MEDICINE

PACES Stations and Acute Scenarios 191

1.1 History-taking 191
  1.1.1 New breathlessness 191
  1.1.2 Solitary pulmonary nodule 193
  1.1.3 Exertional dyspnoea with daily sputum 195
  1.1.4 Dyspnoea and fine inspiratory crackles 197
  1.1.5 Nocturnal cough 199
  1.1.6 Daytime sleepiness and morning headache 202
  1.1.7 Lung cancer with asbestos exposure 204
  1.1.8 Breathlessness with a normal chest radiograph 206

1.2 Clinical examination 209
  1.2.1 Coarse crackles: bronchiectasis 209
  1.2.2 Fine crackles: interstitial lung disease 210
  1.2.3 Stridor 212
  1.2.4 Pleural effusion 213
  1.2.5 Wheeze and crackles: chronic obstructive pulmonary disease 215
  1.2.6 Cor pulmonale 216
  1.2.7 Pneumonectomy/ lobectomy 217
  1.2.8 Apical signs: old tuberculosis 218
  1.2.9 Cystic fibrosis 219
1.3 Communication skills and ethics 220
  1.3.1 Lifestyle modification 220
  1.3.2 Possible cancer 221
  1.3.3 Potentially life-threatening illness 222
  1.3.4 Sudden unexplained death 224
  1.3.5 Intubation for ventilation 225
  1.3.6 Patient refusing ventilation 226
1.4 Acute scenarios 228
  1.4.1 Pleuritic chest pain 228
  1.4.2 Unexplained hypoxia 232
  1.4.3 Haemoptysis and weight loss 234
  1.4.4 Pleural effusion and fever 237
  1.4.5 Lobar collapse in non-smoker 239
  1.4.6 Upper airway obstruction 241

Diseases and Treatments 243

2.1 Upper airway 243
  2.1.1 Sleep apnoea 243
2.2 Atopy and asthma 245
  2.2.1 Allergic rhinitis 245
  2.2.2 Asthma 246
2.3 Chronic obstructive pulmonary disease 251
2.4 Bronchiectasis 253

2.5 Cystic fibrosis 256
2.6 Occupational lung disease 258
  2.6.1 Asbestosis and the pneumoconioses 258
2.7 Diffuse parenchymal lung disease 261
  2.7.1 Usual interstitial pneumonia 261
  2.7.2 Cryptogenic organising pneumonia 262
  2.7.3 Bronchiolitis obliterans 263
2.8 Miscellaneous conditions 264
  2.8.1 Extrinsic allergic alveolitis 264
  2.8.2 Sarcoidosis 265
  2.8.3 Respiratory complications of rheumatoid arthritis 267
  2.8.4 Pulmonary vasculitis 269
  2.8.5 Pulmonary eosinophilia 270
  2.8.6 Iatrogenic lung disease 272
  2.8.7 Smoke inhalation 274
  2.8.8 Sickle cell disease and the lung 276
  2.8.9 Human immunodeficiency virus and the lung 278
2.9 Malignancy 279
  2.9.1 Lung cancer 279
  2.9.2 Mesothelioma 283
  2.9.3 Mediastinal tumours 285
2.10 Disorders of the chest wall and diaphragm 287
2.11 Complications of respiratory disease 288
  2.11.1 Chronic respiratory failure 288
  2.11.2 Cor pulmonale 289
2.12 Treatments in respiratory disease 290
  2.12.1 Domiciliary oxygen therapy 290
  2.12.2 Continuous positive airways pressure 292
  2.12.3 Non-invasive ventilation 292
2.13 Lung transplantation 294

Investigations and Practical Procedures 297
3.1 Arterial blood gas sampling 297
3.2 Aspiration of pleural effusion or pneumothorax 298
3.3 Pleural biopsy 298
3.4 Intercostal tube insertion 300
3.5 Fibreoptic bronchoscopy and transbronchial biopsy 302
  3.5.1 Fibreoptic bronchoscopy 302
  3.5.2 Transbronchial biopsy 302
3.6 Interpretation of clinical data 302
  3.6.1 Arterial blood gases 302
  3.6.2 Lung function tests 304
  3.6.3 Overnight oximetry 306
  3.6.4 Chest radiograph 306
  3.6.5 Computed tomography scan of the thorax 307

Self-assessment 312

Gastroenterology and Hepatology

GASTROENTEROLOGY AND HEPATOLOGY

PACES Stations and Acute Scenarios 3

1.1 History-taking 3
  1.1.1 Heartburn and dyspepsia 3
  1.1.2 Dysphagia and feeding difficulties 5
  1.1.3 Chronic diarrhoea 8
  1.1.4 Rectal bleeding 10
  1.1.5 Weight loss 14
  1.1.6 Chronic abdominal pain 16
  1.1.7 Abnormal liver function tests 18
  1.1.8 Abdominal swelling 21
1.2 Clinical examination 24
  1.2.1 Inflammatory bowel disease 24
  1.2.2 Chronic liver disease 24
  1.2.3 Splenomegaly 25
  1.2.4 Abdominal swelling 26
1.3 Communication skills and ethics 27
  1.3.1 A decision about feeding 27
  1.3.2 Limitation of management 29
  1.3.3 Limitation of investigation 30
  1.3.4 A patient who does not want to give a history 31
1.4 Acute scenarios 32
  1.4.1 Nausea and vomiting 32
  1.4.2 Acute diarrhoea 36
  1.4.3 Haematemesis and melaena 39
  1.4.4 Acute abdominal pain 46
  1.4.5 Jaundice 50
  1.4.6 Acute liver failure 54

Diseases and Treatments 60
2.1 Oesophageal disease 60
  2.1.1 Gastro-oesophageal reflux disease 60
  2.1.2 Achalasia and oesophageal dysmotility 62
  2.1.3 Oesophageal cancer and Barrett's oesophagus 63
2.2 Gastric disease 66
  2.2.1 Peptic ulceration and *Helicobacter pylori* 66
  2.2.2 Gastric carcinoma 68
  2.2.3 Rare gastric tumours 69
  2.2.4 Rare causes of gastrointestinal haemorrhage 70

2.3 Small bowel disease 71
- 2.3.1 Malabsorption 71
  - 2.3.1.1 Bacterial overgrowth 71
  - 2.3.1.2 Other causes of malabsorption 72
- 2.3.2 Coeliac disease 73

2.4 Pancreatic disease 75
- 2.4.1 Acute pancreatitis 75
- 2.4.2 Chronic pancreatitis 78
- 2.4.3 Pancreatic cancer 80
- 2.4.4 Neuroendocrine tumours 82

2.5 Biliary disease 83
- 2.5.1 Choledocholithiasis 83
- 2.5.2 Primary biliary cirrhosis 85
- 2.5.3 Primary sclerosing cholangitis 87
- 2.5.4 Intrahepatic cholestasis 89
- 2.5.5 Cholangiocarcinoma 89

2.6 Infectious diseases 92
- 2.6.1 Food poisoning and gastroenteritis 92
- 2.6.2 Bacterial dysentery 93
- 2.6.3 Antibiotic-associated diarrhoea 94
- 2.6.4 Parasitic infestations of the intestine 94
- 2.6.5 Intestinal and liver amoebiasis 95
- 2.6.6 Intestinal features of HIV infection 95

2.7 Inflammatory bowel disease 95
- 2.7.1 Crohn's disease 95
- 2.7.2 Ulcerative colitis 98
- 2.7.3 Microscopic colitis 101

2.8 Functional bowel disorders 101

2.9 Large bowel disorders 103
- 2.9.1 Adenomatous polyps of the colon 103
- 2.9.2 Colorectal carcinoma 104
- 2.9.3 Diverticular disease 107
- 2.9.4 Intestinal ischaemia 108
- 2.9.5 Anorectal diseases 109

2.10 Liver disease 109
- 2.10.1 Acute viral hepatitis 109
  - 2.10.1.1 Hepatitis A 109
  - 2.10.1.2 Other acute viral hepatitis 112
- 2.10.2 Chronic viral hepatitis 113
  - 2.10.2.1 Hepatitis B 113
  - 2.10.2.2 Hepatitis C 114
- 2.10.3 Acute liver failure 115
- 2.10.4 Alcohol-related liver disease 116
- 2.10.5 Drugs and the liver 118
  - 2.10.5.1 Hepatic drug toxicity 118
  - 2.10.5.2 Drugs and chronic liver disease 120
- 2.10.6 Chronic liver disease and cirrhosis 120
- 2.10.7 Focal liver lesion 124
- 2.10.8 Liver transplantation 127

2.11 Nutrition 129
- 2.11.1 Defining nutrition 129
- 2.11.2 Protein–calorie malnutrition 133
- 2.11.3 Obesity 133
- 2.11.4 Enteral and parenteral nutrition and special diets 134

Investigations and Practical Procedures 136

- 3.1 General investigations 136
- 3.2 Tests of gastrointestinal and liver function 137
- 3.3 Diagnostic and therapeutic endoscopy 138
- 3.4 Diagnostic and therapeutic radiology 139
- 3.5 Rigid sigmoidoscopy and rectal biopsy 140
- 3.6 Paracentesis 143
- 3.7 Liver biopsy 144

Self-assessment 147

Neurology, Ophthalmology and Psychiatry

NEUROLOGY

PACES Stations and Acute Scenarios 3

1.1 History-taking 3
- 1.1.1 Episodic headache 3
- 1.1.2 Facial pain 6
- 1.1.3 Funny turns/blackouts 8
- 1.1.4 Increasing seizure frequency 11
- 1.1.5 Numb toes 12
- 1.1.6 Tremor 15
- 1.1.7 Memory problems 17
- 1.1.8 Chorea 19
- 1.1.9 Muscle weakness and pain 20
- 1.1.10 Sleep disorders 21
- 1.1.11 Dysphagia 24
- 1.1.12 Visual hallucinations 26

1.2 Clinical examination 27
- 1.2.1 Numb toes and foot drop 27
- 1.2.2 Weakness in one leg 28
- 1.2.3 Spastic legs 32
- 1.2.4 Gait disturbance 33
- 1.2.5 Cerebellar syndrome 36
- 1.2.6 Weak arm/hand 37
- 1.2.7 Proximal muscle weakness 40
- 1.2.8 Muscle wasting 41
- 1.2.9 Hemiplegia 42
- 1.2.10 Tremor 44
- 1.2.11 Visual field defect 45
- 1.2.12 Unequal pupils 47
- 1.2.13 Ptosis 48
- 1.2.14 Abnormal ocular movements 51
- 1.2.15 Facial weakness 53
- 1.2.16 Lower cranial nerve assessment 55
- 1.2.17 Speech disturbance 57

1.3 Communication skills and ethics 60

1.3.1 Genetic implications 60

1.3.2 Explanation of the diagnosis of Alzheimer's disease 61

1.3.3 Prognosis after stroke 62

1.3.4 Conversion disorder 63

1.3.5 Explaining the diagnosis of multiple sclerosis 64

1.4 Acute scenarios 65

1.4.1 Acute weakness of legs 65

1.4.2 Acute ischaemic stroke 67

1.4.3 Subarachnoid haemorrhage 71

1.4.4 Status epilepticus 73

1.4.5 Encephalopathy/coma 78

Diseases and Treatments 81

2.1 Peripheral neuropathies and diseases of the lower motor neuron 81

2.1.1 Peripheral neuropathies 81

2.1.2 Guillain–Barré syndrome 85

2.1.3 Motor neuron disease 87

2.2 Diseases of muscle 89

2.2.1 Metabolic muscle disease 89

2.2.2 Inflammatory muscle disease 91

2.2.3 Inherited dystrophies (myopathies) 91

2.2.4 Channelopathies 93

2.2.5 Myasthenia gravis 93

2.3 Extrapyramidal disorders 95

2.3.1 Parkinson's disease 95

2.4 Dementia 99

2.4.1 Alzheimer's disease 99

2.5 Multiple sclerosis 101

2.6 Headache 104

2.6.1 Migraine 104

2.6.2 Trigeminal neuralgia 107

2.6.3 Cluster headache 108

2.6.4 Tension-type headache 109

2.7 Epilepsy 110

2.8 Cerebrovascular disease 116

2.8.1 Stroke 116

2.8.2 Transient ischaemic attacks 120

2.8.3 Intracerebral haemorrhage 122

2.8.4 Subarachnoid haemorrhage 125

2.9 Brain tumours 127

2.10 Neurological complications of infection 131

2.10.1 New variant Creutzfeldt–Jakob disease 131

2.11 Neurological complications of systemic disease 132

2.11.1 Paraneoplastic conditions 132

2.12 Neuropharmacology 133

Investigations and Practical Procedures 139

3.1 Neuropsychometry 139

3.2 Lumbar puncture 140

3.3 Neurophysiology 142

3.3.1 Electroencephalography 142

3.3.2 Evoked potentials 142

3.3.3 Electromyography 142

3.3.4 Nerve conduction studies 143

3.4 Neuroimaging 143

3.4.1 Computed tomography and computed tomography angiography 143

3.4.2 Magnetic resonance imaging and magnetic resonance angiography 144

3.4.3 Angiography 145

3.5 Single-photon emission computed tomography and positron emission tomography 145

3.6 Carotid Dopplers 147

Self-assessment 148

OPHTHALMOLOGY

PACES Stations and Acute Scenarios 161

1.1 Clinical scenarios 161

1.1.1 Examination of the eye 161

1.2 Acute scenarios 164

1.2.1 An acutely painful red eye 164

1.2.2 Two painful red eyes and a systemic disorder 166

1.2.3 Acute painless loss of vision in one eye 168

1.2.4 Acute painful loss of vision in a young woman 170

1.2.5 Acute loss of vision in an elderly man 171

Diseases and Treatments 173

2.1 Iritis 173

2.2 Scleritis 174

2.3 Retinal artery occlusion 175

2.4 Retinal vein occlusion 178

2.5 Optic neuritis 179

2.6 Ischaemic optic neuropathy in giant-cell arteritis 180

2.7 Diabetic retinopathy 181

Investigations and Practical Procedures 186

3.1 Fluorescein angiography 186

3.2 Temporal artery biopsy 186

Self-assessment 188

PSYCHIATRY

PACES Stations and Acute Scenarios 195

1.1 History-taking 195

1.1.1 Eating disorders 195

1.1.2 Medically unexplained symptoms 197

1.2 **Communication skills and ethics 199**
  1.2.1 Panic attack and hyperventilation 199
  1.2.2 Deliberate self-harm 200
  1.2.3 Medically unexplained symptoms 201
1.3 **Acute scenarios 202**
  1.3.1 Acute confusional state 202
  1.3.2 Panic attack and hyperventilation 205
  1.3.3 Deliberate self-harm 207
  1.3.4 The alcoholic in hospital 208
  1.3.5 Drug abuser in hospital 210
  1.3.6 The frightening patient 212

Diseases and Treatments 215

2.1 **Dissociative disorders 215**
2.2 **Dementia 215**
2.3 **Schizophrenia and antipsychotic drugs 217**
  2.3.1 Schizophrenia 217
  2.3.2 Antipsychotics 218
2.4 **Personality disorder 220**
2.5 **Psychiatric presentation of physical disease 221**
2.6 **Psychological reactions to physical illness (adjustment disorders) 222**
2.7 **Anxiety disorders 223**
  2.7.1 Generalised anxiety disorder 225
  2.7.2 Panic disorder 226
  2.7.3 Phobic anxiety disorders 228
2.8 **Obsessive–compulsive disorder 229**
2.9 **Acute stress reactions and post-traumatic stress disorder 231**
  2.9.1 Acute stress reaction 231
  2.9.2 Post-traumatic stress disorder 231
2.10 **Puerperal disorders 233**
  2.10.1 Maternity blues 233
  2.10.2 Postnatal depressive disorder 233
  2.10.3 Puerperal psychosis 233
2.11 **Depression 235**
2.12 **Bipolar affective disorder 237**
2.13 **Delusional disorder 238**
2.14 **The Mental Health Act 1983 239**

Self-assessment 241

Endocrinology

ENDOCRINOLOGY

PACES Stations and Acute Scenarios 3

1.1 **History-taking 3**
  1.1.1 Hypercalcaemia 3
  1.1.2 Polyuria 5
  1.1.3 Faints, sweats and palpitations 8
  1.1.4 Gynaecomastia 12
  1.1.5 Hirsutism 14
  1.1.6 Post-pill amenorrhoea 16
  1.1.7 A short girl with no periods 17
  1.1.8 Young man who has 'not developed' 20
  1.1.9 Depression and diabetes 21
  1.1.10 Acromegaly 23
  1.1.11 Relentless weight gain 24
  1.1.12 Weight loss 26
  1.1.13 Tiredness and lethargy 29
  1.1.14 Flushing and diarrhoea 32
  1.1.15 Avoiding another coronary 34
  1.1.16 High blood pressure and low serum potassium 37
  1.1.17 Tiredness, weight loss and amenorrhoea 39
1.2 **Clinical examination 42**
  1.2.1 Amenorrhoea and low blood pressure 42
  1.2.2 Young man who has 'not developed' 43
  1.2.3 Depression and diabetes 45
  1.2.4 Acromegaly 45
  1.2.5 Weight loss and gritty eyes 47
  1.2.6 Tiredness and lethargy 48
  1.2.7 Hypertension and a lump in the neck 48
1.3 **Communication skills and ethics 50**
  1.3.1 Explaining an uncertain outcome 50
  1.3.2 The possibility of cancer 51
  1.3.3 No medical cause for hirsutism 52
  1.3.4 A short girl with no periods 53
  1.3.5 Simple obesity, not a problem with 'the glands' 54
  1.3.6 I don't want to take the tablets 55
1.4 **Acute scenarios 56**
  1.4.1 Coma with hyponatraemia 56
  1.4.2 Hypercalcaemic and confused 60
  1.4.3 Thyrotoxic crisis 61
  1.4.4 Addisonian crisis 63
  1.4.5 'Off legs' 65

Diseases and Treatments 68

2.1 **Hypothalamic and pituitary diseases 68**
  2.1.1 Cushing's syndrome 68
  2.1.2 Acromegaly 71
  2.1.3 Hyperprolactinaemia 73
  2.1.4 Non-functioning pituitary tumours 76
  2.1.5 Pituitary apoplexy 77
  2.1.6 Craniopharyngioma 78
  2.1.7 Diabetes insipidus 80
  2.1.8 Hypopituitarism and hormone replacement 83

2.2 Adrenal disease 85
- **2.2.1** Cushing's syndrome 85
- **2.2.2** Primary hyperaldosteronism 85
- **2.2.3** Virilising tumours 87
- **2.2.4** Phaeochromocytoma 89
- **2.2.5** Congenital adrenal hyperplasia 92
- **2.2.6** Primary adrenal insufficiency 94

2.3 Thyroid disease 97
- **2.3.1** Hypothyroidism 97
- **2.3.2** Thyrotoxicosis 100
- **2.3.3** Thyroid nodules and goitre 105
- **2.3.4** Thyroid malignancy 107

2.4 Reproductive disorders 107
- **2.4.1** Delayed growth and puberty 107
- **2.4.2** Male hypogonadism 111
- **2.4.3** Oligomenorrhoea/ amenorrhoea and premature menopause 113
- **2.4.4** Turner's syndrome 115
- **2.4.5** Polycystic ovarian syndrome 116
- **2.4.6** Hirsutism 118
- **2.4.7** Erectile dysfunction 120
- **2.4.8** Infertility 123

2.5 Metabolic and bone diseases 125
- **2.5.1** Hyperlipidaemia/ dyslipidaemia 125
- **2.5.2** Porphyria 128
- **2.5.3** Haemochromatosis 130
- **2.5.4** Osteoporosis 131
- **2.5.5** Osteomalacia 134
- **2.5.6** Paget's disease 136
- **2.5.7** Hyperparathyroidism 137
- **2.5.8** Hypercalcaemia 140
- **2.5.9** Hypocalcaemia 141

2.6 Diabetes mellitus 143
- **2.6.1** Management of hyperglycaemic emergencies 145
- **2.6.2** Management of hypoglycaemic emergencies 147
- **2.6.3** Short- and long-term management of diabetes 147
- **2.6.4** Complications 153
- **2.6.5** Important information for patients 160

2.7 Other endocrine disorders 162
- **2.7.1** Multiple endocrine neoplasia 162
- **2.7.2** Autoimmune polyglandular endocrinopathies 163
- **2.7.3** Ectopic hormone syndromes 164

Investigations and Practical Procedures 165

3.1 Stimulation tests 165
- **3.1.1** Short Synacthen test 165
- **3.1.2** Corticotrophin-releasing hormone test 166
- **3.1.3** Thyrotrophin-releasing hormone test 166
- **3.1.4** Gonadotrophin-releasing hormone test 167
- **3.1.5** Insulin tolerance test 167
- **3.1.6** Pentagastrin stimulation test 168
- **3.1.7** Oral glucose tolerance test 169

3.2 Suppression tests 169
- **3.2.1** Overnight dexamethasone suppression test 169
- **3.2.2** Low-dose dexamethasone suppression test 170
- **3.2.3** High-dose dexamethasone suppression test 170
- **3.2.4** Oral glucose tolerance test in acromegaly 171

3.3 Other investigations 171
- **3.3.1** Thyroid function tests 171
- **3.3.2** Water deprivation test 172

Self-assessment 174

Nephrology

NEPHROLOGY

PACES Stations and Acute Scenarios 3

1.1 History-taking 3
- **1.1.1** Dipstick haematuria 3
- **1.1.2** Pregnancy with renal disease 5
- **1.1.3** A swollen young woman 8
- **1.1.4** Rheumatoid arthritis with swollen legs 11
- **1.1.5** A blood test shows moderate renal failure 13
- **1.1.6** Diabetes with impaired renal function 16
- **1.1.7** Atherosclerosis and renal failure 18
- **1.1.8** Recurrent loin pain 20

1.2 Clinical examination 22
- **1.2.1** Polycystic kidneys 22
- **1.2.2** Transplant kidney 23

1.3 Communication skills and ethics 23
- **1.3.1** Renal disease in pregnancy 23
- **1.3.2** A new diagnosis of amyloidosis 24
- **1.3.3** Is dialysis appropriate? 25

1.4 Acute scenarios 26
- **1.4.1** A worrying potassium level 26
- **1.4.2** Postoperative acute renal failure 30
- **1.4.3** Renal impairment and a multisystem disease 33
- **1.4.4** Renal impairment and fever 36
- **1.4.5** Renal failure and haemoptysis 38
- **1.4.6** Renal colic 41
- **1.4.7** Backache and renal failure 43
- **1.4.8** Renal failure and coma 47

Diseases and Treatments 49

2.1 Major renal syndromes 49
2.1.1 Acute renal failure 49
2.1.2 Chronic renal failure 51
2.1.3 End-stage renal failure 58
2.1.4 Nephrotic syndromes 60
2.2 Renal replacement therapy 64
2.2.1 Haemodialysis 64
2.2.2 Peritoneal dialysis 66
2.2.3 Renal transplantation 69
2.3 Glomerular diseases 72
2.3.1 Primary glomerular disease 72
2.3.2 Secondary glomerular disease 79
2.4 Tubulointerstitial diseases 81
2.4.1 Acute tubular necrosis 81
2.4.2 Acute interstitial nephritis 82
2.4.3 Chronic interstitial nephritis 82
2.4.4 Specific tubulointerstitial disorders 83
2.5 Diseases of renal vessels 86
2.5.1 Renovascular disease 86
2.5.2 Cholesterol atheroembolisation 88
2.6 Postrenal problems 89
2.6.1 Obstructive uropathy 89
2.6.2 Stones 90
2.6.3 Retroperitonal fibrosis or periaortitis 91
2.6.4 Urinary tract infection 92
2.7 The kidney in systemic disease 92
2.7.1 Myeloma 92
2.7.2 Amyloidosis 93
2.7.3 Thrombotic microangiopathy (haemolytic–uraemic syndrome) 94
2.7.4 Sickle cell disease 95
2.7.5 Autoimmune rheumatic disorders 95
2.7.6 Systemic vasculitis 97
2.7.7 Diabetic nephropathy 99
2.7.8 Hypertension 101
2.7.9 Sarcoidosis 102
2.7.10 Hepatorenal syndrome 102
2.7.11 Pregnancy and the kidney 103
2.8 Genetic renal conditions 104
2.8.1 Autosomal dominant polycystic kidney disease 104
2.8.2 Alport's syndrome 106
2.8.3 X-linked hypophosphataemic vitamin-D resistant rickets 106

Investigations and Practical Procedures 108

3.1 Examination of the urine 108
3.1.1 Urinalysis 108
3.1.2 Urine microscopy 109
3.2 Estimation of glomerular filtration rate 109
3.3 Imaging the renal tract 110
3.4 Renal biopsy 114

Self-assessment 116

Rheumatology and Clinical Immunology

RHEUMATOLOGY AND CLINICAL IMMUNOLOGY

PACES Stations and Acute Scenarios 3

1.1 History-taking 3
1.1.1 Recurrent chest infections 3
1.1.2 Recurrent meningitis 5
1.1.3 Recurrent facial swelling and abdominal pain 7
1.1.4 Recurrent skin abscesses 9
1.1.5 Flushing and skin rash 12
1.1.6 Drug-induced anaphylaxis 14
1.1.7 Arthralgia, purpuric rash and renal impairment 16
1.1.8 Arthralgia and photosensitive rash 19
1.1.9 Cold fingers and difficulty swallowing 23
1.1.10 Dry eyes and fatigue 25
1.1.11 Breathlessness and weakness 27
1.1.12 Low back pain 30
1.1.13 Chronic back pain 32
1.1.14 Recurrent joint pain and stiffness 33
1.1.15 Foot drop and weight loss in a patient with rheumatoid arthritis 35
1.1.16 Fever, myalgia, arthralgia and elevated acute-phase indices 38
1.1.17 Non-rheumatoid pain and stiffness 40
1.1.18 Widespread pain 42
1.2 Clinical examination 44
1.2.1 Hands (general) 44
1.2.2 Non-rheumatoid pain and stiffness: generalised osteoarthritis 45
1.2.3 Rheumatoid arthritis 46
1.2.4 Psoriatic arthritis 47
1.2.5 Systemic sclerosis 49
1.2.6 Chronic tophaceous gout 49
1.2.7 Ankylosing spondylitis 50
1.2.8 Deformity of bone: Paget's disease 51
1.2.9 Marfan's syndrome 51
1.3 Communication skills and ethics 52
1.3.1 Collapse during a restaurant meal 52
1.3.2 Cold fingers and difficulty swallowing 54
1.3.3 Back pain 55
1.3.4 Widespread pain 56
1.3.5 Explain a recommendation to start a disease-modifying antirheumatic drug 57

1.4 Acute scenarios 59

1.4.1 Fulminant septicaemia in an asplenic woman 59

1.4.2 Collapse during a restaurant meal 61

1.4.3 Systemic lupus erythematosus and confusion 64

1.4.4 Acute hot joints 66

1.4.5 A crush fracture 69

Diseases and Treatments 72

2.1 Immunodeficiency 72

2.1.1 Primary antibody deficiency 72

2.1.2 Combined T-cell and B-cell defects 75

2.1.3 Chronic granulomatous disease 77

2.1.4 Cytokine and cytokine-receptor deficiencies 78

2.1.5 Terminal pathway complement deficiency 80

2.1.6 Hyposplenism 81

2.2 Allergy 82

2.2.1 Anaphylaxis 82

2.2.2 Mastocytosis 84

2.2.3 Nut allergy 85

2.2.4 Drug allergy 87

2.3 Rheumatology 88

2.3.1 Carpal tunnel syndrome 88

2.3.2 Osteoarthritis 89

2.3.3 Rheumatoid arthritis 91

2.3.4 Seronegative spondyloarthropathies 94

2.3.5 Idiopathic inflammatory myopathies 98

2.3.6 Crystal arthritis: gout 99

2.3.7 Calcium pyrophosphate deposition disease 101

2.3.8 Fibromyalgia 101

2.4 Autoimmune rheumatic diseases 103

2.4.1 Systemic lupus erythematosus 103

2.4.2 Sjögren's syndrome 105

2.4.3 Systemic sclerosis (scleroderma) 106

2.5 Vasculitides 109

2.5.1 Giant-cell arteritis and polymyalgia rheumatica 109

2.5.2 Wegener's granulomatosis 111

2.5.3 Polyarteritis nodosa 113

2.5.4 Cryoglobulinaemic vasculitis 114

2.5.5 Behçet's disease 115

2.5.6 Takayasu's arteritis 117

2.5.7 Systemic Still's disease 119

Investigations and Practical Procedures 121

3.1 Assessment of acute-phase response 121

3.1.1 Erythrocyte sedimentation rate 121

3.1.2 C-reactive protein 121

3.2 Serological investigation of autoimmune rheumatic disease 122

3.2.1 Antibodies to nuclear antigens 122

3.2.2 Antibodies to double-stranded DNA 123

3.2.3 Antibodies to extractable nuclear antigens 124

3.2.4 Rheumatoid factor 125

3.2.5 Antineutrophil cytoplasmic antibody 125

3.2.6 Serum complement concentrations 125

3.3 Suspected immune deficiency in adults 126

3.4 Imaging in rheumatological disease 129

3.4.1 Plain radiology 129

3.4.2 Bone densitometry 130

3.4.3 Magnetic resonance imaging 131

3.4.4 Nuclear medicine 131

3.4.5 Ultrasound 132

3.5 Arthrocentesis 132

3.6 Corticosteroid injection techniques 133

3.7 Immunoglobulin replacement 135

Self-assessment 138

INDEX

Note: page numbers in *italics* refer to figures, those in **bold** refer to tables.

A

Abbreviated Mental Test score 26, 141, 178–9
abdominal aortic aneurysm 13, 22, 30
abdominal bloating/distension 65, 80
abdominal confusion 130–1
abdominal examination 22, 130
  checklist 23
  failure to thrive 131
  surgical scars 16
abdominal system 12, 20–5
  examiner's mark-sheet 20
  face and neck 21, 24
  foot of the bed examination 20
  gastroentrological/hepatological cases 20
  haemato-oncological cases 20–1
  hands 20
  palpation 20, 22–24
  percussion 20, 22–24
  presentation of findings 23–4
  renal case **21**
abdominojugular test 29
accessory nerve (XI)
  examination 44
  lesions 44
ACE inhibitors
  heart failure 126
  risks of 126
acetylcholinesterase inhibitors 164
aches and pains 119–21
  history 119–20, **120**
    medications 120
  investigations 120–1
  management 121
  referral letter 119
acoustic neuroma **44**
acromegaly 56
acupressure 79
acupuncture 79, 86
  site of action *83*
Adams-Stokes attack 117, **118**
Addison's disease 56, **112**
adhesions **80**, 90
Adie's pupil 39, **40**
advance directives 176
age-related changes 147
aids for living 166–8
  assistive technology 168
  kitchen aids 166–7, *166*, *167*
  walking aids **134**, 154, 167
airway obstruction 75
alcohol
  falls related to **153**

and urinary incontinence **115**
alcohol abuse, elderly patients 108, 109, 113
alcoholic cerebellar degeneration **47**
alcohol withdrawal
  confusion caused by **94**, **112**
  fine tremor 21
alendronate 121
allodynia **82**
alopecia **55**, *136*
alpha-blockers, and urinary incontinence **115**
Alport's syndrome 168
Alzheimer's disease 147, 162
  undernutrition in 171
  see also confusion; dementia
amitriptyline hydrochloride 62, 73
  neuropathic pain 86
amlodipine 119
anaemia 16, 21, 75, 88, 183, 186
  blood transfusion 75
  and breathlessness **74**
analgesia/analgesics 84–6
  bowel obstruction 91
  diamorphine hydrochloride 81, 85
  falls related to **153**
  fentanyl 85
  methadone hydrochloride 85
  morphine *see* morphine
  neuropathic pain 86
  opioids *see* opioids; and individual drugs
  oxycodone hydrochloride 85
  palliative care 71–4
  prescribing rules *61*, 84
  sites of action *83*
analgesic ladder *61*, 84
anasarca 148
angina, and immobility **114**
angiotensin receptor blockers, heart failure 126
angle of Louis 28
angular cheilitis 21
anisocoria **40**
ankle
  clonus 50–1
  oedema 14, 15, 17, 26, 30
ankylosing spondylitis 26
anorexia 75, 171
antalgic gait **49**
anticoagulation 75, 126
anticonvulsants
  falls related to **153**
  neuropathic pain 86
antidepressants, and urinary incontinence **115**

antiemetics 76, 78–9, **78**, 81, 88–9
  bowel obstruction 91
  prophylactic 76
antihistamines, antiemetic **78**, 81
antipsychotics
  falls related to **153**
  and urinary incontinence **115**
antisecretory agents, bowel obstruction 91
antispasmodics 86
anxiety 91–2
  breathlessness **74**, 87, 99, 102
  coping strategies 92
  management of 75
  nausea and vomiting 79
  treatment 92
aortic dissection **118**
aortic incompetence 27, 30, 32, 33
aortic regurgitation **33**
  auscultation **33**
aortic sclerosis 131
  auscultation **32**
aortic stenosis 27, **32**, **118**, 131
  auscultation **32**
  carotid pulse in 29
aortic valve disease, auscultation **32**
Apert's syndrome 168
apex
  displaced **32**, **33**
  double impulse **32**
  heaving **32**
  tapping **33**
  thrill **32**
apex beat, palpation 29, **30**
arachis oil enema 90
Argyll Robertson pupil 39, **40**
arms
  dermatomes *47*
  joint position test 47
  motor power **46**
    MRC grading scale **46**
  neurological examination 46–9
  root and nerve lesions **51**
  sensory and motor deficits **51**
  tremor **48**
  vibration sense 48
arrhythmias
  atrial fibrillation 16, 27, **27**, 30, **32**, **33**, *108*, 123, 131, 183, 186, 208
  atrial flutter **27**, 108, *108*
arterial blood gases, confusion 114
arteries
  brachial 28
  carotid 16, 29, 30

arthritis 108
  immobility **114**
  inflammatory **122**
  osteoarthritis **107**, 114, **120**, 136
  rheumatoid **18**, **25**, 55, 114
ascites 13, 20, **20–2**, 23, **23**, 24, 31, **32**, 74, 77, 88
  and bowel obstruction **80**
assistive technology 168
ataxia **44**
athetosis **45**
atopic dermatitis **55**
atorvastatin 120
atrial extrasystole **27**
atrial fibrillation 16, 27, **27**, 30, **32**, **33**, *108*, 123, 131, 183, 186, 208
atrial flutter **27**, 108, *108*
atrial myxoma **118**, *125*
atrial septal defect **34**
Attendance Allowance 164, 175, 183, 186
  Special Rules 175
A-type nerve fibres 82
auscultation, chest 17, 29–34
axillary crutches **134**
axillary nerve **48**

B

back pain 181, 185
  elderly patients 121–7
    causes of **122**
    drug history 124
    investigations 125
    management 125–7
    social history 123
baclofen 86
Barthel Activities of Daily Living Index 166, 179–80
basal cell carcinoma **55**
Becker's muscular dystrophy **49**
bell, auscultation with 29
Bell's palsy **43**
benefits 174–5
  Attendance Allowance 175
  Carer's Allowance 175
  Disability Living Allowance 174–5
benzodiazepines 86
  anxiety 75, 99, 102
  breathlessness 73, 75
  confusion 94
  falls related to **153**
  terminal agitation 98, 101
  and urinary incontinence **115**
beta-blockers 126
  slow pulse 27
bisacodyl 90
  suppositories 90
bisphosphonates, bone pain 86
bitemporal hemianopia **39**
blackouts 117
  and driving 119

blind spot
  enlarged **39**
  testing 38
blood-brain barrier 113
blood gases, arterial, confusion 114
blood pressure 27–30, 53, 109
blood transfusion 75
body mass index 170, 172
bone pain 75, 99, 101, 102, 115
  bisphosphonates 86
  NSAIDs 86
bony metastases 62, 72, *84*
borborygmi 65
bowel obstruction 63–5, 76, 79–81, 90–1, 100, 102
  aetiology **80**, 90, *91*
  clinical presentation 90
  complete 81
  epidemiology 90
  ethical decision making 69–70
  nausea and vomiting 69–70, 98, 101
  subacute 81
  treatment
    analgesics 91
    antiemetics 91
    antisecretory agents 91
    bypass surgery 69–70, 81, 91
    corticosteroids 91
    interventional techniques 91
    laxatives 91
    nasogastric tubes 91
bowel sounds 77, 80
brachial pulse 27–9
bradycardia 27
brain metastases 76, 77
  confusion caused by **94**
brain tumour **39**
breaking bad news 70–1
breast cancer 98, 101
  nausea and vomiting 99, 101
  pain 61–3, 65–6, 71–4
breathlessness 72, 73, 87–8, 100, 102, 122
  acute 74–5
  aetiology **74**, 87, *87*
  anxiety **74**, 87, 99, 102
  clinical presentation 87
  epidemiology 87
  ethical decision making 66–7
  fluctuating 74
  investigations 88
  nocturnal 122
  physical signs 87–8
  treatment 88, **88**
Broca's area 142
bronchial obstruction **74**
bronchiectasis 5, 15, 128, 130
  diagnosis 16
  physical findings **18**
bronchospasm 88
bronzed diabetes **21**
B-type nerve fibres 82
Burch colposuspension 157

C

cachexia **21**, **47**, 72, 75, 77, 80, *171*
caffeine, and urinary incontinence **115**
cancer
  bony metastases 62, 72, *84*
  bowel obstruction 63–5, 69–70
  breast 61–3, 65–6, 71–4
  cachexia **47**, 72, 75, 77, 80
  cerebral metastases 76, 77
  colorectal 69–70, **120**
  constipation 63–5, 69–70, 76–9, 89–90
  hypercalcaemia of malignancy 76, 77, 80
  lung 66–7, 70–1, 74–5
  nausea and vomiting 67–9
  ovarian 67–9, 76–9
  pain 61–3, 65–6, 71–4, 82
  prostate **120**, 127
candidiasis **55**
caput medusa **21**
carbon monoxide poisoning **118**
  confusion **112**
cardiac failure
  and immobility **114**
  right-sided 26
cardiac surgery 26
cardiomegaly *124*
cardiovascular drugs, falls related to **153**
cardiovascular system 26–34
  auscultation 29–34
  blood pressure 27–30
  brachial pulse 27–9
  chest inspection 29
  examiner's mark-sheet **26**
  foot of the bed examination 26
  hands 27–30
  jugular venous pressure 28–30
  palpation of apex beat and precordium 29, **30**
  palpation of carotid arteries 29, 30
  presentation of findings 30–3, **31–3**
  radial pulse 27, **27**, 30
cardioverter defibrillators 29
Carer's Allowance 175
carotid arteries, palpation 16, 29, 30
carotid bruits 29
carotid pulse 13, **29**
carotid sinus
  hypersensitivity **118**
  massage 109–10
carotid stenosis 110, **118**
cauda equina syndrome **122**, 135
cellulitis 111, 135
central cyanosis 16, 30
central nervous system 35–52
  arms 35, 36
  cranial nerve examination 36, 45, 52
  examiner's mark-sheet **35**
  foot of the bed examination 35, 36
  higher cortical function 35

central nervous system (*continued*)
   legs 35, 36, 48–52
      presentation of findings 51–2
central scotoma 38, **39**
cerebellar ataxia 133
cerebellar disease **45**
cerebellar gait **49**
cerebellar signs **47**
cerebellopontine angle lesions 43, **44**
cerebral anoxia **45**
cerebral metastases 76, 77
cerebral palsy **45**
cerebrovascular accident *see* stroke
Charcot-Marie-Tooth disease **49**
Charcot's joints 55
Charcot's triad 181–2, 185
chemoreceptor trigger zone **79**
chemotherapy, palliative 67–9
chest
   assessment of expansion 16
   examination 31
   percussion and auscultation 17
chest pain 98, 101, 128
   breast cancer 61–3, 65–6, 71–4
chest X-ray, cardiomegaly *124*
cholangitis 182, 185
chorea **45**
chronic obstructive pulmonary disease
   74, 75, 129, 130
   physical findings **18**
ciliary ganglion *38*
clonazepam, neuropathic pain 86
Clostridium difficile 148
clubbing 16, **18**, 20, 21, 23, 27, 30, 32,
   34, 47, 53, 130
coarctation of aorta **34**
co-codamol *61*
   confusion caused by 113
co-danthramer 62, 65, 90
codeine *61*
cognitive assessment 178–80
   Abbreviated Mental Test score 35, 141,
      178–9
   Mini-Mental State Examination 163, 179
cognitive impairment **107**, 108, 111
   see also confusion
colic 81
collapse 116–19, 139–41, 143–6
   causes **118**
   examination 144
   history 117–18
   investigation 118–19, 144
   management 119, 144–5
   referral letter 116
collapsing pulse 27
colonic inertia 63
colorectal carcinoma **120**
   bowel obstruction 69–70
communication skills and ethics 3, 10,
   10, 11
   examiner's mark-sheet **11**
   key requirements **7**

community nurses 97
community palliative care team 65, 70
compression stockings 144
concussion, and confusion **112**
conductive deafness **44**, 168
confusion 93–4, 98, 101, 108
   abdominal 130–1
   causes **94**, **112**
      cardiovascular 132
      dermatological 135–6
      endocrine 136
      hypercalcaemia 93, **94**, 98, 101, **112**
      neurological 134–5
      ophthalmological 136–7
   cognitive and language assessment 141
   discharge home 138–9
   examination 141
   history 111, 113, 141
      medication 111–12, 184, 186
      smoking and alcohol 113
      social 113
   investigation 93–4, **94**, 113–14, 142
   management 114, 142
   planned discharge 143
   preventive measures 142
   recent onset 110–14
   referral letter 110–11
   respiratory 129–30
   sudden onset 141–3
   treatment 94
Confusion Assessment Method 179
congenital cardiac disease 31
   atrial septal defect **34**
   coarctation of aorta **34**
   Eisenmenger's syndrome **35**
   patent ductus arteriosus **34**
   tetralogy of Fallot **34**
   ventricular septal defect **34**
congestive cardiac failure **74**
conjunctiva, pallor 17
constipation 89–90, 99, 101
   aetiology 89
   cancer-related 69–70, 76–81, 89–90
   causes **64**
   clinical presentation 89
   confusion caused by **94**
   drug-induced 64
   elderly patients 63–5, 89
   epidemiology 89
   follow-up 64
   history 63–4
   history-taking 63–5
   investigations 64
   management 64
   opioid-induced **85**
   overflow diarrhoea 65, 89, 158
   physical signs 90
   treatment 78, 90
coordination 35, 36, 45, 46, 48
corneal reflex *43*, 43
   loss of **43**

coronary artery bypass graft 26
coronary ischaemia 8
cor pulmonale 15, 17, 30
Corrigan's pulse **33**
corticosteroids
   bowel obstruction 91
   neuropathic pain 86
   risk of gastrointestinal bleeding 86
   side effects, confusion **94**
   site of action *83*
cough 74, 87
   nocturnal 122
cough syncope **118**
cranial nerves
   accessory (XI)
      examination 44
      lesions **44**
   examination 36–46
   facial (VII), examination **43**
   glossopharyngeal (IX)
      examination 45
      lesions of **45**
   hypoglossal (XII)
      examination 45
      lesions of **45**
   olfactory (I), examination 36, 45
   optic (II) *37*
      examination 45
   trigeminal (V), examination 41, 45
   vagus (X)
      examination 45
      lesions of **45**
   vestibulocochlear (VIII), examination **45**
craniopharyngioma **39**
C-reactive protein 109, 113, 120
creatine kinase 109
C-type nerve fibres 82
Cushing's syndrome 56
cutlery 166, *167*
cyanosis 16, 17, 27, **34**, 53, 72, 75
   central 16, 30
   peripheral 16, 27
cyclizine **78**, 81, 89, 98, 101
cyclooxygenase-2 inhibitors 136
cystic fibrosis 16, **18**
cystometry 156

D

D-dimer 72–3, 113
deafness 168–70
   aetiology 168
   clinical presentation 169
   complications 169–70
   conductive **44**, 168
   epidemiology 169
   investigations 169
   patient information 170
   physical signs 169
   Rinne's test 43, 169
   sensorineural 43, 44, **44**, 168

deafness (*continued*)
  treatment 169
  Weber's test 43, 44, 169
deep vein thrombosis 72, 74
delta frame **134**
dementia **94**, **107**, 111, 153, 162–4
  aetiology 162–3
  clinical presentation 163
  complications 164
  differential diagnosis 163
  disease associations 164
  epidemiology 163
  and immobility **114**
  patient/carer information 164
  physical signs 163
  prevention 164
  prognosis 164
  treatment 163–4
  see also cognitive impairment;
    confusion
depression 92–3, 99, 102, 111
  clinical presentation 92–3, *93*
  diagnosis in healthy population 92
  failure to diagnose 92
  and immobility **114**
  prevalence 92
  treatment 93
  skin examination 135–6
desmopressin, urinary incontinence 157
dexamethasone 73, 75, **78**, 81
  bowel obstruction 91
  stridor 88
dextrocardia 29
diabetes mellitus 111, **112**
  type 2 183–4, 186
diabetic ulcer **55**
diamorphine hydrochloride 81, 85
diaphragm, auscultation with 29
diarrhoea, overflow 65, 89, 158
diastolic heart murmurs **32**
diclofenac sodium 62, 73
digoxin 126
  toxicity 111
dihydrocodeine *61*
Diogenes syndrome 108
diplopia 40, **41**, 119
dipstick urine test 113, 116
Disability Living Allowance 174–5
disorientation 115
diuretics
  heart failure 126
  and urinary incontinence **115**
dizziness 7
  and falls 108
docusate sodium 90
domperidone **78**, 89, 98, 101
donepezil 164, 184, 186
do not attempt resuscitation orders
    150–1
dress code for PACES 5
driving, blackouts 119

drop attacks 117
dry mouth, opioid-induced **85**
Duchenne's muscular dystrophy **50**
duloxetine 156–7
Dupuytren's contracture **21**
dying patients *see* end of life care;
    palliative care
dysarthria 35, **36**, 44, **47**, 135, 142
dyspareunia 156
dysphagia 172, 185, 187
dysphasia 35, **36**, 135, 142
dysphonia 44, 135
dyspnoea *see* breathlessness
dystonia **45**
dysuria 115

E

Edinger-Westphal nucleus *38*
effort syncope 117
Eisenmenger's syndrome **34**
ejection systolic murmur 131
elbow crutches **134**
elder abuse 108
elderly patients
  aches and pains 119–21
  age-related changes 147
  alcohol abuse 108, 109, 113
  altered response to disease 148
  background to disease *147*
  benefits 174–5
  collapse 116–19
  confusion *see* confusion
  constipation 63–5, 89
  differential diagnosis 148
  disease susceptibility 147–8
  drowsiness/tiredness 127
  examination 149–50
  expectations 148–9
  faecal incontinence 157–8
  failure to thrive 127–9
  falls 107–10
  health and social services provision
      149
  hearing impairment 168–70
  history-taking 149
  hypothermia 158–61
  immobility 114–16
  investigations 150
  legal aspects of care 175–6
  malnutrition 170–4
  management 150
  multiple pathologies 147
  prescribing 148, 161–2
    drug charts 161–2
    starting new drugs 162
  rehabilitation 165–6
  risk factors 147
  social problems 148
  swollen legs and back pain 121–7
  urinary incontinence 114–16

electroencephalography 109
emotional pain 82
encephalitis, confusion **112**
end of life care 70–1, 94–6, 100, 102,
    145
  changing care focus 94–5
  communication 95
  Gold Standards Framework 96
  holistic 96
  Liverpool Care Pathway 96
  peaceful death 97, *97*
  place of 96
  planning 94
  prescribing 95
  respiratory secretions 95–6
  symptom control 95
  terminal agitation 95, **95**, **96**
  withholding/withdrawing treatment 95
  see also palliative care
end of life decisions 150
endocarditis 27
  infectious 132
endocrine system 56
Enduring Power of Attorney 164, 176
enemas 90
epilepsy 108
  postictal confusion **94**, **112**
erythema ab igne 136, *137*
erythema multiforme **55**
erythema nodosum **55**
erythrocyte sedimentation rate, raised
    120
examination 3, 5, 12–14
  explanation of findings 13
  presentation of findings 14
  timing of 12
exophthalmos 56
eye movements 39, 40, **41**, 45, 52
  lateral gaze pathways *41*
  saccades 40
eyes 58
  thyrotoxicosis **45**, **58**

F

face and neck, examination 16, 21, 24
facial nerve (VII), examination 43, **43**
facial weakness **44**
faecal incontinence 157–8
  aetiology 157
  complications 158
  epidemiology 158
  investigation 158
  physical signs 158
  treatment 158
failure to thrive 127–9
  abdominal 131
  history 128
  investigation 128
  management 128–9
  prognosis 128

falls 107–10, 151–4, 181, 185
  aetiology 151, **152**
    medication-related 153, **153**
  alcohol abuse 108, 109
  cardiovascular causes 131–2
  clinical presentation 151
  complications 154
  epidemiology 151
  history 107–9
    medications 109
    past medical 108
    social 108
  investigation 109–10, **152**
    blood tests 109
    cardiac tests 109
    neurological tests 109
  investigations 153
  locomotor causes 136
  management 110, **152**, 154
  neurological causes 132–4
  patient autonomy 137–8
  prodrome 108
  referral letter 107
  risk factors **107**
  SPLATT acronym 108
fear of falling syndrome 110
feet, painful **114**
feminisation **21**
femoral nerve **51**
fentanyl patch 85, 100, 103
festinant gait **49**
fever 74
fits see seizures
fluid thrill 23
focal neurological deficit 77
folate deficiency 21
foot of the bed examination
  abdominal system 20
  respiratory system 15
foot drop 132
fourth nerve palsy **41**
Friedreich's ataxia **47**
functional assessment 178–80
fundoscopy 52
fungal infection, skin **55**
furosemide 119

G

gabapentin, neuropathic pain 86, 98, 101
gag reflex 44
gait abnormalities **50**, 108, 132–4
  cerebellar ataxia 133
  myopathic gait 133
  parkinsonian gait 132, 153
  scissors gait 132
  sensory ataxia **49**, 133
  spastic hemiplegic gait 132
  steppage gait/foot drop 132
galantamine 164

GALS examination 55, **56**
Geriatric Depression Scale 179
geriatrics see elderly patients
giant cell arteritis 119, **120**
glaucoma **39**
gliclazide, side effects 111–12
glossitis, atrophic 21
glossopharyngeal nerve (IX)
  examination 45
  lesions of **45**
glycerol suppositories 90
glyceryl trinitrate 26
glycopyrronium bromide, respiratory secretions 96
goitre 56
Gold Standards Framework 96
gout 55
gouty tophi **55**
granisetron **78**, 98, 99, 101, 102
Graves' disease 56
gutter frame **134**
gynaecomastia **21**

H

haemochromatosis, hyperpigmentation **21**
haemoptysis 72, 74, 87, 128
Hallpike manoeuvre 153
hallucinations, opioid-induced **85**
haloperidol **78**
  confusion 94, 142
  terminal agitation **96**
hands 16–18, 20, **21**, 23, 27, 30
  clubbing 17, **17**, **21**, 27, 130
  examination 17, **17**, 23, 30, 46
  koilonychia 20
  metabolic flap 24, 53, 130
  splinter haemorrhage 27
  tremor 20, 36
head injury, and confusion **112**
hearing aids 169
hearing impairment see deafness
heart block, second-degree **27**
heart failure 88, 132
  causes of 123
  management 126
heart murmurs
  diastolic **32**
  loud 31
  systolic 31, **32**, **33**
  third heart sound 31
heel-shin test 50
heliox 88
hemiparesis 135
hemiplegia **36**
hemiplegic gait **49**
Henoch-Schönlein purpura **55**
hepatojugular test 29
hepatomegaly 21, 24, 75, 131
  causes **25**

hepatosplenomegaly, causes **25**
hereditary haemorrhagic telangiectasia 21
hereditary motor sensory neuropathy **49**
herpes simplex **55**
herpes zoster **55**, 135
  loss of sensation **43**
higher cortical function assessment 35
hip replacement 111
history-taking 6–9
  beginning the consultation 6–7
  checking information 7
  commencement of 6–7
  directed questions 8
  examiner's mark-sheet **7**
  exploration of main problems 9
  family history 9
  functional enquiry 9
  medical and social background 8
  medication 9
  past medical history 9
  'sensitive' issues 9
  social aspects 8
  social history 9
hoarseness 128
holistic care 96
homonymous hemianopia **39**, 137
Horner's syndrome **18**, 40, **40**, **45**
Hospice at Home scheme 97
hospital care, costs of *141*
Huntington's disease 36, **45**
hydralazine 126
hydration 81
hydrocephalus, normal-pressure 114, 162
hydronephrosis 67–9, 77
hyoscine butylbromide 81
hyoscine hydrobromide **78**
  bowel obstruction 91
  respiratory secretions 95–6
hyperalgesia **82**
hypercalcaemia
  confusion caused by 93, **94**, 98, 101, **112**
  of malignancy 76, 77, 80
hyperglycaemia, and confusion **112**
hyperpathia **82**
hyperpigmentation **21**
hypersomnia 92
hypertension, in stroke 144
hyperthermia 161
hyperthyroidism 136
hypertrophic cardiomyopathy **29**
  auscultation **32**
  carotid pulse in 29
hypertrophic obstructive cardiomyopathy **118**
hypertrophic pulmonary osteoarthropathy 128

hypoalbuminaemia **122**
hypoglossal nerve (XII)
  examination 45
  lesions of **45**
hypoglycaemia
  and collapse **118**
  and confusion **112**
  gliclazide-induced 111–12
hypokalaemia 77, 80
hyponatraemia 183, 186
  confusion caused by **94**
hypoproteinaemia 74
hypostatic pneumonia 110
hypotension
  acute event leading to **107**
  orthostatic **118**
  postural **107**, 117, 119
hypothermia 158–61
  aetiology 159
  clinical presentation 159
  complications 160
  and confusion **112**
  ECG changes *160*
  epidemiology 159
  investigations 159–60
  pathophysiology 159
  physical signs 159
  post-fall 110
  prevention 161
  prognosis 160
  treatment 160
hypothyroidism 56, 136
hypoxia
  confusion caused by **94**, **112**
  and epileptic fits 117
HYVET 147

I

immobility 114–16
  causes **114**
    neurological 135
  history 114–15
    psychiatric 115
  musculoskeletal 114–15
  neurological 114
incontinence 108
  faecal 157–8
  urinary 114–16, 155–7
infection
  confusion caused by **94**, **112**
  urinary tract 142
insomnia 92
intention tremor **45**
intermediate care 143
interstitial lung disease, physical findings
    16
investigations
  choice of 178
  justification for 178
involuntary movement 45, **45**, 46, 49

iritis **40**
irregular pulse 27, **27**
ischaemia **118**
ischaemic heart disease 26, 108, 111
isoniazid 135

J

jaundice 20, **21**, 23, 24, 80
  causes of **148**
jaw jerk **43**
joint position sense
  arm 48
  leg 47, 50, 51
jugular venous pressure 28, 30
  angle of Louis 28
  external 28
  hepatojugular test 29
  internal 29
  raised 29, **33**
jugular venous pulse 28

K

ketamine, neuropathic pain 86
kettle tipper 166, *167*
key holders 167, *168*
kidneys 130
  enlarged 22, **23**
    causes **26**
  polycystic 23
kitchen aids 166–7, *166*, *167*
koilonychia 20, 23, 55
Korsakoff's psychosis 174
kyphosis 17, 109, 132

L

lactulose 90
Lambert-Eaton myasthenic syndrome
    120
lateral geniculate body *38*
laxatives 78, 81, 90, 99, 101
  bowel obstruction 91
  combination 65, 90
    co-danthramer 62, 65, 90
  osmotic 90
    lactulose 90
    magnesium hydroxide 81
    polyethylene glycol 65
  rectal preparations 90
  softeners 65, 90
    docusate sodium 90
    liquid paraffin 90
  stimulant 65, 90
    bisacodyl 90
    senna 78, 90
    sodium picosulphate 90
Leber's hereditary optic atrophy **39**
left ventricular aneurysm *125*
left ventricular hypertrophy **30**

legs
  dermatomes *51*
  joint position sense 47, 48, 50, 51
  motor power **47**
  muscle wasting **49**
  neurological examination 12, 49, 51
  oedema **31**, 72, 74, 121–7, 136
  root and nerve lesions 14, **48**
  sensory and motor deficits **48**, 51
  vibration sense 48, 51
leg ulcer **55**
leuconychia **22**, **55**
levomepromazine **78**
  confusion 94
  terminal agitation **96**
Lewy body disease 162
lichen planus **55**
lidocaine patches 86
liquid paraffin 90
lisinopril, side effects 111
liver, palpation **13**
liver disease
  chronic 20–1, 23–5, 131
    signs of **21**
liver failure, confusion caused by **94**
Liverpool Care Pathway 96
living wills 176
lobectomy, physical findings **18**
local anaesthetics, site of action *83*
locomotor system 55
Looser's zone 182, 186
lorazapam **78**
lorazepam 75
  confusion 94, 142
  terminal agitation **96**
loss of consciousness 108
low-molecular-weight heparin 73, 75, 98,
    101
lumbar spondylosis **122**
lung cancer
  breathlessness 66–7, 74–5
  end of life care 70–1
  palliative care 74–5
lung disease, and immobility **114**
lymphadenopathy 18, 75, 130
lymphangitis carcinomatosis **74**, 75, 87,
    87
lymphoedema 135–6
lymphoma **120**

M

Macmillan nurses 97
macular disease **39**
magnesium hydroxide 81
malnutrition 170–4, 182–3, 186
  aetiology 170
  cachexia **47**, 72, 75, 77, 80, *171*
  complications 171, 172, *173*
  epidemiology 170
  investigations 172

malnutrition (*continued*)
  obesity 170, 172–3
  physical signs 171–2
  prevention 173
  prognosis 173
  treatment 172
  underlying cause 172
Marfan's syndrome 27
Marie Curie nurses 97
median nerve 47, **48**
memantine 164
membrane-stabilising drugs 86
memory impairment 115, 184, 186
meningitis, confusion **112**
mental capacity 175
Mental Capacity Act (2005) 176
Mental Health Act 143
mesothelioma 129, 130
metabolic flap 16–18, 20, 23, 24, 53, 130
metastatic cancer
  bone 62, 72, *84*
  brain 76, 77
methadone hydrochloride 85
metoclopramide hydrochloride 62, 78, **78**, 89, 98, 101
micturition syncope **118**
midazolam
  confusion 94
  terminal agitation **96**
Mini-Mental State Examination 163, 179
mitral facies 28, **32**, **33**
mitral regurgitation 29, **32**
  auscultation **32**
mitral stenosis 30, 31, **118**
  auscultation **33**
mitral valve disease, mixed, auscultation **31**
mitral valve prolapse, auscultation **32**
mood assessment 178–80
morphine *61*, 62, 84, 98, 101
  breakthrough dose 84, 99, 101
  commencing therapy 65–6
  dose titration 84, 99, 102
  fears about 85–6
  modified-release 84
  parenteral 85
  side effects 66, 77
motor neuron disease 36, 49, **114**
multiple sclerosis **37**, **48**
multisystem atrophy **118**
muscle wasting, leg **49**
muscular dystrophy **36**, **49**
muscular power, arms **46**
musculoskeletal pain 72
myeloma **120**
myoclonic jerks, opioid-induced **85**
myopathic gait 133
myopathy **114**, 115
myositis **114**
myotonic dystrophy **36**
'myxoedema madness' **112**

N

nails, conditions of **55**
nasogastric tubes 81, 91
nausea and vomiting 88–9
  acute 76–9
  aetiology 88, *89*
  antiemetics 76, 78–9, **78**, 81, 88–9
  bowel obstruction 69–70, 98, 101
  breast cancer 99, 101
  epidemiology 88
  neural mechanisms **79**, *89*
  opioid-induced **85**
  ovarian cancer 67–9
necrobiosis lipoidica diabeticorum **55**
nephropathy 111
nephrotic syndrome 130
nerve blocks 86
nerve fibres, pain-related 82
nerves
  axillary **48**
  femoral **51**
  median 47, **48**
  optic *37*
  peroneal **50**
  radial **48**
  short ciliary *38*
  tibial **50**
  ulnar **46**
neurocardiogenic syncope 117, **118**
  mechanism of 119
neurofibromatosis **55**
neuropathic pain 62, 72, **82**, 98, 101
  co-analgesics 86
  membrane-stabilising drugs 86
Neurotips 42
nightmares, opioid-induced **85**
nitrates 126
nitrofurantoin 135
nociception **82**
nociceptors 82
normal-pressure hydrocephalus 114, 162
NSAIDs 73
  bone pain 86
  risk of gastrointestinal bleeding 86, 111
  site of action *83*
  see also individual drugs
nutrition, parenteral 70, 81
nystagmus **36**, 47, 50, 52

O

obesity 170, 172–3, 182, 186
occupational therapist 146
octreotide, bowel obstruction 91
oedema
  ankle 14, 15, 17, 26, 30
  legs **31**, 72, 74
  peripheral 121–7, 136
    causes of **122**
    investigations 124–5, *124*

    management 125–7
  sacral **31**
oesophageal carcinoma 100, 103
olecranon bursitis **55**
olfactory nerve (I), examination 45
ophthalmoplegia 41, 42, 58
opioids *61*, 62, 84–5
  bone pain 99, 102
  breathlessness 73, 75
  epidural 86
  fears about 85–6
  intrathecal 86
  parenteral 85
  side effects 63, 72, 85, **85**
    confusion **94**
  site of action *83*
  stepwise approach 63
  see also individual drugs
optic atrophy **47**
optic nerve (II) *38*
  examination 38
optic neuritis **39**
organomegaly 77
  causes **25**
  palpation for 22
  see also individual organs
orthopnoea 122
orthostatic hypotension **118**
osmotic laxatives 90
  lactulose 90
  magnesium hydroxide 81
  polyethylene glycol 65
osteoarthritis **107**, 114, **120**, 136
osteomalacia 173–4, 182, 186
  causes 173
  clinical features 173
  radiology 173
  treatment 173
osteoporosis 107, 108, 109, 110
  and back pain **122**
  prophylaxis 121
otosclerosis 168
ototoxic drugs 168
ovarian cancer 67–9, 76–9
overflow diarrhoea 65, 89, 158
overflow incontinence 115, **155**
oxybutynin, urinary incontinence 116, 157
oxycodone hydrochloride 85
  parenteral 85

P

pacemakers 29
PACES stations 3
  abdominal system 12, 20–5
    examination 20
    examiner's mark-sheet **20**
    face and neck 21, 24
    foot of the bed examination 20
    gastroentrological/hepatological cases **8**

PACES stations (*continued*)
  haemato-oncological cases 20, **21**
  hands 20
  palpation 22
  percussion 22
  presentation of findings 23–4
  renal case **21**
cardiovascular system 26–34
  auscultation 29–34
  blood pressure 27–30
  brachial pulse 27–9
  chest inspection 29
  examiner's mark-sheet **26**
  face and neck 24
  foot of the bed examination 26
  hands 27–30
  jugular venous pressure 28–30
  palpation of apex beat and
    precordium 29, **30**
  palpation of carotid arteries 29, 30
  presentation of findings 30–3, **31–3**
  radial pulse 27, **27**, 30
carousel **3**
central nervous system 35–52
  arms 35, 36
  cranial nerve examination 36, 45, 52
  examiner's mark-sheet **35**
  foot of the bed examination 35, 36
  higher cortical function 35
  legs 35, 36, 48–52
  presentation of findings 51–2, **52**
communication skills and ethics 3, 10,
  10, **11**
  examiner's mark-sheet **11**
  key requirements **11**
dress code 5
endocrine system 56
examination 3, 5, 12–14
  explanation of findings 13
  presentation of findings 14
  timing of 12
eyes 58
history-taking
  checking information 7
  commencement of 6–7
  directed questions 8
  examiner's mark-sheet **7**
  exploration of main problems 7
  family history 9
  functional enquiry 9
  medical and social background 8
  medication 9
  past medical history 9
  'sensitive' issues 9
  social aspects 8
  social history 9
locomotor system 55
  examiner's mark-sheet **54**
respiratory system 15–19
  chest and assessment of expansion 16
  examiner's mark-sheet **15**

face and neck 16
  hands 16, **17**
  percussion and auscultation 17
  presentation of findings 17
  trachea 16
rules of thumb 5
pain 82–6
  acute 71–4
  aetiology 82
  assessment 61–3, 83
  breaththrough 73, 99, 101
  cancer-related 61–3, 65–6, 71–4, 82
  characterization of 72
  clinical presentation 83, *83*
  epidemiology 82
  ethical decision making 65–6
  history 62
  investigation 62
  management 62–3
  musculoskeletal 72
  neuroanatomy of *83*
  neuropathic 62, 72, **82**
  perception of 82
  physical signs 83–4
  referral letter 61
  referred 84
  somatic **82**
  tenesmus 80
  terminology **82**
  total pain model 61, 63, *83*
  treatment *see* analgesia/analgesics
  visceral **82**
painful feet **114**
pain sensation 42
palate, high arched 28
palliative care 67–9, 100, 102
  analgesia 71–4
  breathlessness 74–5
  community nurses 97
  hospital teams 97
  inpatient units 96–7
  nausea and vomiting 67–70, 76–9
  specialist services 96–7
  see also end of life care
pallor 28
palmar erythema **21**
palpation
  abdomen 20, 22–4
  carotid arteries 16, 29, 30
  liver 13
papilloedema **39**, 77, 137
paracetamol *61*, 73
  site of action *83*
paraneoplastic syndrome **47**
paranoid delusional state **94**
paraplegic gait **49**
parasternal heave 29
parenteral nutrition 70, 81
Parinaud's midbrain syndrome 39
parkinsonian gait 132, 153
parkinsonism 134–5

Parkinson's disease **36**, **45**, 49, 135
  confusion **112**
  dementia in 162
  falls in 108
  immobility **114**
  medication, falls related to **153**
  urge incontinence 114
parotid gland, swelling 21
past medical history 9
patent ductus arteriosus **34**
peak flow 5, 17
pes carinatum 16
pectus excavatum 16
pelvic mass 67–9, 76–9
percussion
  abdomen 20, 22–4
  chest 17
percutaneous endoscopic gastrostomy
  145
pericardial effusion **74**, 88
peripheral cyanosis 16, 27
peripheral neuropathy **36**, **114**
peripheral vascular disease, and
  immobility **114**
peristalsis, visible 77, 80
peroneal nerves **50**
pes cavus **47**
petichiae 28
phenytoin 135
phosphate enema 90
physiotherapist 146
pin prick 42, 47, 50
pituitary tumour **39**
pityriasis **55**
pleural effusion **31**, 72, 73, **74**, 75, 88
  physical findings **18**
pleural rub 75, 88
pleurodesis 73, 75
pneumonectomy, physical findings
  18
pneumonia 74
  hypostatic 110
pneumothorax 74, **74**
  traumatic *87*
poisoning, carbon monoxide **112**, **118**
polio **49**
polycystic kidneys 130, 131
polyethylene glycol 65
polymyalgia 115
polymyalgia rheumatica 119, **120**
  management 121
polymyositis 115, **120**
polypharmacy **107**, 148
polypoid tumour **80**
posterior commissure *38*
postictal confusion **94**, **112**
postural hypotension 117, 119
  and falls **107**, 108
postural sway 107
postural tremor **45**
potato peeler 167, *167*

Power of Attorney 176
precordium, palpation 29, **30**
prednisolone 121
Preferred Place of Care project 96
presbyacusis 168
prescribing
    elderly patients 148, 161–2
    end of life care 95
pressure area care 144
primary biliary cirrhosis 131
prostate cancer **120**, 127
psoriasis **55**
psoriatic arthropathy 55
psychosocial pain 82
ptosis 36, 40, **41**
pulmonary embolus 72, 73, 74, **74**, 98, 101, **118**
    and immobility 111
pulmonary hypertension **30**, 118
pulmonary regurgitation, auscultation **33**
pulmonary stenosis **118**
pulse 17
    brachial 27–9
    cannon *a* wave 27
    carotid 13, **29**
    collapsing **27**, 28
    Corrigan's **33**
    irregular 27, **27**
    jugular venous 28
    radial 27
    slow rising **32**
pulse pressure
    low **32**
    wide **32**, **33**
pupil, abnormalities of **40**
pupillary responses 38, 45
    afferent pupillary defect 38, 39
    near response 39
purpura **21**, **55**
pyramidal weakness 46
pyrexia *see* fever

Q

quadrupod **134**

R

radial nerve **48**
radial pulse 27
radiotherapy
    fibrosis induced by 90
    palliative 73, 86
raised intracranial pressure 76, **112**
Ramsay Hunt syndrome **43**
rectal examination 77, 80, 131
rectal obstruction 63
recurrent laryngeal nerve palsy 44
red reflex 58
referred pain 84
rehabilitation 145–6, 165–6, 184–5, 187
    aids for living 166–8

day units 166
discharge planning 166
    process 165
    setting 165
    specialist units 166
    team 165
relatives, breaking bad news 70–1
renal failure 67–9
    nausea and vomiting 76
residential care, costs of *141*
respiratory confusion 129–30
respiratory depression, opioid-induced **85**
respiratory secretions 95–6
respiratory system 15–19
    chest and assessment of expansion 16
    crackles 130
    examiner's mark-sheet **15**
    face and neck 16
    foot of the bed examination 15
    hands 16, **17**
    percussion and auscultation 17
    presentation of findings 17
    trachea 16
resting tremor **45**
rhabdomyolysis 109
rheumatic heart disease 123
rheumatoid arthritis **18**, **25**, 55
rheumatoid nodules **55**
rib fractures 72, 73, 109
right ventricular heave **33**
Rinne's test 43, 169
risedronate 121
rivastigmine 164
rollator **134**, 167
Romberg's test 49, **49**, 183, 186
rosacea **55**
Roth's spots 132

S

sacral oedema **31**
salbutamol 88
scabies **55**
scissors gait 132
scleroderma 15, 16, 18
scoliosis 16, **47**, 115
scotoma 38, **39**
scratch marks **21**
sedation
    confused patients 142
    opioid-induced **85**
sedatives, confusion caused by **94**
seizures 184, 186
    causes of **148**
selective serotonin reuptake inhibitors 93
senile squalor syndrome 108
senna 78, 90, 92, 99, 101
sensation, testing for 41
sensorineural deafness **44**, 168
sensory ataxia **49**, 133

sensory inattention 47
septic shock **118**
Shy-Drager syndrome 131, 134
sinus arrhythmia **27**
sinus rhythm 16, 17
sixth nerve palsy **41**, 42
smell, sense of 36, 45
social aspects of patient's condition 8
social worker 146
sodium citrate enema 90
sodium picosulphate 90, 92
somatic pain **82**
spastic hemiplegic gait 132
spastic paraparesis **47**
speech/language therapist 146
spider naevi **21**, 24
spinal cord compression 135, 181, 185
spinal cord lesions **36**
spinal stenosis **122**
spiritual pain 82
spirometry 5, 17
spironolactone 126
spleen 130
splenomegaly **21**, 22, 24, **25**, 131
    causes **25**
    palpation for **21**
splinter haemorrhage 27
sputum 15, 128, 130
statins, muscle pain 115
stents, bowel obstruction 91
steppage/equine gait **49**
steppage gait 132
sternocleidomastoids
    palpation 44
    tautness of 28
sticks **134**, 167
stimulant laxatives 65, 90
    bisacodyl 90
    senna 78, 90
    sodium picosulphate 90
stool culture 64
STRATIFY risk assessment 180
stress incontinence 115, 116, **155**, 156–7
stridor 75, 88
stroke 43, 49, 108, *109*, **114**, 143–6
    confusion **112**
    end of life care 145
    hypertension in 144
    inability to swallow 145
    options for discharge 146
    recovery from 145
    rehabilitation 145–6, 165–6
subclavian steal **118**
subdural haematoma 108, 111, 135
suicidal thoughts 99, 102
superior colliculus *38*
superior vena cava, obstruction **74**, 75, 87, 88
support groups 92
suppositories 90
swollen legs 121–7

syncope 108, 117
  cough **118**
  of effort 117
  micturition **118**
  neurocardiogenic 117, **118**, 119
  see also collapse
syphilis serology 113
systemic lupus erythematosus **120**
systemic sclerosis 55
systolic heart murmurs 31, **32**

T

tachycardia 27, 30
Tai Chi 110, 154
tamponade **118**
tap turner 166, *166*
telecare 168
tenesmus 80
TENS 86
  site of action *83*
terminal agitation **95**, 98, 101
  treatment **96**
terminal illness 70–1
testamentary capacity 175–6
testicular atrophy **21**
tetralogy of Fallot **34**
third nerve palsy 39, **40**, *40*, **41**
thyroid diseases
  hyperthyroidism 136
  hypothyroidism 136
thyroid function tests 113
thyrotoxicosis **45**, **58**
tibial nerves 50
tilt-table testing 110
tinnitus **44**
tissue paper skin **21**
tolterodine, urinary incontinence 116, 157
tongue, examination 45
tongue biting 108, 117
trachea, examination of 17
tramadol *61*
transcutaneous nerve stimulation *see*
    TENS
trapezius muscle, examination 44
tremor **45**
  hands 20, 36
  intention **45**
  postural **45**
  resting **45**
tricuspid incompetence **33**
tricyclic antidepressants 93
  falls related to **153**
  neuropathic pain 86
trigeminal nerve (V)
  abnormalities of **43**
  examination 45
  sensory distribution *42*

tripod **134**
troponin 109, 124
tuberculosis 128
tumours
  brain **39**
  pituitary **39**
  polypoid **80**
tunnel vision **39**

U

ulcer
  diabetic **55**
  venous ulcer **55**
ulnar nerve **46**
'Up & Go' test 180
upper airway obstruction, physical
    findings **18**
uraemia, confusion caused by **94**
urge incontinence 115, 116, **155**, 157
urinary incontinence 114–16, 155–7
  aetiology and pathophysiology 155–6
    age-related changes 155
    gender-related factors 155–6
  clinical presentation 156
  complications 157
  drug history 115–16, **115**
  epidemiology 156
  examination 156
  functional and iatrogenic **155**
  history 115
  investigation 116, 156
  management 116
    exercises 156
    intermittent self-catheterisation 157
    pads and pants 157
  mixed **155**
  overflow 115, **155**
  persistent 157
  referral letter 114
  risk factors 156
  stress 115, 116, **155**, 156–7
  in syncope 117
  urge 115, 116, **155**, 157
urinary retention 181, 185
  confusion caused by **94**
urinary tract infection 142
urodynamic investigation 116, 156
Usher's syndrome 169

V

vagus nerve (X)
  examination 45
  lesions of **45**
valproic acid, neuropathic pain 86
valvular heart disease
  aortic stenosis 27, **32**, **118**, 131

confusion 132
  mitral stenosis **30**, 31, **118**
varicose eczema **55**
vascular dementia 162
veins, superior vena cava **74**, 75, 87
venlafaxine 93
venting gastrostomy 91
ventricular extrasystole 27
ventricular septal defect **30**, **32**
vertebrobasilar insufficiency 117, **118**
vertigo **44**, 108
vestibulocochlear nerve (VIII),
    examination 45
vibration sense
  arm 48
  leg 48, 51
visceral pain **82**
visual acuity 37, **39**, **45**
  reduced **52**
visual fields 37, **37**, 38, **39**, 40, **45**
visual impairment 111
  and falls **107**, 108
visual inattention 37
vitamin B_1 (thiamine), deficiency 174
vitamin B_{12} deficiency 21
vitamin C, deficiency 172
vitamin D, deficiency 171
vitamin K, deficiency 171
vitiligo **55**, 136, *137*
vocal fremitus 17
vocal resonance 17
vomiting centre **79**, 89

W

waddling gait **49**
walking aids **134**, 154, 167
Weber's test 43, 169
weight loss 75, 92
  see also failure to thrive
Wernicke's area 142
Wernicke's encephalopathy **112**, 174,
    183, 186
wheelchairs 167
wheezing 74
whispering pectoriloquy 17
Wilson's disease **45**
withholding/withdrawing treatment
  95

X

xanthelasma **55**

Z

Zimmer frames **134**, 167
zoledronic acid 99, 102